黏膜免疫学与病毒学

Mucosal Immunology and Virology

〔美〕S.K.蒂林 编著

国 泰 王军志 等 译

科学出版社

北 京

图字：01-2012-8045 号

内 容 简 介

本书从介绍病毒入侵机体，到展示黏膜免疫系统在防御中所起的作用，结合临床表现阐明其机理，为寻找有效的预防和治疗措施提供科学依据。全书共七章，第1章简述了黏膜免疫在防卫病毒性疾病中的作用；第2章主述肛门与生殖道黏膜免疫和病毒学；第3、4章阐述了消化道黏膜免疫和病毒学；第5、7章主要阐述病毒性疾病的口腔和眼部表现；第6章是普通呼吸道病毒和肺部黏膜免疫。

本书对从事免疫学、病毒学及相关学科的研究人员、教师、研究生均有一定参考价值。

Translation from English language edition: Mucosal Immunology and Virology by Stephen K. Tyring

Copyright © 2006 Springer London

Springer London is a part of Springer Science+Business Media

All Rights Reserved

图书在版编目（CIP）数据

黏膜免疫学与病毒学/(美)蒂林(Tyring, S. K.)编著；国泰，王军志等译.—北京：科学出版社，2013
Mucosal Immunology and Virology
ISBN 978-7-03-036007-6

Ⅰ.①黏… Ⅱ.①蒂… ②国… ③王… Ⅲ.①黏膜—免疫学②人体病毒学 Ⅳ.①R392②R373

中国版本图书馆CIP数据核字（2012）第265464号

责任编辑：罗 静 夏 梁 刘 晶 / 责任校对：林青梅
责任印制：徐晓晨 / 封面设计：美光制版

科学出版社 出版
北京东黄城根北街16号
邮政编码：100717
http://www.sciencep.com

北京建宏印刷有限公司 印刷
科学出版社发行 各地新华书店经销

*

2013年1月第 一 版　开本：787×1092 1/16
2021年1月第五次印刷　印张：16 1/2
字数：391 000

定价：108.00元
（如有印装质量问题，我社负责调换）

感谢李莹博士（MSD）、谭业双医生（郧阳医学院）、Sherry X.H.G.（NYU），在本书的翻译和校对过程中给予的帮助，感谢谷金莲老师对中文初稿的通阅！感谢"863"计划（新型轮状病毒疫苗研发及其综合技术支持平台2006AA02A206）、艾滋病和病毒性肝炎等重大传染病防治国家科技重大专项（艾滋病、乙型肝炎、结核病及新突发传染病诊断试剂的质量评价技术及标准品研究2012ZX10004702）以及"863"计划（腮腺炎减毒活疫苗等病毒性疫苗关键技术及产品研发2012AA02A404）为本书出版提供的支持！

译者名单

国　泰　王军志　杜加亮　刘悦越　刘　艳　于晴川
李　东　米旭光　高加梅　范行良　张　瑞　于振行
苏　悦　付涌水　李琦涵　郭舒杨　兰志岭　姚　昕
张向颖　李肖锋

序 一

黏膜免疫自20世纪60年代提出以来，越来越受到人们的重视，它在机体抵御微生物入侵的过程中起到至关重要的作用。经过几十年的发展，黏膜免疫的研究取得了长足的进步，也成为新型疫苗研发的重要方向。针对我国缺乏比较系统阐述黏膜免疫学相关书籍的这一情况，中国食品药品检定研究院肠道病毒疫苗室的科研人员组织编译了《黏膜免疫学与病毒学》一书。

中国食品药品检定研究院是国家食品药品监督管理局的直属事业单位，是国家检验药品生物制品质量的法定机构和最高技术仲裁机构。六十多年来，为预防性和治疗用生物制品质量控制工作，降低流行病发病率，以及提升行业综合水平作出诸多贡献。特别是近几年，技术能力水平被WHO和国际同行认可，为我国生物制品质量提高奠定了坚实的基础。

2012年3月，中国食品药品检定研究院正式成立了肠道病毒疫苗室，使病毒及其相关产品的研究和质量控制与黏膜免疫学基础知识紧密结合，学科设置和职能划分更加清晰合理，从体制上为科研和检验工作驶入快车道提供了系统的保障，也为该学科的远期发展搭建了系统和科学的基础平台。

《黏膜免疫学与病毒学》主要对黏膜免疫系统的构成及免疫特征、功能性组分及其作用机制和黏膜免疫系统的调节三方面中的热点进行了系统性的描述，是我国黏膜免疫研究领域为数不多的书籍，为医疗、预防领域和检定检验系统工作的科研人员提供基础性参考资料。

2012年6月28日

序 二

黏膜免疫系统是全身免疫系统的一个重要组成部分，由黏膜局部的黏膜相关淋巴组织（MALT）和免疫细胞组成，前者是黏膜免疫应答的诱导和活化部位；后者则是黏膜免疫的效应部位。它们构成机体与外环境间一道有效的防御屏障，对进入的病原体产生应答，抵抗它们对机体的侵袭，覆盖在胃肠道、呼吸道、泌尿生殖道及一些外分泌腺的黏膜面积超过 $400m^2$，是大部分病原体进入人体的主要门户，而且人体黏膜免疫细胞占所有免疫细胞的 80%，因此黏膜免疫在机体免疫中占有非常重要的地位。机体抵抗病原微生物感染的免疫机制主要包括固有免疫或称天然免疫（非特异性免疫）与获得性免疫（特异性免疫），前者提供了对新抗原的迅速反应，并奠定了获得性免疫反应的基础，固有免疫对病原体是非特异的，没有记忆性，而获得性免疫是抗原特异的，疾病恢复后保留记忆，提供再感染时的防御。该书以消化道黏膜免疫和常见病毒为例，较详细地阐述了参与黏膜天然免疫的体液因子、受体及 T、B 细胞所起的作用；消化道中诱导获得性免疫的部位、效应部位。全书共分七章，第一章简述了黏膜免疫在防卫病毒性疾病中的作用；第二章主述肛门与生殖道黏膜免疫和病毒学；第三、四章阐述了消化道黏膜免疫和病毒学；第五、七章主要阐述病毒性疾病的口腔和眼部表现；第六章是普通呼吸道病毒和肺部黏膜免疫。该书通过病毒入侵机体后，黏膜免疫系统在防御中所起的作用，结合临床表现阐明其机理，为寻找有效的预防和治疗措施提供科学依据。

传染病一直是人类健康的威胁者，尽管许多可用疫苗预防的疾病在发达国家已经得到了控制，但对于一些贫困国家来说，这些疾病仍然是主要的公众健康问题，因此，获得更多的高效疫苗越来越受到人们的关注。最近几年，研发黏膜疫苗成为一个新热点。

该书对从事免疫学、病毒学及相关学科的研究人员、教师、研究生均有一定参考价值。

沈倍奋

2011 年 12 月 28 日

目 录

序一
序二

第1章　黏膜免疫在病毒性疾病中的保护作用　　　　　　　　　　1
　　　　Vandana Madkan, Karan Sra, and Stephen K. Tyring
　　参考文献　　　　　　　　　　　　　　　　　　　　　　　　4

第2章　肛门生殖器黏膜免疫学和病毒学　　　　　　　　　　　　6
　　　　Anthony Simmons
　　黏膜表面免疫系统的挑战　　　　　　　　　　　　　　　　　7
　　黏膜部位的固有免疫和适应性免疫　　　　　　　　　　　　　10
　　病毒感染免疫应答机制　　　　　　　　　　　　　　　　　　11
　　黏膜免疫和外周免疫之间的相互作用　　　　　　　　　　　　13
　　黏膜免疫的细胞和分子　　　　　　　　　　　　　　　　　　13
　　生殖器部位的主要病毒感染　　　　　　　　　　　　　　　　13
　　总结　　　　　　　　　　　　　　　　　　　　　　　　　　19
　　参考文献　　　　　　　　　　　　　　　　　　　　　　　　19

第3章　胃肠道黏膜免疫学　　　　　　　　　　　　　　　　　　23
　　　　David A. Bland, Carlos A. Barrera, and Victor E. Reyes
　　胃肠道黏膜的固有免疫防御　　　　　　　　　　　　　　　　24
　　中间免疫程序　　　　　　　　　　　　　　　　　　　　　　31
　　适应性免疫应答　　　　　　　　　　　　　　　　　　　　　32
　　胃肠道的常见感染及免疫应答　　　　　　　　　　　　　　　39
　　胃肠道的显性免疫应答　　　　　　　　　　　　　　　　　　47
　　总结　　　　　　　　　　　　　　　　　　　　　　　　　　50
　　参考文献　　　　　　　　　　　　　　　　　　　　　　　　51

第4章	胃肠道病毒学	59
	Richard L. Ward, Xi Jiang, Tibor Farkas, and Dorsey M. Bass	
	胃肠道病毒	59
	轮状病毒	60
	杯状病毒	75
	星形病毒	88
	参考文献	92
第5章	病毒性疾病的口腔表现	111
	Denis P. Lynch	
	疱疹病毒	111
	HPV	124
	口腔疣	124
	尖锐湿疣	125
	局灶性上皮增生症	126
	HPV 与口腔疣的关系	127
	副黏病毒	128
	柯萨奇病毒	129
	疱疹性咽峡炎	130
	人类免疫缺陷病毒	131
	参考文献	149
第6章	常见呼吸道病毒及肺部黏膜免疫	189
	David B. Huang	
	导致呼吸道感染的常见病毒	189
	肺部黏膜免疫	202
	总结	204
	参考文献	205
第7章	病毒性疾病的眼部表现	212
	Steven Yeh and Mitchell P. Weikert	
	单纯疱疹病毒 1 型和 2 型	213
	水痘 - 带状疱疹病毒	216
	EB 病毒	220
	巨细胞病毒	221
	人类疱疹病毒 -8	224
	传染性软疣	225
	人乳头瘤病毒	227

腺病毒	228
非特异性滤泡性结膜炎	230
人类免疫缺陷病毒	230
麻疹	232
腮腺炎	233
风疹	233
小核糖核酸病毒	234
总结	235
参考文献	235
索引	247

第1章
黏膜免疫在病毒性疾病中的保护作用

Vandana Madkan, Karan Sra, and Stephen K. Tyring

研究黏膜免疫为洞悉每天都要抵御其遭遇的大量病毒和其他病原体的人体错综复杂的系统提供了令人惊奇的途径。黏膜总表面积比一个半网球场还大[1,2],是一层内衬于与外界相通的腔体或通道并能分泌黏液的膜,黏膜主要定位在胃肠道、泌尿生殖道和呼吸道,是病原入侵的门户。事实上,除极少数病原体通过节肢动物或其他动物的叮咬、注射、输血等途径入侵机体以外,绝大多数病原体都是通过黏膜入侵的[1]。身体依靠存于黏膜内的免疫细胞和抗体抵御暴露生物体的攻击,因此,人体内胃肠道黏膜组织中的淋巴细胞比其他所有淋巴器官(外周免疫系统的组成成分)的总和还多就不足为奇了[3]。

世界上很多严重的疾病都是通过黏膜感染传播的。世界卫生组织2004年公布的《世界卫生报告》显示,90%以上感染性疾病死亡病例由以下6种病变引起的:下呼吸道感染、艾滋病(AIDS)、腹泻、结核、疟疾及麻疹,合计每年造成1300万人死亡[4]。上述6种感染性疾病中,除疟疾截然不同之外,其他5种均主要由病原体通过黏膜感染[3]。甚至某些曾经认为是非感染性的疾病,如某些癌症,现在显示也存在感染性病因。例如,宫颈癌是发展中国家女性最为常见的癌症之一,现在已知它与人类乳头瘤病毒感染有关,通过肛门生殖道黏膜感染传播[1]。

然而,奇怪的是,尽管占压倒性数量的感染性病原体是通过黏膜表面入侵人体的,但迄今已研制的大部分疫苗设计却是针对外周免疫系统。与黏膜免疫系统地位等同的外周免疫系统,由骨髓、淋巴结和脾组成,通过淋巴液将外来抗原提呈给淋巴结。外周免疫系统与进入身体的病原体抗衡并阻止其致病。然而,黏膜免疫系统则是通过黏膜屏障战胜病原体并阻止感染发生[5]。虽然大多数疫苗,包括所有传统推荐的儿童期疫苗都是通过注射施用的,可以刺激外周免疫系统,但是并不清楚它们是否会提供足够的以分泌型免疫球蛋白A(secretory immunoglobulin A,sIgA)等为判断指标的黏膜免疫[6]。

例如,对比脊髓灰质炎灭活疫苗(inactive poliovirus vaccine,IPV)和口服脊髓灰质炎疫苗(oral poliovirus vaccine,OPV)免疫反应后,研究人员发现单独注射IPV不能引起黏膜免疫反应,但如将IPV施用于已经接触过OPV抗原的个体,则可产生充分的黏膜免疫应答[7]。自然感染脊髓灰质炎病毒或口服 OPV 后,暴露的个体黏膜表面都会出现分泌型 IgA。但是只有在机体自然感染或口服接种后,IPV 已接种者才能产生强的 IgA。如果没有以前的感染,IPV 已接种者依然可能通过黏膜途径感染脊髓灰质炎病毒。如果 IPV 已接种者被暴露和感染,他们可以无临床症状,但仍可将疾病传播给未完全免疫者。这一发现对人类彻底根除脊髓灰质炎具有极其重要的意义。在 IPV 已接种者的社区,IPV 已接种者同低接种率的人群接触时,仍可传播脊髓灰质炎病毒,而后者体内并没有对疾病的黏膜和外周保护,如此造成的脊髓灰质炎病毒的流行可能会毁掉人的性命。未接种脊髓灰质炎病毒疫苗者与已接种疫苗的人群接触[7],导致了这种情形于 1978 年和 1992 年在荷兰的一个小的宗教社区发生。由于完全由口服接种的免疫本身就会具有一定的发病率,因此以 OPV 初免且以 IPV 加强的方法解决为宜。

随着对免疫系统以及对外周免疫和黏膜免疫的复杂相互作用有了更深入的认识,改良疫苗成为新的研究方向。由于黏膜防御比外周免疫系统对防止感染更有优势,而且传统疫苗并不能提供黏膜免疫防护,几个新的靶向黏膜应答的疫苗正在研究。如上所述,通过黏膜传播的肠道传染病可以引起惊人的发病率和死亡率,发展中国家情况尤甚。在世界范围内,肠道传染病每年可导致 200 万儿童死亡,其中有 400 人发生在美国[8]。病原体可能包括病毒(如轮状病毒和诺如病毒)、侵袭性细菌(如大肠杆菌和志贺氏菌),以及毒素细菌(包括霍乱)。用于预防霍乱弧菌感染的注射型疫苗已确定很大程度上无效[9]。但霍乱弧菌会造成重症腹泻暴发和偶发性流行,研发黏膜疫苗的尝试已经启动。现有的口服霍乱疫苗显示有效且可产生群体保护[10]。目前最常用的霍乱疫苗(Dukoral)是由重组霍乱毒素亚基和灭活的全细胞霍乱弧菌组成的,疫苗可以刺激肠道黏膜产生 sIgA[9]。

轮状病毒是引发感染性腹泻的最常见病原体。在感染性腹泻导致的死亡病例中轮状病毒腹泻占 20%[8]。全球范围内,每年该病毒感染可导致约 50 万儿童死亡[9],在美国高发于冬季。两种新型口服减毒活疫苗正在研制,尝试减少每年遭此困扰的人数。Rotarix 和 RotaTeq 都是弱毒口服病毒疫苗并在一定的群体中有效,目前正在进行进一步的临床试验[9]。

肠道感染是引起世界范围内儿童死亡的第二大病因,而位于首位的则是呼吸道感染。也许最为众所周知的感染下呼吸道的病原体是流感病毒。由于其天然变异性和基因突变,流感病毒每年都会引发流行甚至是大流行,致使几百万人死亡。据统计,仅在美国每年流感流行导致 2 万人死亡,数万人住院[11],对工业化国家也是巨大的经济负担。几年来,美国已针对流感病毒实施了标准免疫接种,发病率和死亡率较高的人群优先接种,如 65 岁以上老人或者长期就医者等。美国市场上最常用流感疫苗是注射型疫苗,作用在产生 IgG 抗体的外周免疫系统,也经证明偶尔有黏膜保护效果[9],但产生的黏膜 IgG 高于 IgA。新批准的更容易使用的流感疫苗 FluMist,通过鼻腔黏膜接种,提供的免疫效果可与自然感染获得的免疫媲美。自然感染能够提供长效的免疫,可在鼻腔洗出物中检测出有 IgA 反应,在下呼吸道中有 IgG 反应,并可以保护病毒再次感染及抵抗抗原性相似的毒株[11]。同样,活病毒疫苗接种也能诱导黏膜及血清中均产生 IgA 和 IgG 应答,然而,灭活疫苗免疫可以获得更高水平的血清应答[11]。

另外，流感减毒活疫苗的副作用比灭活疫苗的更久更严重。尽管美国每年都接种大量的流感灭活疫苗，但除注射部位的局部反应以外，很少有其他副反应症状。在研究人群中减毒活疫苗接种显示安全有效[11]，但短期的症状包括咳嗽、打喷嚏、恶心及呕吐等其他全身症状也偶见报道。另外，人们担心可能会出现因人类污染造成活病毒基因改变及继发于接种部位的中枢神经系统（central nervous system，CNS）不良副反应。尽管对于两种疫苗的优缺点需进一步研究，但减毒活疫苗接种还是有本质优势的。例如，一些病毒（像流感病毒），会发生抗原漂移和转变，产生新的病毒株。患者在一生中都可能需要接种活疫苗来加强免疫，虽然如此但其仍比灭活疫苗年接种的总量要少。除了可以提供根本的黏膜保护，FluMist还有其他优点。2004年注射型流感疫苗紧缺，每次到货时，公共卫生诊所门口就排满了老人和慢性病患者。而经黏膜的疫苗的一个主要优点就是容易接种，就流感病毒和相关黏膜疫苗来讲，患者可以自行接种FluMist。甚至还有额外的优点就是，大量本来因为害怕打针而拒绝接种的患者在不使用针头的情况下可能会重新考虑接种了。

少数疾病可能有这样的特征——会毁灭整个村庄并导致劳动力死亡，从而破坏一个国家的经济基础。在这个意义上，人类免疫缺陷病毒（human immunodeficiency virus，HIV）是目前不发达国家所面临的最大威胁。据估计，在非洲撒哈拉沙漠以南的一些国家，大约60%的15岁青少年承受着HIV流行的严重打击，因而会在60岁以前死亡[4]。目前一些新药使控制疾病进程有了希望，但仅仅限于能够负担得起药费的患者。像乌干达、印度和泰国这些国家，HIV阳性个体主要是性工作者和他们的直接接触者，他们一般都无法负担高昂的抗逆转录治疗费用。虽然目前完全没有可用的疫苗，但通过阻断肛门生殖道黏膜接触传播可能是抑制该疾病肆虐的最好方法。人们正致力于针对口腔和鼻腔黏膜的疫苗，因为早期研究显示在该部位免疫的反应可产生对其他黏膜部位的保护，但机制还不清楚[12]。另外，日本研究者发现将HIV gp160脂质体经鼻接种至一组小鼠，可以在黏膜和全身部位观察到有效的HIV特异性免疫。通过ELISA在血清、唾液、粪便提取物和阴道洗出物可检测出HIV特异性抗体。上述研究使用的小鼠包括Th1和Th2细胞缺陷型及无免疫细胞缺陷的"野生型"鼠，每型都有恰当的黏膜反应[12]。

黏膜接种仅仅是抵御HIV的先锋医疗技术的一方面。目前正研发局部黏膜使用的杀微生物剂，这种化合物可吸附生理性液体中的HIV-1，以防止病毒接触靶细胞。如制药工业中用于胶囊外薄衣的醋酸纤维素酞酸素（cellulose acetate phthalate，CAP）具有局部杀微生物剂的作用。当遇到HIV后，能使其包膜糖蛋白脱落从而失去感染能力[13]。其他化合物如二苦杏仁酸醚钠，甚至宿主自己的β-防御素，对HIV和单纯疱疹病毒（herpes simplex virus，HSV）都具有抵御能力[14,15]。

虽然人疱疹病毒HSV-1和HSV-2对人类的经济危害小于HIV，也不是导致健康成人死亡的常见原因，但疫苗可以帮助降低病毒传播，从而减轻其他方面正常成人的心理损伤，并可能会减少因疱疹性脑炎而死亡的新生儿数量。早期研究显示，注射型的重组糖蛋白（gD）疫苗对接种前体内没有HSV-1和HSV-2抗体的女性能提供抵抗HSV-2感染的保护作用，但对于接种前体内有HSV-1抗体的女性无保护作用，对于男性，不管其体内有无HSV-1抗体均无保护作用。这种免疫不一致性的原因虽然未被完全阐明，但引出一种假说：

因女性比男性具有更大的黏膜表面，如女性阴道对比男性生殖器区域，所以疫苗刺激黏膜免疫给女性提供更好的保护作用[16]。深入研究发现，之前感染过 HSV-1 可以对 HSV-2 有保护作用，然而这种保护作用也依赖于在某处黏膜表面作为刺激物的两种病毒的感染位点，决定能否对其他表面提供保护作用。Bernstein 等研究发现接种疱疹病毒疫苗对于非生殖器疱疹患者复发人数的降低和增加没有影响[17]。

黏膜免疫的机制复杂，至今尚未完全清楚。我们使用各种方式极力调节黏膜免疫系统去预防感染和疾病。然而，黏膜免疫不仅可以预防常见的和严重的传染病，在防止自身免疫性疾病方面也有作用[5,9]。虽然这种作用迄今没有在人类研究的报道，但是用抗原口服刺激事实上可导致抗原耐受。给特定的大鼠种群（一种实验性自身免疫性脑脊髓炎多发性硬化动物模型）喂食髓磷脂碱蛋白，可诱发大鼠对髓磷脂碱蛋白产生免疫耐受[18]。据猜测，可能对肠黏膜反复高剂量的抗原刺激会引发若干机制，从而抑制了潜在损伤性免疫反应[19]。依施用剂量的不同，这些反应包括自身反应性 T 细胞的凋亡和失能[9]。因此，黏膜免疫学研究不仅可用于减少感染性疾病，还可以用于预防自身免疫性相关病症。

相反地，我们也渴望能诱导出针对非感染性抗原的免疫反应。如避孕疫苗，研究人员试图通过接种疫苗诱导免疫反应，从而使男性和（或）女性产生抗人类精子抗体[2]。30% 不孕夫妇的黏液分泌物中存在精子抗体，避孕疫苗原理与此相类似。虽然存在争议，但这方面的研究需要建立在对黏膜免疫系统有更广阔的认识的基础之上。

参 考 文 献

[1] Hoft DF, Eickhoff CS. Type 1 immunity provides both optimal mucosal and systemic protection against a mucosally invasive, intracellular pathogen. Infect Immun 2005;73:4934–4940.

[2] Seipp R. Mucosal Immunity and Vaccines. 2005. Retrieved from the World Wide Web July 02, 2005: http://www.bioteach.ubc.ca/Biomedicine/mucosalimmunity/.

[3] Russell MW. Mucosal immunity. Chapter 5: 64–80. In New Bacterial Vaccines (Eds. Ellis, R.W. and Brodeur, B.R.) Eurekah.com, Georgetown TX and Kluwer Academic/ Plenum, New York. 2003.

[4] Davey S. Infectious Diseases are the biggest killers of the young. 1999,World Health Organization. Retrieved from the World Wide Web July 08, 2005: http://www.who.int/infectious-disease-report/pages/ch1text.html.

[5] Anderson AO. Peripheral and Mucosal Immunity: Critical Issues for Oral Vaccine Design. 2004. Retrieved from the World Wide Web July 14, 2005: http://www.geocities.com/artnscience/crossregulation.html.

[6] Ogra PL. Mucosal immunity: Some historical perspective on host-pathogen interactions and implications for mucosal vaccines. Immunol Cell Biol 2003;81:23–33.

[7] Herremans TM, Reimerink JH, Buisman AM, Kimman TJ, Koopmans MP. Induction of mucosal immunity by inactivated poliovirus vaccine is dependent on previous mucosal contact with live virus. J Immunol 1999;162: 5011–5018.

[8] Frye RE, Tamer MA.Diarrhea. 2005. Retrieved from the World Wide Web July 28, 2005: http://www.emedicine.com/ped/topic583.htm.

[9] Holmgren J, Czerkinsky C.Mucosal immunity and vaccines. Nat Med 2005;11:45–53.

[10] Lucas ME, Deen JL, Seidlein L, et al. Effectiveness of mass oral cholera vaccination in Beira,

Mozambique. N Engl J Med 2005;352:757–767.

[11] Cox RJ, Brokstad KA, Ogra P. Influenza virus: immunity and vaccination strategies. Comparison of the immune response to inactivated and live, attenuated influenza vaccines. Scand J Immunol 2004;59:1–15.

[12] Sakaue G, Hiroi T, Nakagawa Y, et al. HIV mucosal vaccine: nasal immunization with gp160-encapsulated hemagglutinating virus of Japan-liposome induces antigen-specific CTLs and neutralizing antibody responses. J Immunol 2003;170:495–502.

[13] Neurath AR, Strick N, Li YY, Debnath AK. Cellulose acetate phthalate, a common pharmaceutical excipient, inactivates HIV-1 and blocks the coreceptor binding site on the virus envelope glycoprotein gp120. BMC Infect Dis 2001;1:17.

[14] Scordi-Bello IA, Mosoian A, He C, et al. Mandelic acid condensation polymer: novel candidate microbicide for prevention of human immunodeficiency virus and herpes simplex virus entry. Antimicrob Agents Chemother 2005;49:3607–3615.

[15] Quinones-Mateu ME, Lederman MM, Feng Z, et al. Human epithelial beta-defensins 2 and 3 inhibit HIV-1 replication. AIDS 2003;17:F39–48.

[16] Stanberry LR, Spruance SL, Cunningham AL, et al. Glycoprotein-D-adjuvant vaccine to prevent genital herpes. N Engl J Med 2002;347:1652–1661.

[17] Bernstein DI, Aoki FY, Tyring SK, et al. Safety and immunogenicity of glycoprotein D-adjuvant genital herpes vaccine. Clin Infect Dis 2005;40:1271–1281.

[18] Whitacre CC, Gienapp IE, Orosz CG, Bitar DM. Oral tolerance in experimental autoimmune encephalomyelitis. III. Evidence for clonal anergy. J Immunol 1991;147:2155–2163.

[19] Wu HY, Weiner HL. Oral Tolerance. Immunol Res 2003;28:265–284.

第2章
肛门生殖器黏膜免疫学和病毒学
Anthony Simmons

目前认为免疫系统划分为两个独立的部分[1]：外周（常常不严密地称之为系统）免疫组织和黏膜相关淋巴组织（mucosa-associated lymphoid tissue，MALT）。虽然依据功能分为两个部分，但其作用却是既彼此独立又相互协同。事实就是，黏膜不仅是机体抵御潜在致病性微生物的物理屏障，还是由不同程度的固有和适应性宿主应答形成的第一道重要防线。在黏膜表面宿主固有和适应性防御重要的生理学意义，造就了黏膜免疫研究处于优先位置。

除了外周免疫与有效疫苗设计具有清晰密切的关系外，动员黏膜免疫系统也能针对一些流行的病毒提供最佳保护。在此简要地回顾一下免疫系统各分支的本质，并说明抵御病原体宿主免疫系统每一分支在组织解剖部位、诱导模式及最后发生作用的各效应细胞间的平衡方面存在的差异。全部的信息表明，在黏膜表面对致病性病毒最有效的反应是由相同部分内的细胞所介导的。免疫系统细分为外周免疫组织和MALT，这样就不会混淆体液和细胞应答之间，或固有免疫和适应性免疫之间的区别（图2.1和图2.2）。事实上，黏膜，

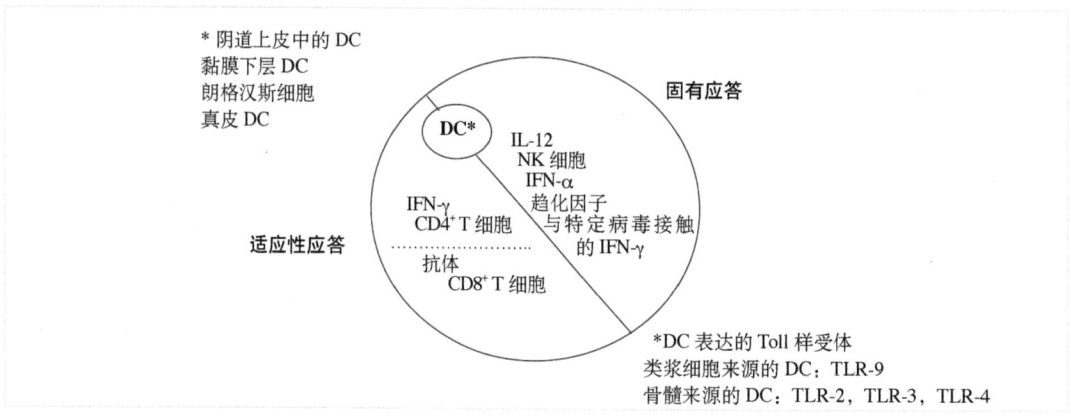

图2.1　固有免疫和适应性免疫系统的相互作用。本图强调了树突状细胞（dentritic cell，DC）可以影响固有免疫和适应性免疫（在不同的组织中方式不同），以及固有应答可能会影响阴道中适应性应答形成环境的某些机制。最近有证据表明黏膜下层的CD11b(⁺)DC可以诱导辅助性T细胞1（Th1）对于HSV-2的应答[7]，而非朗格汉斯细胞。阴道上皮附近的淋巴结感染后出现了分泌IFN-γ的CD11c(⁺)DC，而后黏膜下层DC被募集到感染部位，这样便刺激了CD4⁺T细胞。似乎没有其他细胞对HSV的肽段进行MHC II类分子提呈。白细胞介素12，IL-12；自然杀伤，NK；Toll样受体，TLR。

包括肛门与生殖道黏膜,是宿主固有和适应性防御的主要部位,同时也有多种细胞和可溶性效应因子的参与。

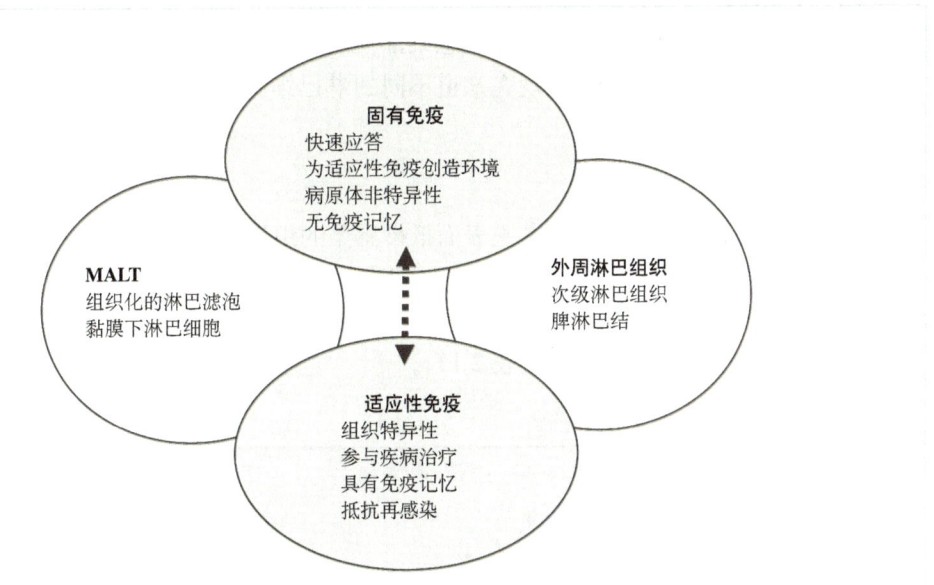

图 2.2　固有免疫和适应性免疫系统形态和功能的区分,以及在不同部位的不同作用。DC 上的 TLR 使固有免疫应答十分快速,并且可以分泌趋化因子和细胞因子,从而募集淋巴细胞至感染区域。

黏膜表面免疫系统的挑战

黏膜是机体内最大的组织器官,其表面积约有 1.5 个网球场大小,约为皮肤面积的 200 倍。绝大多数的病原体必须首先通过黏膜屏障,才能进入宿主造成感染。当然,血源性传播包括蚊虫叮咬、注射、输血等,是病毒在宿主间传播的另外一条除黏膜外唯一的途径。黏膜屏障包括全部胃肠道、呼吸道和泌尿生殖道。本文中的"肛门生殖道"是指性传播传染病发生的重要黏膜组件,疾病包括单纯疱疹病毒(herpes simplex virus,HSV)和人乳头瘤病毒(human papilloma virus,HPV)。由于对人类免疫缺陷病毒(human immunodeficiency virus,HIV)免疫应答并没有确切地涉及黏膜免疫,因此本章不考虑 HIV。HIV 或者是 HIV 感染的细胞一般通过肛门生殖道黏膜的破损处进入宿主体内,并且感染是全身性。当然,因为 HIV 导致的免疫力受损而引起其他病毒在肛门生殖道的感染,同样会产生灾难性的后果。

外周免疫系统

免疫应答遍布全身。外来抗原和骨髓来源免疫细胞首次在机体进化出的特定部位相接触,以达到保护机体的目的。根据解剖学术语,外周免疫系统是指骨髓、淋巴结和脾脏。外周免疫的关键组件是将抗原运送至淋巴结的淋巴系统。中枢神经系统内没有普通淋巴系统,因此在解剖学上与其他组织有明显的区分,不十分严密地称为免疫"豁免"部位。就免疫而言，中枢神经系统显然是特殊的部位，但在此不做详细陈述。

从历史角度看，由于病毒感染都有全身性阶段，所以抗病毒免疫途径一直关注于刺激外周适应性免疫，并认为是抵御病毒完美可行的策略，如腮腺炎、麻疹、风疹和脊髓灰质炎。但是上述策略对保护以黏膜为原发感染部位的却并不成功，主要的例子有单纯疱疹、乳头瘤病毒感染和传染性软疣。现在知道不同的淋巴细胞群会循环优先定居于一个或另外的免疫部位（如外周或黏膜）。

黏膜免疫系统

黏膜免疫包括了保护宿主在黏膜表面抵御感染的组织、细胞和可溶性效应分子的网络。黏膜免疫最重要的是大约有80%激活的B细胞并不存在于传统的次级淋巴组织中，如脾脏和淋巴结，而是集聚在MALT内[2]。并且，MALT中包含了一系列解剖单位，免疫组织相关的每个位点都有自己的名称（表2.1）。

表2.1 黏膜免疫系统的多样性：蛋白质和主要分支

	名称	缩写	描述
蛋白质	免疫球蛋白	Ig	抗体：IgA、IgG、IgM三型
	分泌型免疫球蛋白A	sIgA	分泌进黏液的黏膜免疫的重要组分
	分泌型免疫球蛋白M	sIgM	IgM，也能跨膜分泌的Ig
	多聚免疫球蛋白受体	pIgR	pIgR在上皮细胞上发现
	多聚IgA/IgM分子	pIgA/IgM	Ig与pIgR结合后的复合物
	分泌成分	SC	与Ig结合，可穿过黏膜
分区	派尔集合淋巴结	PP结	肠壁主要次级诱导区
	黏膜相关淋巴组织	MALT	黏膜免疫组织的统称
	上皮内淋巴细胞	IEL	常在上皮细胞中发现的一类细胞
	肠道相关淋巴组织	GALT	包括PP结和阑尾（次级淋巴组织）
	鼻相关淋巴组织	NALT	包括扁桃体和腺样体（次级淋巴组织）
	涎腺导管相关淋巴组织	SALT	含大量IEL；固有应答的一部分
	结膜相关淋巴组织	CALT	与LDALT联合保护眼睛
	泪液排泄相关淋巴组织	LDALT	在维护眼表面完整方面扮演主要角色
	喉相关淋巴组织	LALT	推测是儿童中的呼吸系统黏膜诱导部位
	支气管相关淋巴组织	BALT	防御吸入的病原体

本书将MALT分为不同的部分，目的并不是避免混淆，而是将功能和解剖部位联系起来，从而有助于科学地交流。在不同部分中，已被广泛研究且最重要的是肠道相关淋巴组织（gut-associated lymphoid tissue，GALT；在第3章讨论）和鼻相关淋巴组织（nasopharyngeal-associated lymphoid tissue，NALT）。在人类和非人灵长类动物中，唾液腺（和唾液导管）相关的MALT都已从解剖学上得到了确证。在人类中，人们发现了唾

液腺中发生常与干燥综合征等自身免疫病有关的淋巴瘤,揭示了唾液腺相关 MALT 的存在。很明显,肺脏经常会接触病原体,40% 儿童和青少年的肺组织中可以确认含有支气管相关淋巴组织(bronchus-associated lymphoid tissue,BALT),但没有证据显示正常的成年人含有 BALT。然而,当肺部发生炎症反应时可形成组织化的淋巴结构,此时 BALT 的作用就凸显出来。

黏膜免疫应答的诱导和效应阶段

宿主对于外来抗原的应答通常分为诱导阶段和效应阶段。免疫的诱导阶段是指通过与同种异体抗原的接触启动淋巴细胞,将它们提呈至所谓的诱导部位,相当于经典的淋巴结和脾脏。然而,黏膜部位免疫应答的诱导不仅发生在引流淋巴结,而且发生在局部淋巴细胞集合中。这些细胞通常位于组织学上可识别的淋巴结构中,如肠壁内的派尔集合淋巴结(Peyer's patch,PP 结)或散在的组织化淋巴滤泡,这些结构位于多种黏膜表面,尤其是肠道相关的黏膜表面。诱导阶段过后,启动的淋巴细胞迁移到局部淋巴结内增殖成熟。在黏膜部位,淋巴细胞的启动将深远影响着由一定黏膜选择性细胞黏附分子参与的淋巴细胞的接续行为,赋予这些细胞能够再进入黏膜部位的能力,这个过程称之为"归巢"。这些黏附分子有时也称为归巢分子。因此,当启动的黏膜淋巴细胞进入淋巴结扩增,继而又重新进入血流时,这些细胞就可以到达效应部位,如多数黏膜固有层。黏膜多处确实都存在淋巴组织,这些淋巴组织在组织形态上容易被认为是淋巴滤泡。但在未感染的生殖道内并未发现此类滤泡。因此,这里显然有个问题:在肛门生殖道黏膜部位更有效的免疫应答,是否由像鼻子这样的远端黏膜部位的免疫所引起呢(图 2.3)?

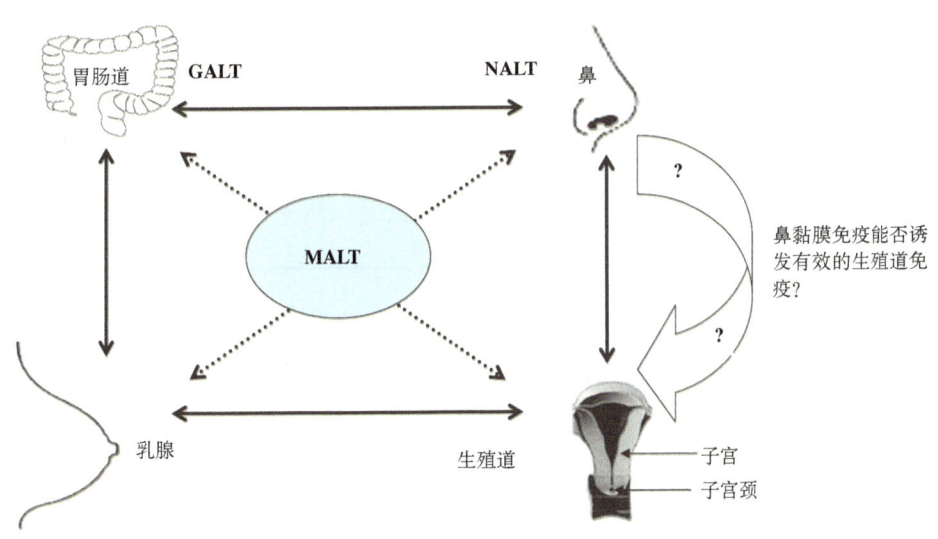

图 2.3 MALT 主要部位。黏膜组织间存在免疫学上相互作用的可能。这幅图强调常见黏膜免疫系统中的免疫可能是保护远端黏膜部位的有效方法。例如,有研究指出基本上鼻的免疫可有效防护生殖器疱疹感染[20]和乳头瘤病毒感染[18]。鼻相关淋巴组织,NALT。

PP 结位于肠道壁内，是最早发现的特殊淋巴组织集合之一。这种组织化的黏膜淋巴系统中有一种类似淋巴结的滤泡结构，不同的是这种结构额外地装配有一种特殊细胞——专门负责跨上皮转运的M细胞[3]。因此，该系统在将外来抗原提呈给 MALT 的过程中起重要作用，在肠道中尤为明显。

其他的一些黏膜部位有弥散的淋巴组织，这些组织目前还未被确认，有待于相关技术的进一步发展。另外，在许多黏膜部位，其复杂的免疫机制还有待于进一步的研究。生殖道黏膜免疫即属于此类。

黏膜部位的固有免疫和适应性免疫

目前，越来越多的证据表明，机体对外来抗原早期适应性应答的产生依赖于该应答诱导阶段所遇到的固有环境（图 2.1 和表 2.2）。然而，该适应性应答也包括 APC 表达的共刺激分子的改变，从而导致细胞因子及其他辅助分子的分泌。

表 2.2 固有免疫和适应性免疫的要素

	关键参与者	关键特征	关键性质
固有应答	不成熟 DC 上皮/内皮细胞 自然杀伤（nature killer，NK）细胞 粒细胞 单核细胞/巨噬细胞系 肥大细胞及嗜碱性粒细胞	快速应答（数分钟）	分子模式识别 种系编码的 受体重排非必需 非克隆 趋化因子、共刺激分子和细胞因子的表达引起相互作用
固有和适应性应答的相互作用	成熟 DC γδ T 细胞 趋化因子 细胞因子 补体蛋白	相互作用使固有环境能影响适应性应答	交叉重叠（沟通）
适应性应答产生	B 细胞（如黏膜 IgA 抗体） T 细胞（辅助性，抑制性，细胞毒性） 补体 趋化因子 细胞因子	记忆性；获得性免疫独有的特征是需要几天时间或抗原的预先暴露	特异抗原识别 基因片段重排对产生特异性是必需的 延迟的

这种情况下就会降低刺激 T 细胞应答阈值[4]。这里主要概括说明的是：病毒初次感染时，宿主固有因子（种系编码）与适应性免疫之间的微妙平衡决定了宿主的抵抗力和康复情况（图 2.1）。

宿主抵御病原微生物的第一道天然防线是物理屏障，包括皮肤和黏膜。通常来说，这是感染必须突破的防线。黏膜细胞的直接感染是避开物理屏障的主要途径。例如，病毒感染多发生于鼻咽部、支气管、胃肠道、结膜、唾液腺、皮肤及本章重点介绍的肛门生殖道等部位的黏膜细胞。由此可知，对于性传播疾病疫苗的研发及其他免疫治疗方法的突破，仍然需要对黏膜表面免疫更加详尽的理解。只有在极少数情况下宿主的皮肤黏膜并不能作为抵御感染的物理屏障。例如，某些节肢动物媒介可以直接将病毒注入宿主的血液中，或者是通过输血或吸毒者共用针头静脉注射等途径直接接触被病毒污染的血液而导致感染。

病毒感染免疫应答机制

固有免疫系统：病原体相关分子模式和 Toll 样受体

固有免疫系统可以使宿主识别广泛的病原体，包括病毒，即使是暴露于先前从未接触过的病原体时，也可迅速产生抗微生物的免疫应答和炎症反应。有证据显示，病原体上有一些结构保守基序 PAMP（pathogen-associated molecular pattern，病原体相关分子模式）。这些保守序列可以被诸如巨噬细胞等具有特定受体家族的细胞识别，就像在超市里使用货物条形码对货物进行识别一样。这些受体（相当于货物条码识别器）被称为 Toll 样受体（Toll-like receptor，TLR）。之所以称之为 TLR 是因为其与 Toll 受体十分类似，而后者则是在 10 年前研究黑腹果蝇（Drosophila melanogaster）的胚胎发育过程中发现的。TLR 在机体抵御病原体和其他毒性刺激时具有十分重要的作用。目前，有 10 种 TLR 被发现并且已经克隆入哺乳动物中，每种 TLR 都识别一套独特的 PAMP（表 2.3）。依赖于配体识别，受体家族可以激活多种信号途径对病毒、细菌、炎症和肿瘤进行抵御。因此，可以利用这些靶位点开发一些新的治疗方法（如 TLR-7 和 TLR-8）。

表 2.3 TLR 及其重要配体

TLR	主要配体
TLR-1	微生物脂蛋白
TLR-2	GPI 锚
TLR-3*	双链 RNA
TLR-4	革兰氏阴性菌的脂多糖
TLR-5	细菌鞭毛蛋白
TLR-6	与 TLR-2 一起作为支原体脂蛋白受体
TLR-7, 8*	未知（与咪唑喹啉药物相互作用）
TLR-9*	未甲基化的 CpG 岛
TLR-10	未知

* 与病毒有特殊关联。

对于病毒而言，目前确定的仅有极少数独特的分子结构可以激活固有免疫系统。在这些分子结构中，有一种是双链 RNA（dsRNA），存在于某些病毒的基因组中，或在另一些病毒复制过程中短暂出现。在哺乳类动物细胞中的 dsRNA 受体是 TLR 家族成员 TLR-3，但是对于 TLR-3 和配体的相互作用机制尚不完全清楚。此外，TLR 受体家族成员 TLR-9 可以对含有非甲基化 CpG 模体的核酸产生应答，包括 HSV DNA[4, 5]。在生殖器疱疹的动物模型小鼠中发现，HSV-2 病毒可以通过 TLR-9 与黏膜的浆细胞样 DC 相互作用[6]。因此，HSV DNA 中大量存在的 CpG 似乎表明"CpG 岛"就是固有免疫细胞识别 HSV-2 的 PAMP。但是研究表明，CD4$^+$ T 细胞识别通过黏膜下 DC 提呈的特殊抗原肽段[7]，这些现象表明了起源于固有免疫应答和适应性免疫应答不同的 DC 细胞群的作用是不同的。很显然，TLR-9 识别 HSV 完整病毒 DNA 的效率要高于识别提取的 DNA。信号通过不同 TLR 引起的细胞应答既有区别又可重叠[8]。例如，TLR-3 主要刺激产生 IFN-β 和多种化学增活素，而 TLR-4 则可刺激 IFN-β 的分泌，同时伴有吞噬作用和炎症反应。

与配体结合后，TLR 可以激活多种信号通路参与抗病毒应答。例如，浆细胞样 DC 上的 TLR-9 识别 HSV-2 的"CpG 岛"后可以刺激产生高水平的 I 型 IFN，具有强大的抗病毒功能。在体内，TLR 介导对 HSV-2 的应答可能需要两种细胞诱导的协同级联反应，首先是受感染的基质细胞，其次是未感染的 DC[9]。两种细胞对于 TLR 引导抗疱疹病毒免疫至产生 Th1 细胞应答都是必需的。

适应性免疫

适应性免疫和固有免疫的主要不同之处在于适应性免疫应答具有抗原特异性和记忆性。因此，适应性免疫不仅参与宿主初次感染微生物和病毒抗原的恢复过程，而且可以预防宿主的再次感染。

传统观点认为，表达 CD8 分子的细胞毒性 T 淋巴细胞（cytotoxic T lymphocyte，CTL）参与从感染到恢复的过程[10~13]。$CD8^+$ T 细胞通过与病毒编码蛋白的相互作用识别感染的细胞。这些蛋白质首先在感染细胞内通过特定机制（蛋白酶体）被裂解成小的肽段，而后再同宿主细胞主要组织相容性复合物（major histocompatibility complex，MHC）基因编码的 I 类分子结合成 MHC-I 类分子-肽段复合物，展示于细胞表面。通过这种机制，循环的淋巴细胞通过自身变化来熟练识别感染部位或肿瘤，并且具有独特的机制区分正常细胞和非正常细胞，如被感染细胞。然而，从感染中恢复的这种 MHC-I 限制的 $CD8^+$ T 细胞依赖性，可导致多种病毒通过不同的协同进化机制逃逸细胞介导的免疫监视。

病毒感染揭示了脊椎动物宿主免疫应答和免疫力的局限性，因为宿主对病毒的抵御恢复和免疫构成了天然和固有防御以及 T、B 细胞参与的适应性免疫应答的重要因素。所以病毒感染有助于阐明免疫应答的三个基本特性，即特异性、耐受性和记忆性。

生殖道黏膜免疫系统

尽管普遍认为泌尿生殖道是黏膜免疫系统的组成部分，但是对生殖道进行深入研究是最近才开展起来的。与其他的典型黏膜部位或外周免疫部位相比，泌尿生殖道免疫系统有其独特的特点。例如，女性泌尿生殖道分泌的抗体不仅来源于局部常驻浆细胞，还来源于血液，这也反映了抗体结构的异质性。又如，女性生殖道的分泌物中含有大量的单体 IgA，主要来源于血液中免疫球蛋白的直接渗出。此外，尤其是在女性生殖道中，免疫活性细胞的分布和特性，以及免疫球蛋白同种型比率、分子形式等方面都受到激素的影响[14~16]。

以上因素可能为 HPV 病毒样颗粒（virus-like particle，VLP）免疫宿主后对生殖器疣产生异乎寻常的保护效果提供了合理的解释，虽然 VLP 不能复制，但可以刺激产生针对病毒衣壳蛋白的抗体[17]。然而，Dupuy 等[18, 19]研究表明鼻腔内接种 HPV-16 的 VLP 或 HPV *L1* 基因可以诱导细胞应答，后者可以在阴道和脾脏内具有细胞毒性及 IFN-γ 分泌能力的淋巴细胞内检测到。

黏膜免疫和外周免疫之间的相互作用

在黏膜免疫的诱导阶段启动的淋巴细胞及 APC 穿越局部淋巴结，为黏膜免疫系统和外周免疫系统之间的相互作用（Cross-Talk）提供了机会（表2.2）。目前出现的一个重要的热点问题是：黏膜免疫是否是保护黏膜感染的最有效方式。关于淋巴细胞启动后循环并归巢至黏膜效应部位的研究已经比较充分，这就使研究者开始探讨一个问题：鼻黏膜免疫是否比系统免疫更能保护机体免于生殖道疱疹病毒[20, 21]和乳头瘤病毒[18]的感染（图2.3）。

黏膜免疫的细胞和分子

黏膜适应性免疫的基础是分泌性抗体。IgA 及少量的 IgM、IgG 分泌进入黏膜表面附着的黏液里，构成了抵御具有潜在侵袭性的病原微生物的第一道特殊防线。如果这道屏障破裂，抗原就会与黏膜内血清来源的 IgG 抗体相遇，形成免疫复合物激活补体，并在局部生成炎症介质。炎症反应的持续发展对宿主是有害的，幸运的是，血清来源的 IgA 和局部组织分泌的单体或双体 IgA 在黏膜基质内对抗原的竞争作用可调节炎症反应。黏膜内的血管内皮细胞选择性表达黏附分子的调节使黏膜免疫系统中 T 细胞和 B 细胞优先渗出。

黏膜分泌型 sIgA（secretory IgA，sIgA）抗体通常缺乏激活补体的特性[22~24]，并且多通过非炎症的机制来排除入侵的病原体。外分泌腺和分泌性黏膜组织含有机体大部分活化的 B 细胞，尤其在肠道固有层至少占有全部 Ig 分泌性免疫细胞的 80%[2]，这是 sIgA 能够成为主要的第一道特异性防线的细胞基础。在所有的外分泌位点中，IgA 分泌细胞主要产生 IgA 二聚体或更大的多聚体（polymeric IgA，pIgA），这些抗体可以通过受体介导的机制进行主动运输来穿过分泌型上皮细胞。据估计，机体每天合成和分泌的 IgA 量比 IgG 和 IgM 总量还高[25]。

生殖器部位的主要病毒感染

单纯疱疹

生殖器疱疹（genital herpes，GH）通常（但并非绝对）是由 HSV-2 感染所致[26~28]。根据型特异性的血清学研究，据估计美国约有 22% 的成年人感染过 HSV-2。不管有没有明显的症状，所有的 HSV 感染者都会经生殖器或其他腰部以下皮区定期排毒，从而导致人群中存在大量因无明显症状而不能诊断的 GH 患者。单纯疱疹的致病机制十分复杂，因为病毒可在皮肤黏膜表面和感觉神经系统之间频繁穿梭。当皮肤或黏膜第一次接触 HSV 时，病毒不仅可以在接触位点造成不明显的原发感染，而且可以同时沿轴突逆行到感觉神经节。在感觉神经元中病毒处于非复制休眠状态，也称潜伏感染，并持续终身。这种潜伏感染的意义是病毒在宿主体内形成了可以周期性激活的病毒基因组库。HSV 在神经节的神经元之间传播后再次活化，并沿着神经以顺轴突运输的方式返回至皮肤黏膜表面，在原发感染的相同皮区引起疾病复发（图 2.4 和图 2.5）。另外，HSV 也可经过皮肤黏膜排毒传染给其他人，但并不产生明显的症状。

因此，HSV 的黏膜免疫面临独特的挑战：不仅要在原发感染时促进宿主的恢复，而且要对从皮肤神经末梢释放的病毒进行快速应答。

总之，单纯疱疹有两个明显的阶段：缺乏特异性免疫力的宿主的原发感染和具有预存免疫的宿主的复发感染。

若感染 HSV-2，女性生殖道内会产生固有免疫和适应性免疫应答。应答可以在宫颈中产生针对病毒的抗体，尽管宫颈和血清 IgG 抗体的特异性十分相似，但宫颈和血清 IgA 的特异性不同，说明宫颈 IgA 在局部产生而 IgG 不在局部产生[29]。在 HSV-1 型血清阳性且新近感染 HSV-2 的女性宫颈部可检测到记忆性抗体应答[30]。一般认为，抗体既可以促进原发感染的恢复，又可以预防复发感染，但是情况并非完全如此。有报道称[31]，在先天性无丙种球蛋白血症的极端病例中，

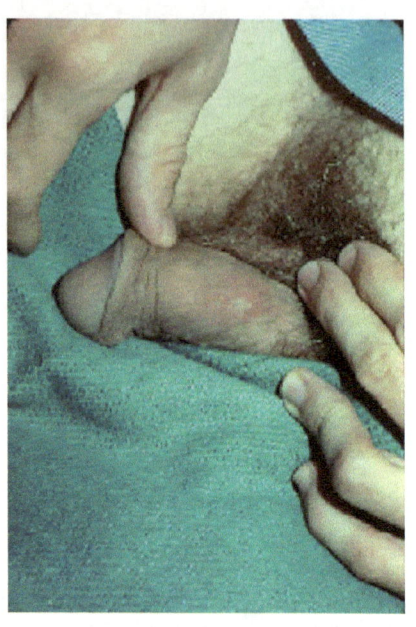

图 2.4 GH 复发造成的阴茎损伤，需细心才能发现的典型形态，宿主黏膜反应可控制其发展。大多数复发症状较轻，所以无法辨认出这是 GH 患者。

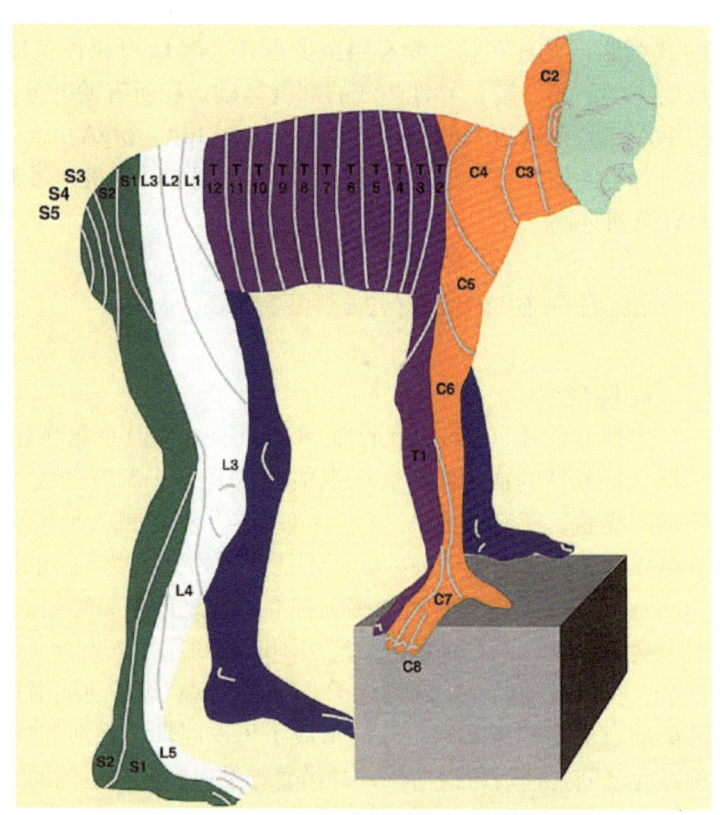

图 2.5 人体皮区图标示出受各自感觉神经节神经支配的皮肤区域。从图中可以很容易地看出，由于生殖器受 S2 和 S3 支配，所以这些神经节的潜伏感染很容易导致臀部、大腿和其他腰部以下部位的复发性损伤。

原发感染通常可以自然恢复，仅有少数顽固性疱疹病例发生明显的疱疹损伤。在这些个体中，病毒感染的复发既不会过于频繁也不会导致严重后果。这种明显异常现象的原因变得更加清晰，并非是由于抗体不能到达病毒隐藏的神经组织那样简单。同时，若不考虑抗原的特异性，活化的淋巴细胞可以轻易透过血脑屏障[32]，而不能攻击HSV感染细胞的失能抗体的分子机制被认为是宿主与大分子DNA病毒共进化产生免疫逃避策略的另一个特例。

HSV可以利用隐性机制使感染的细胞逃逸抗体介导的免疫应答。尽管宿主产生了强大的全身性的病毒特异性抗体应答[33]，但是HSV仍能够在拥有预存免疫的宿主体内持续存在，并且在皮肤黏膜表面引起复发（图2.4），这种现象进一步证明了HSV进化出了可以逃逸抗体介导的防御机制。相反，出现临床症状的原发感染显得更加严重（图2.6）。病毒逃逸的分子机制是HSV-1编码的两种糖蛋白gC和gE可分别与补体和免疫球蛋白的Fc段相互作用[34,35]。这些特性对于固有免疫和获得性免疫都有重大影响，包括干扰补体的组分C1q、C3、C5和备解素，并且可以阻断抗体介导的细胞依赖的细胞毒作用。但是，全身性抗体有助于阻止HSV在新生儿间的致命性传播[36]。

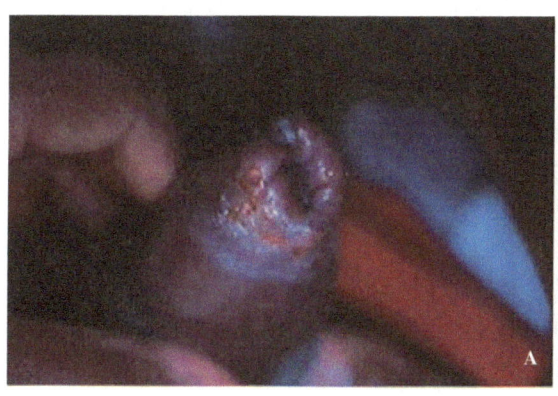
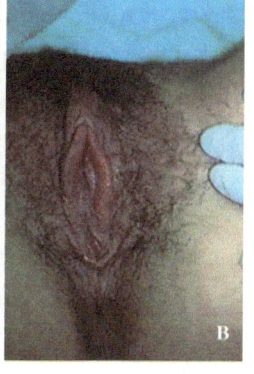

图2.6 A.免疫正常的男性原发GH，显示中等肿胀（龟头炎）；B.女性患者的原发GH症状显示两侧弥漫性损伤（Source: Courtesy of S. Tyring）。

生殖器HSV感染的恢复及对T细胞的依赖

疾病或药物可导致细胞介导免疫的选择性抑制，从而使患者免疫功能低下。几十年前就认识到在单纯疱疹恢复过程中，细胞介导的免疫机制占主要作用[28]。在后续的动物研究中得出了相同的结论，并对部分机制的揭示进行了漫长的探讨[37]。AIDS的全球大流行给我们提供了生动的例子（图2.7），在AIDS流行区，HSV难以治愈且威胁生命。持续性感染的患者在治疗过程中，若不能治愈急性感染，易使HSV进化出耐药株，对抗病毒药物如阿昔洛韦及其衍生物等具有抵抗作用（图2.8）。

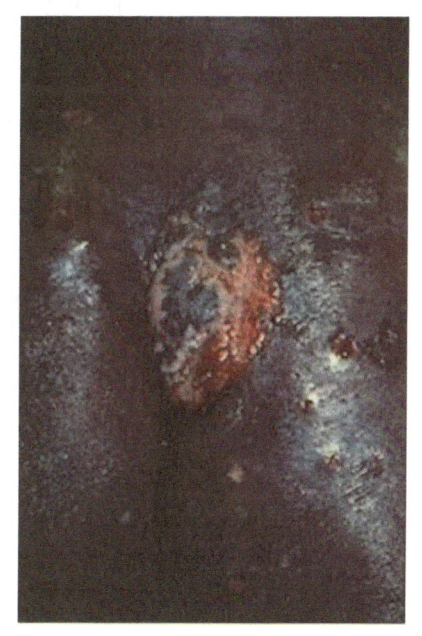

图2.7 HIV阳性患者臀部的HSV复发。损伤的消退依赖于完整的（黏膜）细胞免疫（Source: Courtesy of S. Tyring）。

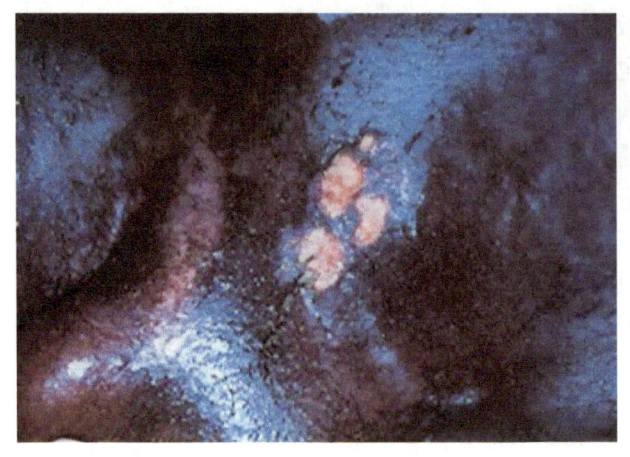

图2.8 生殖器区域的持续性皮肤黏膜损伤是免疫受损患者对所使用的抗病毒药物耐药的特征。此图显示阿昔洛韦耐药性HSV导致的腹股沟顽固损伤,且此HIV感染患者的免疫系统无法根除这种损伤。长期药物压力下的病毒生长会导致耐药,这类耐药多由编码病毒胸苷激酶(thymidine kinase,TK)的基因突变导致,通过磷酸化阿昔洛韦阻止其影响HSV复制。意外的是,TK突变的病毒不能从潜伏期再活化,因此它在一般人群中不易存活(Source: Courtesy of S. Tyring)。

复发性单纯疱疹

HSV可导致在原发感染的同一皮区的皮肤黏膜部位再次出现水疱样损伤。

与单纯体液防御缺陷的患者相比,细胞免疫损伤的宿主若感染主要引起生殖器皮肤和黏膜症状的普通性传播传染病,其后果更加严重。例如,很长时间以来人们认为在白血病或其他疾病(尤其是HIV感染,图2.7),或是药物治疗导致黏膜T细胞功能受损的患者中,HSV是导致严重的进行性溃疡和致命性皮肤溃疡的病因。

生殖器疣

乳头瘤病毒是世界上导致性传播感染的最常见病毒之一。免疫系统经常不能消除生殖道内的HPV感染,则可能产生肉眼不可见的生殖器疣。迄今确定的100多种HPV型别中,大约有30种是通过性接触传播的。大多数的HPV感染与HSV一样都是无害的,其中许多HPV的感染者是没有症状的。但是,一些HPV的感染则可导致生殖器疣的发生,好发部位多是阴道、宫颈、外阴、阴茎和直肠。少数HPV的感染会有异常的宫颈涂片,并且少数几个型别(尤其是HPV-16和HPV-18)与宫颈、外阴、阴道、肛门或阴茎的癌症相关。

据美国社会健康协会(American Social Health Association)估计,在美国至少有2000万HPV感染者,并且每年通过性接触增加约550万的新患者,新发感染的流行呈上升趋势[38]。生殖器HPV感染可通过与感染者进行口交、阴道性交或肛交的直接接触过程中传播。在与HPV感

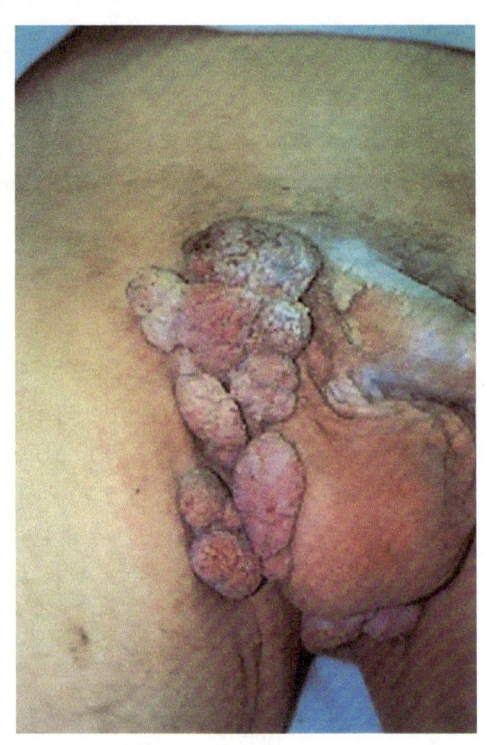

图2.9 生殖器疣在细胞介导的免疫受损的HIV患者中不受控制地生长(Source: Courtesy of S. Tyring)。

染者有过性接触的人中,约 2/3 在 3 个月内发生生殖器疣。在女性中,疣多发于阴道、宫颈或肛周。男性生殖器疣的发病率较低,多位于龟头、阴茎、阴囊或肛周部位。与 HPV 患者进行口交后也有可能发生口腔或咽喉部疣,但是非常罕见。

缺乏炎症是疣的一大特征,但在疣消解时的基底部可观察到组织学上的炎症反应和疣在免疫受损患者中的行为不受控制的现象。这些都说明尽管过程较长,但宿主应答仍在疣的控制中起重要作用。若宿主的免疫功能受损,HPV 的感染也会变得严重且难以根除(图 2.9)。

在 HIV 感染者和免疫功能受损患者中,疣持续存在并且发展成为肿瘤的概率增加,因此要对这些患者实行密切监测。需要开展的常规筛查至少应该包括每年一次宫颈涂片和外生殖器外观检查。出于大量原因的考虑包括监狱释放人员的随访护理不良,现行的实施标准要求,每 6 个月对监禁中的女性 HIV 感染者进行一次宫颈涂片观察。大多数的医疗机构有能力进行现场阴道镜检查,一些学者建议,阴道镜应该作为 HIV 合并 HPV 感染患者的基本检查。在对继发模糊性宫颈炎症的人群进行检查时,宫颈涂片诊断的准确性会下降。宫颈涂片异常的患者都应该做阴道镜检查,包括非典型和低度非典型增生病变。所有非典型增生的患者都应该进行积极治疗。

Buschke 和 Llöwenstein 巨大湿疣(giant condyloma of Buschke and Löwenstein, GCBL)极可能是一个典型的例子:宿主的免疫系统不能控制 HPV 感染。GCBL 是一种好发于阴茎的局部破坏性的疣状损伤,但也可发生于肛门生殖器区其他部位(图 2.10)。GCBL 通常被认为是疣状癌和口腔乳头瘤病毒的局部变异。

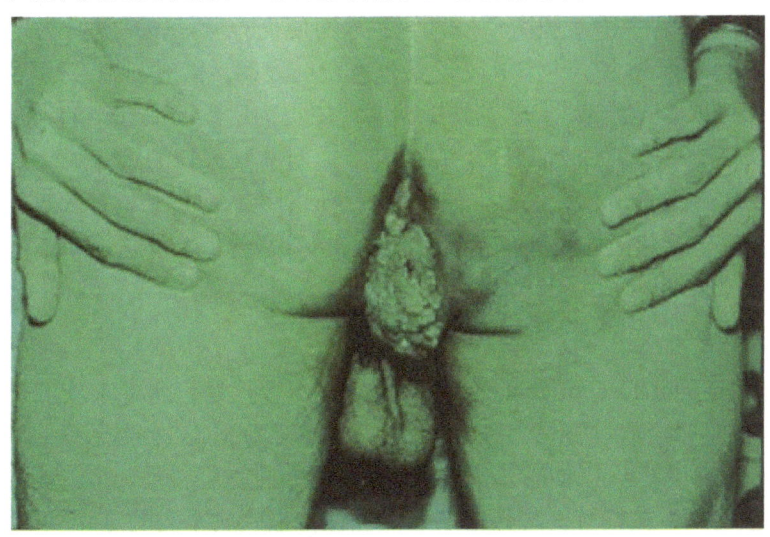

图 2.10 Buschke 和 Llöwenstein 巨大湿疣。不受控制的 HPV 感染的可能症状,可以认为是黏膜免疫的失败(Source: Courtesy of S. Tyring)。

虽然 GCBL 的发病机制并不确定,但是有一种假说倾向于乳头瘤病毒感染,因为在损伤处可发现 HPV-6、HPV-11、HPV-16、HPV-18、甚至 HPV-54 型的共存[39]。虽然 HPV-6 和 HPV-11 的 E6 蛋白与肿瘤抑制蛋白 P53 的结合能力低于 HPV-16 和 HPV-18,但是在理论上可以加速降解 P53 蛋白,E6 蛋白还可以抑制 P53 的转录。另一种发病机制的假说是 P53 蛋白的自发变异导致克隆化细胞增殖。有若干报道,如一项针对 GCBL 及鳞状细胞癌的研究结果表明，生殖器疣中 P53 过量表达。但一项近期研究推论出，尽管 P53 的确过量表达，但并不存在突变。其他与 GCBL 发病机制有关的因素包括长期的化学接触、长期刺激及不良的卫生条件。

尽管 GCBL 生长缓慢且很少转移，但是其对邻近的组织破坏性极强。GCBL 最常出现的部位是龟头，但也可发生于任何肛门生殖器黏膜表面，如外阴、阴道、直肠、阴囊和膀胱。GCBL 经常会被误诊为顽固性尖锐湿疣。幸运的是，美国的 GCBL 发病率较低，在阴茎癌患者中的占比不足 24%，同时阴茎癌的发病数只占男性恶性肿瘤总数的 0.3%~0.5%。然而，大约有 50% 的阴茎低分化度鳞状细胞癌的病因是疣状癌。GCBL 在阴茎以外的部位发作较少见，发生在肛周、外阴或膀胱部位的 GCBL 的报道不足 100 例。

对于黏膜免疫在 HPV 相关的宫颈疾病中的作用，我们现在的认识非常浅显。自然感染 HPV 的患者可产生血清抗衣壳抗体，但是无论在 HIV 阳性或阴性女性体内，这些抗体都不能保护机体免受 HPV 再次感染，这可能是由于自然 HPV 感染所产生的抗体浓度太低[41]。难以理解的是，通过鼻腔接种 HPV-16 的 VLP（尽管其不能复制），就可诱导阴道内特异性的 IFN-γ 分泌型 CD4[+] T 细胞和 CD8[+] CTL 的产生[18]。VLP 虽然不复制，但可以诱导机体产生高水平的抗体，从而保护女性免于 HPV-16 的感染及 HPV-16 相关的上皮瘤的形成[17]。这些结论提示两点：① VLP 可以诱导细胞及体液免疫应答；② 鼻腔免疫可以作为有效的免疫策略来保护 HPV 在远端黏膜的感染，这一点与 HSV 类似。

在保护生殖器黏膜抵御 HPV 感染的过程中，固有免疫起着十分重要的作用。免疫调节化合物咪喹莫特可以通过 IL-7 刺激免疫系统，从而使疣有所好转。这有力地提示了固有免疫对于疣的控制有十分重要的作用[42]。最近有研究表明，同时利用 CTL 表位和表皮下注射咪喹莫特，可以大量激活 CD8[+] T 细胞使其产生更为广泛的活性，如促进淋巴细胞增殖、提高细胞的杀伤性及增加细胞因子的生成[43]。对咪喹莫特的进一步研究发现，其可在表皮 DC 的表面与 TLR-7 相互作用，但是这种作用对于抗病毒适应性免疫的影响尚不清楚。在血清和黏膜分泌物中依赖抗原刺激所维持的高滴度抗体，或抗原激活的 T 细胞与记忆性最为密切。

传染性软疣

传染性软疣病毒（molluscum contagiosum virus，MCV）是痘病毒家族的一员，可产生一个或多个小的皮肤损伤，通常数月后可自愈。曾经认为 MCV 主要感染儿童，现在成人生殖器的 MCV 感染慢慢浮出水面[44]。传染性软疣通过性途径传播，方式为皮肤或黏膜与患者活动期的损伤处直接接触。与其他的病毒性性传播疾病不同的是，MCV 有时也可通过一些物体进行传播，如接触过病损的毛巾和衣物等。与患者在同一泳池游泳或同一浴池洗浴都可能造成 MCV 感染。此外，MCV 也可通过自我接种传播，因此，MCV 的分批损害很具有特征性。病毒的潜伏期为 1 周至 6 个月，平均为 2 个月。

皮肤的破损处多位于大腿、臀部、腹股沟及下腹部，偶尔也会出现在外生殖器和肛周部位。病变发展缓慢，多为肉色或灰白色，并且通常不会引起太大的问题。病变可持续 2 周至 4 年，平均为 2 年。尽管病变处会有瘙痒或压痛，但是对于免疫能力正常的患者而言不会产生更大的损伤。病变可复发，但尚不清楚是由于再次感染或亚临床感染的恶化还是潜伏感染的再度活化所致。

传染性软疣与免疫系统

在感染 HIV 的患者中，传染性软疣呈进行性发展，其临床特点不够典型[45, 46]。病变处损伤较大，呈疣状且明显过度角质化（图 2.11）。有研究表明，免疫刺激物（如咪喹莫特）对疣有一定的控制作用[47]。最后还发现 MCV 可以编码与 CD150 类似的蛋白质[48]，后者是激活抗病毒免疫中关键细胞因子 IFN-γ 通路中的主要受体。原有的潜在保护机制认为，黏膜处原有的或快速招募来的细胞可以快速清除病原体。但上述 MCV 中病毒和宿主共进化的现象似乎提供了推翻这一机制的例证。因此，关于黏膜免疫参与 MCV 的控制的结论毋庸置疑，但是其特殊的机制却还不清楚。最近有报道显示测得了 MCV 的全长序列，这可能会促进其黏膜保护机制及更多的治疗方法的研究。

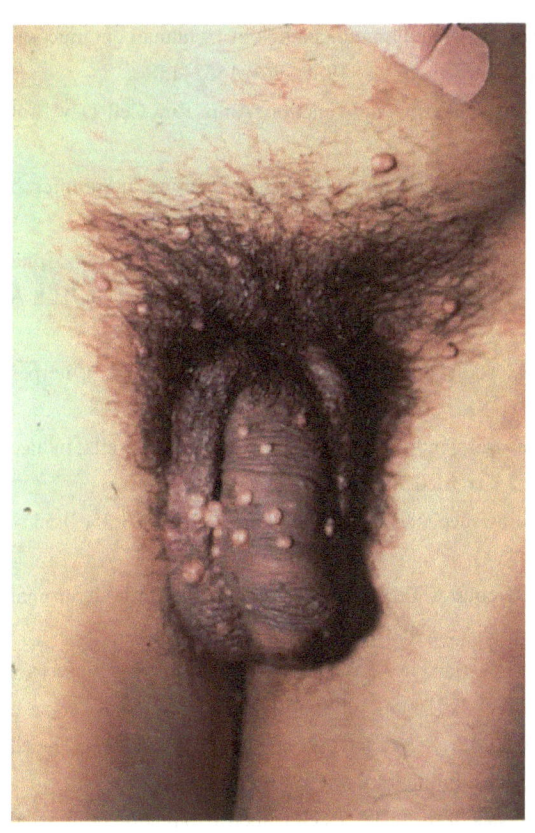

图 2.11 HIV 阳性患者传染性软疣造成的生殖器和下肢的广泛损伤，证明了免疫系统对疾病控制的重要性（Source: Courtesy of S. Tyring）。

总结

黏膜免疫系统很大程度上独立于系统免疫，以保护人体最大的器官（包括胃肠道和生殖器的皮肤与黏膜）免受病原微生物的侵害。总的来讲，黏膜免疫系统面积有一个半网球场大。在黏膜免疫中既有固有免疫也有适应性免疫，只是两者的免疫细胞略有不同。例如，具有重要的调节作用的上皮内淋巴细胞，其 T 细胞受体常含有 γδ 链而非 αβ 链。80%激活的淋巴细胞都位于黏膜组织中，而不是位于经典的二级淋巴器官，如淋巴结和脾脏。在黏膜部位激活的淋巴细胞进入引流淋巴结，并配备了归巢受体，一旦这些淋巴细胞离开了淋巴结，通过胸导管进入血液循环，归巢受体可使这些淋巴细胞优先进入黏膜效应部位。在生殖道内它们主要以独立的上皮内淋巴细胞存在，而非组织化淋巴滤泡。尽管传统观点认为生殖道黏膜作为第一线防御主要是由特异性抗体的分泌产生的，但是目前较倾向于固有免疫和 T 细胞介导的免疫机制发挥更重要的作用，如在 HSV、HPV、MCV 等病毒的感染过程中。

参 考 文 献

[1] Abraham R, Ogra PL. Mucosal microenvironment and mucosal response. Am J Trop Med Hyg 1994;50(5 suppl):3–9.

[2] Brandtzaeg P, Halstensen TS, Kett K, et al. Immunobiology and immunopathology of human gut mucosa: humoral immunity and intraepithelial lymphocytes. Gastroenterology 1989;97(6):1562–1584.

[3] Kraehenbuhl JP, Neutra MR. Epithelial M cells: differentiation and function. Annu Rev Cell Dev Biol 2000; 16:301–332.

[4] Herbst MM, Pyles RB. Immunostimulatory CpG treatment for genital HSV-2 infections. J Antimicrob Chemother 2003;52(6):887–889.

[5] Hochrein H, Schlatter B, O'Keeffe M, et al. Herpes simplex virus type-1 induces IFN-alpha production via Toll-like receptor 9-dependent and -independent pathways. Proc Natl Acad Sci U S A 2004;101(31):11416–11421.

[6] Lund J, Sato A, Akira S, Medzhitov R, Iwasaki A. Tolllike receptor 9-mediated recognition of herpes simplex virus-2 by plasmacytoid dendritic cells. J Exp Med 2003;198(3):513–520.

[7] Zhao X, Deak E, Soderberg K, et al. Vaginal submucosal dendritic cells, but not Langerhans cells, induce protective Th1 responses to herpes simplex virus-2. J Exp Med 2003;197(2):153–162.

[8] Akira S, Sato S. Toll-like receptors and their signaling mechanisms. Scand J Infect Dis 2003;35(9):555–562.

[9] Sato A, Iwasaki A. Induction of antiviral immunity requires Toll-like receptor signaling in both stromal and dendritic cell compartments. Proc Natl Acad Sci USA 2004;101(46):16274–16279.

[10] Doherty PC, Christensen JP, Belz GT, Stevenson PG, Sangster MY. Dissecting the host response to a gammaherpesvirus. Philos Trans R Soc Lond B Biol Sci 2001; 356(1408):581–593.

[11] Doherty PC, Topham DJ, Tripp RA, Cardin RD, Brooks JW, Stevenson PG. Effector $CD4^+$ and $CD8^+$ T-cell mechanisms in the control of respiratory virus infections. Immunol Rev 1997;159:105–117.

[12] Doherty PC, Riberdy JM, Belz GT. Quantitative analysis of the $CD8^+$ T-cell response to readily eliminated and persistent viruses. Philos Trans R Soc Lond B Biol Sci 2000;355(1400):1093–1101.

[13] Stevenson PG, Belz GT, Altman JD, Doherty PC. Changing patterns of dominance in the $CD8^+$ T cell response during acute and persistent murine gammaherpesvirus infection. Eur J Immunol 1999;29(4):1059–1067.

[14] Richardson J, Kaushic C, Wira CR. Estradiol regulation of secretory component: expression by rat uterine epithelial cells. J Steroid Biochem Mol Biol 1993; 47(1–6):143–149.

[15] Richardson JM, Kaushic C, Wira CR. Polymeric immunoglobin (Ig) receptor production and IgA transcytosis in polarized primary cultures of mature rat uterine epithelial cells. Biol Reprod 1995;53(3):488–498.

[16] Kaushic C, Richardson JM, Wira CR. Regulation of polymeric immunoglobulin A receptor messenger ribonucleic acid expression in rodent uteri: effect of sex hormones. Endocrinology 1995;136(7):2836–2844.

[17] Koutsky LA, Ault KA, Wheeler CM, et al. A controlled trial of a human papillomavirus type 16 vaccine. N Engl J Med 2002;347(21):1645–1651.

[18] Dupuy C, Buzoni-Gatel D, Touze A, Bout D, Coursaget P. Nasal immunization of mice with human papillomavirus type 16 (HPV-16) virus-like particles or with the HPV-16 L1 gene elicits specific cytotoxic T lymphocytes in vaginal draining lymph nodes. J Virol 1999;73(11):9063–9071.

[19] Dupuy C, Buzoni-Gatel D, Touze A, Le Cann P, Bout D, Coursaget P. Cell mediated immunity induced in mice by HPV 16 L1 virus-like particles. Microb Pathog 1997; 22(4):219–225.

[20] Milligan GN, Dudley-McClain KL, Chu CF, Young CG. Efficacy of genital T cell responses to herpes simplex virus type 2 resulting from immunization of the nasal mucosa. Virology 2004;318(2):507–515.

[21] Gallichan WS, Johnson DC, Graham FL, Rosenthal KL. Mucosal immunity and protection after intranasal immunization with recombinant adenovirus expressing herpes simplex virus glycoprotein B. J Infect Dis 1993;168(3):622–629.

[22] Mestecky J, Russell MW, Jackson S, Brown TA. The human IgA system: a reassessment. Clin Immunol Immunopathol 1986;40(1):105–114.

[23] Brandtzaeg P, Baklien K, Bjerke K,Rognum TO, Scott H, Valnes K. Nature and properties of the human gastrointestinal immune system. In: Miller K, Nicklin S, eds. Immunology of the Gastrointestinal Tract. Boca Raton, FL: CRC Press, 1987:1–86.

[24] Kilian M, Russell MW. Function of mucosal immunoglobulins. In: Ogra PL, Mestecky J, Lamm ME, Strober W,McGhee JR, Bienenstock J, eds.Handbook of Mucosal Immunology. Orlando, FL: Academic Press, 1994:127–137.

[25] Conley ME, Delacroix DL. Intravascular and mucosal immunoglobulin A: two separate but related systems of immune defense? Ann Intern Med 1987;106(6):892–899.

[26] Ashley R, Benedetti J, Corey L. Humoral immune response to HSV-1 and HSV-2 viral proteins in patients with primary genital herpes. J Med Virol 1985;17(2): 153–166.

[27] Corey L, Adams HG, Brown ZA, Holmes KK. Genital herpes simplex virus infections: clinical manifestations, course, and complications. Ann Intern Med 1983; 98(1):958–972.

[28] Simmons A, Osman MN, Stanberry LR. Genital Herpes. In: Gorbach SL, Bartlett JG, Blacklow NR, eds. Infectious Diseases. Philadelphia: Lippincott Williams & Wilkins, 2004:904–915.

[29] Brandtzaeg P. Mucosal immunity in the female genital tract. J Reprod Immunol 1997;36(1–2):23–50.

[30] Ashley R, Wald A, Corey L. Cervical antibodies in patients with oral herpes simplex virus type 1 (HSV-1) infection: local anamnestic responses after genital HSV-2 infection. J Virol 1994;68(8):5284–5286.

[31] Kraemer CK, Benvenuto C, Weber CW, Zampese MS, Cestari TF. Chronic cutaneous herpes simplex in a patient with hypogammaglobulinemia. Skin Med 2004; 3(2):111–113.

[32] Irani DN,Griffin DE.Regulation of lymphocyte homing into the brain during viral encephalitis at various stages of infection. J Immunol 1996;156(10):3850–3857.

[33] Lubinski JM, Jiang M, Hook L, et al. Herpes simplex virus type 1 evades the effects of antibody and complement in vivo. J Virol 2002;76(18):9232–9241.

[34] Kostavasili I, Sahu A, Friedman HM, Eisenberg RJ, Cohen GH, Lambris JD. Mechanism of complement inactivation by glycoprotein C of herpes simplex virus. J Immunol 1997;158(4):1763–1771.

[35] Weeks BS, Sundaresan P, Nagashunmugam T, Kang E, Friedman HM. The herpes simplex virus-1 glycoprotein E (gE) mediates IgG binding and cell-to-cell spread through distinct gE domains. Biochem Biophys Res Commun 1997;235(1):31–35.

[36] Ashley RL, Dalessio J, Burchett S, et al. Herpes simplex virus-2 (HSV-2) type-specific antibody correlates of protection in infants exposed to HSV-2 at birth. J Clin Invest 1992;90(2):511–514.

[37] Simmons A, Tscharke D, Speck P. The role of immune mechanisms in control of herpes simplex virus infection of the peripheral nervous system. Curr Top Microbiol Immunol 1992;179:31–56.

[38] Koshiol JE, Laurent SA, Pimenta JM. Rate and predictors of new genital warts claims and genital wartsrelated healthcare utilization among privately insured patients in the United States. Sex Transm Dis 2004; 31(12):748–752.

[39] Haycox CL. Kuypers J. Krieger JN. Role of human papillomavirus typing in diagnosis and clinical decision making for a giant verrucous genital lesion. Urology 1999;53(3):627–630.

[40] Pilotti S. Donghi R. D'Amato L, et al. HPV detection and p53 alteration in squamous cell verrucous

malignancies of the lower genital tract. Diagn Mol Pathol 1993;2(4): 248–256.

[41] Viscidi RP, Snyder B, Cu-Uvin S, et al. Human papillomavirus capsid antibody response to natural infection and risk of subsequent HPV infection in HIV-positive and HIV-negative women. Cancer Epidemiol Biomarkers Prev 2005;14(1):283–288.

[42] Smith KJ, Hamza S, Skelton H. The imidazoquinolines and their place in the therapy of cutaneous disease. Expert Opin Pharmacother 2003;4(7):1105–1119.

[43] Rechtsteiner G, Warger T, Osterloh P, Schild H, Radsak MP. Cutting edge: priming of CTL by transcutaneous peptide immunization with imiquimod. J Immunol 2005;174(5):2476–2480.

[44] Laxmisha C, Thappa DM, Jaisankar TJ. Clinical profile of molluscum contagiosum in children versus adults. Dermatol Online J 2003;9(5):1.

[45] Smith KJ, Skelton H. Molluscum contagiosum: recent advances in pathogenic mechanisms, and new therapies. Am J Clin Dermatol 2002;3(8):535–545.

[46] Smith KJ, Skelton HG, Yeager J, et al. Cutaneous findings in HIV-1-positive patients: a 42-month prospective study. Military Medical Consortium for the Advancement of Retroviral Research (MMCARR). J Am Acad Dermatol 1994;31(5 pt 1):746–754.

[47] Hengge UR, Cusini M. Topical immunomodulators for the treatment of external genital warts, cutaneous warts and molluscum contagiosum. Br J Dermatol 2003; 149(suppl 66):15–19.

[48] Sidorenko SP, Clark EA. The dual-function CD150 receptor subfamily: the viral attraction. Nat Immunol 2003;4(1):19–24.

第3章
胃肠道黏膜免疫学

David A. Bland, Carlos A. Barrera, and Victor E. Reyes

试想一下，除了原核生物之外，假如地球表面上的其他物质都是肉眼看不见的话，那么地球上无处不在的可见细菌附着在不可见的"物体"上，人们看世间万物便如幽灵般存在。

因此，人类进化形成的复杂的免疫系统使我们能够与微生物共存。持续暴露于细菌的皮肤和气道准备好了抵御或中和细菌不断攻击的工具。然而，没有一种组织比胃肠道（gastrointestinal，GI）黏膜暴露于包括细菌在内的更多种类的外界物质之中。从出生开始，我们的胃肠道黏膜就不断地遭到各种外来抗原的攻击，如食物性抗原、正常菌群和病原体。由于胃肠道黏膜表面覆盖一层上皮细胞，具有复杂的隐窝和绒毛结构，表面积极其大，因此容易成为许多传染性病原体定植和入侵的部位。某些病原体定植于上皮表面，而另一些病原体则定植于上皮屏障内部或穿过上皮屏障侵入人体。黏膜免疫系统不仅必须识别这些病原体，而且同时也必须忽略共生菌群和食物性抗原。因此，胃肠道的局部免疫系统是高度特异性的，对保障人类健康至关重要，这一点毫无疑问。

与很多病毒一样，许多肠道细菌进化出能够有效逃避或破坏宿主免疫应答的机制。此外，定居在人胃肠道的共生菌群增加了局部免疫应答的复杂性，一方面这种局部免疫应答可对病原体起到基本的防御作用，另一方面宿主免疫系统对共生菌群产生的不适当免疫防御可引发疾病。

虽然胃肠道黏膜免疫系统的结构和功能与更高级的免疫系统相似，但肠道中的诱导部位（inductive site）和效应部位（effector site）使得胃肠道免疫系统能够对特有的肠道细菌的攻击作出适当的应答。另外，近期研究表明，黏膜免疫系统的调控可能比预想的更加分散。特定免疫区与免疫细胞协同作用的特征使免疫模式的概念发生了变化，如肠相关淋巴组织（gut-associated lymphoid tissue，GALT）与非GALT免疫细胞（如肠道上皮内淋巴细胞）的协同作用。在黏膜免疫系统范畴内，固有免疫系统与适应性免疫系统的相互作用和集中免疫调控等概念正受到质疑。另外，我们已知道一种特殊的T细胞群特异性地归巢于胃肠道。正是这些特异性的免疫细胞与肠道的结构细胞共同作用，形成了针对肠道病原体的免疫防御系统。

本章内容概述了构成胃肠道固有免疫应答与适应性免疫应答的元素及其如何在具有代表性的感染反应中发挥作用。胃肠道黏膜反应必须能够通过对共生菌群及食物性抗原形成免疫抑制来将有害抗原与之区分。若不幸发生过度的免疫防御，则会引发食物过敏和炎性肠病（inflammatory bowel disease，IBD）等常见的临床疾病。

胃肠道黏膜的固有免疫防御

黏膜免疫的一个重要作用就是其中的固有免疫能够保护宿主胃肠道表面免受抗原的攻击。固有免疫屏障包括由杯状细胞分泌的黏液形成的物理屏障，它们覆盖于上皮细胞表面提供保护作用。潜在病原体可能会陷入黏液中，从而无法感染上皮细胞。除了黏液，一系列蛋白水解酶，如胰蛋白酶、糜蛋白酶、胃蛋白酶，与胆盐和强酸一起也能够抵御潜在病原体入侵。另外，还有其他一些重要的非细胞性体液因子参与到黏膜表面的固有免疫防御之中。黏膜上皮一直被认为是阻止病原体入侵的物理屏障，然而近10年的研究结果显示它对于宿主的保护作用比预想的更加重要。多项独立的研究结果提供的证据表明黏膜上皮可能直接影响着适应性免疫应答，这部分内容将在下文中进行介绍。

胃肠道上皮

黏膜上皮的结构和功能

上皮细胞屏障是选择性渗透的，这种组织结构不仅可以防止未完全消化的食物、细菌和细菌产物毫无控制地进入宿主体内，而且还可以调节液体和电解质的吸收及分泌。柱状上皮细胞的顶端表面有紧密连接和黏着连接，它们可以将细胞间隙与肠腔分隔。细胞之间的黏附结构是由蛋白复合物组成的，如封闭蛋白、封闭小带-1和封闭小带-2（zonula occluden，ZO-1和ZO-2）及Claudin封闭蛋白家族成员。这些连接蛋白受到炎性产物和免疫应答的调节。例如，促炎性细胞因子能够下调连接蛋白组分ZO-1的表达，如γ-干扰素（interferon-γ，IFN-γ）（图3.1）。这种时间依赖性下调与跨上皮电阻的显著降低有关，后者可由甘露醇通量的上升来验证。在人类IBD中，紧密连接蛋白中的封闭蛋白表达减少，提示在活动性IBD中，上皮细胞中封闭蛋白表达的下调可增强细胞间的通透性和中性粒细胞的渗出[2]。

当上皮细胞层受到损伤时，能够分泌一些影响上皮细胞增殖、迁移和创伤愈合的上皮细胞因子。例如，表皮生长因子（epidermal growth factor，EGF）可以通过促进转化生长因子-β（transforming growth factor-β，TGF-β）[3]、成纤维细胞生长因子（fibroblast growth factor，FGF）、肝细胞生长因子（hepatocyte growth factor，HGF）和小肠三叶因子（intestinal trefoil factor，ITF）的分泌而发挥部分作用。ITF向上皮细胞顶端分泌，它的功能是增加上皮细胞向损伤部位的迁移[4]。

在上皮细胞层受到感染或侵袭的过程中，免疫细胞或炎症细胞向侵袭部位的皮下间隙迁移增加。例如，在针对细菌感染的应答过程中，人肠道上皮细胞分泌的介质，如趋化因子，对于激活急性黏膜炎症反应是必不可少的。在这种情况下，大量的肠道侵袭性细菌和一些非侵袭性的细菌性病原体与上皮细胞膜相互作用，并诱导上皮细胞上调有效的趋化因子的分泌和释放，以促进中性粒细胞（如CXCL1/GROα、CXCL2/GROβ、CXCL5/ENA78和CXCL8/IL-8）[5,6]、单核细胞/巨噬细胞（如CCL2/MCP-1）[6,7]和未成熟的表达CCR6

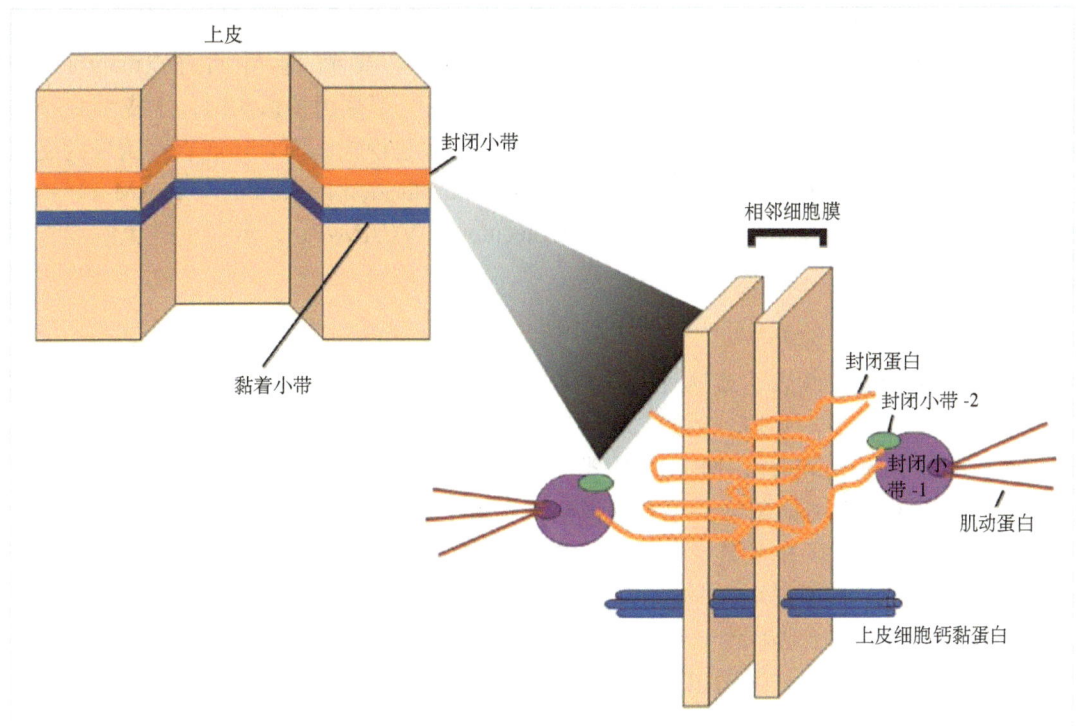

图 3.1 肠道上皮细胞的连接复合物。跨膜封闭蛋白是封闭小带（ZO）的封闭蛋白，它直接与 ZO-1 相互作用。ZO 在上皮细胞的顶端表面形成嵴线，将细胞连接在一起。这种黏着小带在毗邻的细胞间形成连续的带状连接，增强了上皮屏障的机械强度。黏着小带由上皮细胞钙黏蛋白组成。

的树突状细胞（dendritic cell，DC）（CCL20/MIP-3α）[8] 向感染部位募集。此外，在炎症状态下，人肠道上皮细胞还能够分泌 IFN-γ 诱导趋化因子（IFN-γ-inducible chemokine），如 CCL9/Mig、CCL10/IP-10、CCL11/I-TAC[9,10]，这些因子可以化学诱导有记忆表型的表达 CXCR3 的 T 细胞及肠道上皮细胞本身分泌 IFN-γ。与前面提到的趋化因子相反，在细菌感染时，IFN-γ 诱导趋化因子 CCL9、CCL10 和 CCL11 的表达不是单独上调，而是协同上调。另外，肠道上皮细胞上调表达和分泌趋化因子的动力学及作用于相似靶点的趋化因子的生物学和功能特性的差异，可能会导致趋化因子形成时间和空间浓度梯度，以促进趋化因子对于肠黏膜中炎症性靶细胞的化学趋向化 [6]。

很多研究已经开始阐明上皮在产生信号过程中的作用，这些信号对黏膜适应性免疫的发育十分重要。就这一点而言，小肠上皮细胞可持续分泌 CCL25/TECK，它的同源受体 CCR9 是由倾向于分布在小肠黏膜的表达 α4β7 的 T 细胞表达 [11,12]。相反地，人结肠上皮细胞并不分泌 CCL25，而分泌 CCL28/MEC，它的同源配体是 CCR10[13,14]。因此，CCR10 表达细胞亚群倾向于分布在肠道中分泌 CCL28 的区域（如结肠和唾液腺）。CCL28 似乎对淋巴细胞亚群分别向小肠和结肠的选择性迁移十分重要。

除了趋化因子，在细菌感染应答中，肠上皮细胞还能表达多种细胞因子。上皮细胞表达的一些细胞因子包括 EBI3、肿瘤坏死因子 -α（tumor necrosis factor-α, TNF-α）、白细胞介素（interleukin，IL）-12p35、IL-15、粒细胞-巨噬细胞集落刺激因子（granulocyte-macrophage colony-stimulating factor，GM-CSF）和巨噬细胞抑制因子（macrophage inhibitory factor，MIF）[5,15~18]。在受到细菌感染或促炎性细胞因子影响时，上皮细胞释放的细胞因子不仅可以影响黏膜组织中免疫细胞的基因表达模式，而且还能直接诱导内皮细胞表达黏附分子，如细胞内黏附分子-1（intracellular adhesion molecule-1，ICAM-1）和血管细胞黏附分子-1（vascular cell adhesion molecule-1，VCAM-1），可以促进免疫细胞和炎症细胞向黏膜聚集[19]。

上皮细胞受体及其功能

上皮细胞能够持续表达或诱导表达对宿主免疫十分重要的受体，这与它在完整黏膜免疫系统中的作用是一致的。例如，胃肠道上皮细胞表达主要组织相容性复合物（major histocompatability complex，MHC）II类分子和非典型MHC I类分子（如CD1d、MICA）[20]及CD86协同刺激分子，这说明胃肠道上皮细胞具有抗原提呈细胞（antigen-presenting cell，APC）的功能。传统的APC能够摄取、处理抗原，并以MHC II类分子复合物的形式完成抗原提呈。协同刺激分子（如CD80和CD86）的表达以及CD28的参与，使APC能够最大限度地激活T细胞。因此，胃肠道上皮细胞可能会摄取肠腔中被蛋白水解酶部分水解的抗原，并通过上皮细胞内蛋白水解酶进一步加工[21]，最后提呈给固有层中的T细胞。

Mayer及其同事的研究表明，在正常情况下，肠道上皮细胞会选择性激活具有抑制活性的$CD8^+$ T细胞，它有助于控制肠道炎症。这种$CD8^+$ T细胞的选择性激活有赖于上皮细胞表达的一种CD8配体，即癌胚抗原（carcinoembryonic antigen，CEA）家族成员gp180[22,23]。然而，有趣的是，IBD患者的肠道上皮细胞缺乏gp180，所以不能激活具有抑制作用的$CD8^+$ T细胞。该研究团队近期的另一项研究表明肠道上皮细胞表达的新型B7家族成员B7h和B7-H1对T细胞有调节活性[24]。

除了表达参与T细胞相互作用的受体，人肠道上皮细胞还能够表达一系列细胞因子受体，这些受体包括公认的IL-1、IL-4、IL-6、IL-7、IL-9、IL-10、IL-15、IL-17、IFN-γ、GM-CSF和TNF-α受体[4,7,19]，以及一些趋化因子受体，如CXCR4、CCR5、CCR6和CX3CR1受体[19,25]。一部分受体表达在上皮细胞的底外侧表面，另一部分表达在细胞顶端或两极。这种表达方式说明上皮细胞的信号转导和功能发挥不仅受肠腔内抗原、细菌及细菌产物的影响，还受到黏膜局部免疫细胞群释放的细胞因子和趋化因子的影响，这就使上皮细胞能发现并对皮下间隙发生的免疫变化作出应答。

虽然有些致病菌能够侵入上皮细胞，直接或通过向细胞分泌细菌产物间接地改变细胞内的信号转导途径[26,27]，如沙门氏菌（*Salmonella*）、志贺氏菌（*Shigella*）、肠侵袭性大肠杆菌（*Escherichia coli*）、耶尔森氏菌（*Yersinia*）和李斯特菌（*Listeria*），但是肠道上皮细胞也能表达Toll样受体（toll-like receptor，TLR），这是一种进化保守的受体家族，通过识别细菌分子的保守部位在固有免疫中发挥作用[28,29]。这些受体将在下文详述。简而言之，上皮细胞可不同程度地表达TLR-2、TLR-3、TLR-4和TLR-5，这表明脂多糖（lipopolysaccharide，LPS）和其他细菌产物，如鞭毛蛋白，能够通过这些受体作用于上皮细胞[30,31]。

在调节免疫细胞和炎症细胞转运中发挥重要作用的另一类重要的膜分子是黏附分子，包括 ICAM-1、淋巴细胞功能相关抗原 -3（lymphocyte function associated antigen-3，LFA-3）（CD58）、钙黏附素和胆糖蛋白（biliary glycoprotein，BGP）[32,33]。例如，肠上皮细胞经过细菌侵袭或激动剂刺激（IFN-γ 或 TNF-α）后可上调 ICAM-1 的表达[29,34]，并且 ICAM-1 的表达具有极性，集中在肠道上皮细胞的顶端表面，其密度在细胞间连接区域最高。研究已经表明 ICAM-1 的水平升高与中性粒细胞的顶端黏附增强相关[34,35]，这可能是由于上调的顶端 ICAM-1 的表达使中性粒细胞从上皮渗出到肠隐窝，从而在该部位形成上皮防御机制。

核因子 NF-κB：肠道上皮细胞固有免疫应答的一种重要调节因子

虽然许多细菌性病原体以不同的方式进入上皮细胞并有不同的细胞内生活方式，但它们都可以激活转录因子 NF-κB（nuclear factor-kappa B）及其靶基因，从而激活肠上皮细胞内的信号转导[36]。因此，人们认为 NF-κB 是上皮细胞信号通路的重要调节因子，该信号通路在启动宿主固有免疫应答抵御微生物感染中是必不可少的。大量的肠道病原体和促炎性细胞因子（如 TNF-α 和 IL-1）只有首先激活 Iκ 激酶（I kappa kinase，IKK）复合物，尤其是 IKKβ 亚基，才能进一步激活 NF-κB。此外，还有一些病原体（如耶尔森氏菌）能够通过它们的 III 型分泌蛋白建立起一种阻止 NF-κB 和其他信号转导通路激活的策略，继而调节宿主炎症反应[37,38]。

过去的 10 年里，许多研究结果揭示了肠道上皮细胞在免疫应答中的重要作用，上皮细胞一方面维持着与外界隔离的物理屏障，另一方面与免疫细胞和炎症细胞一起防止感染和上皮损伤。肠道上皮细胞通过分泌抗微生物肽和其他抗微生物产物及启动黏膜固有免疫必需的信号分子等作用，在宿主肠腔内防御机制中发挥关键作用，同时，肠道上皮细胞还可通过将适宜的细胞群聚集到肠道黏膜为宿主的适应性免疫应答创造条件。

固有体液因子

抗微生物肽

人们在对植物和昆虫抗微生物特性的研究中发现了一个进化保守的蛋白家族，此后实际上在所有的多细胞生物体中也发现了这种蛋白质，包括人类。由于该蛋白家族具有广泛的多样性，所以试图对这种肽进行分类不太成功，因此只能根据它们的二级结构和大小进行简单的分类。此类分子被称为阳离子抗微生物肽（cationic antimicrobial peptide，CAMP），它们具有抗病毒、真菌和细菌性病原体的能力。目前，人们对 CAMP 的抗细菌特性了解得最为清楚。CAMP 与细菌相互作用时最令人关注的可能是细菌很难产生对 CAMP 的耐受。实际上，目前大量研究团队致力于将抗微生物肽作为下一代抗生素。

细菌胞膜与多细胞微生物胞膜的组成不同，抗微生物肽就是根据这种基本的差异而设计的，所以抗微生物肽能有效阻断细菌感染。大多数细菌双层胞膜的外层由大量带负电荷的磷脂类基团构成，而植物和动物的胞膜外层由不带电荷的脂类构成。利用这一特性，具有不同一级结构的 CAMP 可以相似的方式发挥作用，这是因为它们的亲水和疏水残基能够形成一致的、不相关联的两性二级结构。

目前有很多假说来解释 CAMP 是用什么方式杀死细菌的，且均以肽与类脂双层膜的相互作用开始，并伴随着细菌包膜的物理性破坏。基于这一点，人们认为可能是 CAMP 导致双层膜上形成小孔，使细胞成分外流。其他理论则认为内化的 CAMP 是通过细菌包膜的致死性去极化作用、水解酶类的激活对细胞壁的降解作用或细胞活性的破坏来杀死细菌的。

CAMP 似乎在胃肠道黏膜固有免疫中发挥着十分重要的作用，因为在唾液、母乳和肠道的上皮细胞及帕内特细胞（Paneth cell）中都存在着 CAMP 分子。

防御素

与 CAMP 相似，防御素（defensin）也是高阳离子蛋白/肽。它们富含精氨酸，分子质量为 3.0～4.5kDa。防御素按照 β 片层结构和含二硫键的半胱氨酸进行分类。虽然人类防御素按照二硫键的排列被分为 α 和 β 两类，但人们在灵长类中还分离出了新型的第三类环型肽，称为 θ- 防御素。防御素首先被合成为前肽，经翻译后修饰，成为有活性的形式。

α- 防御素全长 29~35 个残基，含有一个三链 β 片层结构。目前已鉴定出 6 种 α- 防御素：人中性粒细胞肽 1～4（human neutrophil peptide，HNP）及人防御素 -5 和人防御素 -6（human defensin，HD）[39]。就像名称所表示的那样，HNP 主要在中性粒细胞中表达，但在 IL-2 存在的情况下，T 细胞和自然杀伤（natural killer，NK）细胞中也分离出了 HNP-1、HNP-2 和 HNP-3[40]。HD-5 和 HD-6 主要在肠道帕内特细胞中表达[41]。

与 α- 防御素不同，β- 防御素全长达 45 个残基，有不同的二硫键（半胱氨酸）配对。目前有 4 种 β- 防御素 [HBD-(1～4)]，绝大多数主要由上皮细胞合成[42]。

防御素除了具有直接抗微生物特性外，还可通过募集和激活白细胞在胃肠道固有免疫应答中发挥重要作用。事实上，直到最近才把防御素和趋化因子（可溶性白细胞募集因子的经典类型）的研究合二为一；基于结构和功能的相似性，许多防御素和趋化因子家族的蛋白质可以作为 CAMP 及免疫效应细胞的趋化激活因子，因此在固有免疫系统和适应性免疫系统之间产生了重要的联系，有利于宿主防御肠道内病原体[43]。

乳铁蛋白

绝大多数的乳铁蛋白（lactoferrin）可以从所有哺乳类动物乳汁中分离，包括人类[44]。也可在外分泌液中检测到，如泪液、唾液、胆汁和胰液。另外，多型核白细胞（polymorphonuclear cell，PMN）是这种铁结合蛋白的主要合成细胞。成熟的人乳铁蛋白（human lactoferrin，hLf）含 692 个氨基酸，折叠成两个凸起：N 端和 C 端突起。每个突起均含有铁结合位点[45]。

除了作为铁的运载体，乳铁蛋白还有非常重要的抗微生物特性[46]。虽然乳铁蛋白通过清除铁来防御细菌感染的特性仍然存在争议，但它的直接抗微生物作用已被证实。乳铁蛋白与 LPS 的 A 部分结合，导致 LPS 从革兰氏阴性菌中分离。对乳铁蛋白和其他已知的 LPS 结合蛋白进行序列比对发现，两者在结构上具有显著的同源性，这种活性被认为对破坏细菌包膜起关键作用。

另外，乳铁蛋白对细菌的另一种直接效应来自于它自身的裂解产物。胃蛋白酶可将乳铁蛋白裂解成一种 N 端衍生肽，即乳铁蛋白 H[47]。虽然机制未明，但是乳铁蛋白 H 可以和革兰氏阴性菌的 LPS 及革兰氏阳性菌的胞壁酸结合。因此，人们提出假说，认为乳铁蛋白 H 会导致细菌胞膜的裂解。

溶菌酶

溶菌酶（lysozyme）是一种高阳离子蛋白质，能够水解细胞壁肽聚糖中的 N- 乙酰胞壁酸（N-acetylmuramic acid，NAM）和 N- 乙酰葡萄糖胺（N-acetylglucosamine，NAG）的 β-1,4 糖苷键，从而破坏特定的革兰氏阳性菌。然而，溶菌酶对许多致病菌并不是非常有效，如溶血性链球菌、李斯特菌和分枝杆菌。这种耐受性是由于细胞壁的肽聚糖组分含有 O- 乙酰基团，它干扰溶菌酶与 NAM-NAG 连接的相互作用。有趣的是，溶菌酶热变性实验表明这种蛋白质实际上能通过激活一种称为胞壁酸酶的细菌自溶酶而间接杀死细菌。

由于许多革兰氏阴性菌拥有一层厚的阴离子外膜，因此溶菌酶通常对这类细菌作用不大。然而，在补体系统存在的情况下，溶菌酶可利用过氧化物酶使细菌的细胞壁穿孔。此外，溶菌酶还可以与乳铁蛋白发生协同作用诱导细菌裂解。

干扰素

干扰素（interferon，IFN）在人类疾病中发挥着关键作用，分为 I 型 IFN（IFN-α 和 IFN-β）和 II 型 IFN（IFN-γ）。目前已证实 I 型 IFN 在炎症、免疫调节和 T 细胞应答中具有重要作用，并且成纤维细胞、上皮细胞及造血源性细胞均能合成 IFN。I 型 IFN 是一种多功能免疫调节性细胞因子，在细胞因子级联反应中发挥重要作用，包括多种抗炎特性。最早发现 IFN 的特性是抗病毒作用，病毒感染的细胞合成 IFN，IFN 分泌后作用于其相邻的细胞，形成一种抗病毒状态。II 型 IFN 由活化的 T 细胞、NK 细胞和巨噬细胞合成。IFN-γ 具有免疫促进作用，能使巨噬细胞进一步活化。也能诱导巨噬细胞、DC 和 B 细胞中 MHC I 类和 MHC II 类分子的表达增强。有趣的是，IFN-γ 促进 MHC 分子表达的效应也会影响抗原向 T 细胞的提呈过程。

血管生成素

血管生成素（angiogenin，Ang）代表了一类新型的在宿主固有防御中发挥重要作用的抗微生物蛋白。炎症发生时，Ang mRNA 表达迅速增加，血清中的蛋白质水平在急性反应期上升[48]。鼠和人的 Ang 基因位于 14 号染色体上[49]。最近的研究表明，不同的 Ang 具有严格的组织分布。Hooper 及其同事[50]指出 Ang4 由肠道表达，受革兰氏阳性菌的诱导。更加明确的是，Ang4 由肠道的帕内特细胞分泌，其分泌形态也具有潜在的抗革兰氏阳性菌的活性。这组研究者还提出 Ang4 是宿主胃肠道上皮固有免疫防御的介质，而该家族的其他成员（如 Ang1）很有可能是宿主全身固有免疫防御中之前尚未被重视的组分。

正常菌群

免疫系统作用的典型描述常是识别"自己"和"非己"。然而，在两种情况下，这种定义并不完全准确。一是免疫系统需要在转化细胞发生癌变前，识别并破坏它们，这也是免疫系统最重要的功能之一。二是黏膜免疫系统必须分清潜在有害的肠道细菌和长期寄居于人体胃肠道的正常、有益的菌群。正常人类肠道含有10万亿～100万亿的细菌，种类超过500种，包括需氧菌和厌氧菌。它们在人类一出生就定植于肠道中。

这些共生菌群在固有黏膜免疫系统中发挥着深远和积极的作用。在无菌环境下出生的动物已被证实免疫系统失调。另外，黏膜相关淋巴组织（mucosa-associated lymphoid tissue，MALT）结构也不能正常发育，如派尔集合淋巴结（Peyer's patch，PP结）。正常菌群对人体防御发挥着多种作用。例如，正常菌群通过与病原体竞争结合位点或必需的营养物质来防止病原体定植。此外，正常菌群还可以分泌某些杀灭或抑制非共生菌的物质来拮抗其他细菌的侵袭。肠道细菌能合成多种抑制或杀灭其他细菌的物质，有相对非特异性的脂肪酸和过氧化物，也有高度特异的杆菌素。而且，正常菌群可刺激某些特定组织的发育，如盲肠和胃肠道中一些特定淋巴组织。与普通动物相比，无菌动物的盲肠体积大、壁薄、液体充盈。另外，与普通动物相比，无菌动物在经受免疫刺激后，其肠道淋巴组织发育不良。正常菌群已被证实的另一作用是刺激交叉反应抗体的合成。已知正常菌群在动物体内作为抗原，可诱导免疫应答。可以想象，针对正常菌群成分产生的极低水平的抗体可以与某些相关病原体发生交叉反应，从而防止感染或侵袭。

TLR

细菌感染的速度对宿主来说是势不可挡的，因此宿主需要一套分子哨兵受体系统，这套系统具有如下特点。①由最先遭遇到病原微生物的宿主细胞表达；②可区别病原体和宿主；③具有启动针对有害微生物的更强的应答。作为早期免疫应答组分，固有免疫细胞是合成这些受体的理想细胞。巨噬细胞和DC表面受体的发现是哺乳动物固有免疫系统研究的里程碑事件，这种受体与之前在果蝇中发现的Toll家族抗微生物受体相似。这个不断扩大的受体家族被称为TLR，它存在于多种人类造血细胞中。而且，在多处胃肠道表面也发现了TLR，这一发现为胃肠道黏膜上皮细胞是免疫细胞的说法提供了支持。TLR家族以模式识别受体（pattern recognition receptor，PRR）的形式对病原体特异性分子模式（pathogen-specific molecular pattern，PAMP）发挥作用，包括CpG DNA基序、肽聚糖、LPS、鞭毛蛋白和其他细菌表面产物或分解产物。

TLR-1 和 TLR-2

TLR-1的发现源于果蝇Toll受体和人IL-1受体存在结构域的同源性。TLR-1在脾脏和外周血细胞（包括巨噬细胞）中表达，TLR-2能识别多种PAMP，包括细菌脂蛋白/脂肽、肽聚糖和糖基磷脂酰肌醇（glycosyl phosphatidyl inositol，GPI），并诱导信号转导。CD14可显著增强TLR-2的信号转导。最近报道显示TLR-1协助TLR-2介导针对微生物脂蛋白和三酰脂肽的应答，因此当LPS不存在时，它们成为抵御革兰氏阳性菌感染的非常重要的哨兵受体[51]。

TLR-3

TLR-3可以识别只存在于病毒中的双链RNA（double-stranded RNA，dsRNA）[52]。因此，

这种 PAMP 受体在黏膜细菌免疫中作用甚微，但是与抗轮状病毒（rotavirus，RV）感染应答具有非常高的相关性，因为 RV 是世界范围内导致严重腹泻的最常见病因。RV 每年可导致约 100 万人死亡，占腹泻死亡人数的 20%~25%，其中 6% 的死亡病例为 5 岁以下儿童[53]。

TLR-4

在抗微生物固有免疫系统中，研究最多的就是革兰氏阴性菌产物 LPS 介导的细胞活化机制。在发现 GPI 锚定膜蛋白 CD14 是 LPS 的受体后，人们开始了对信号转导协同受体的研究。事实上，由于 CD14 没有胞浆区，因此不能启动信号转导。之后，人们发现 CD14 能够与 TLR-4 协同作用，与 LPS 结合，TLR-4 提供细胞活化所必需的胞浆转导信号。TLR-4 在功能上与 LPS 相互作用需要一种称为 MD-2 的可溶性分泌型分子。由于肠道上皮细胞并不表达 CD14，所以 MD-2 在肠道中就更为重要。

TLR-5

TLR-5 识别革兰氏阳性菌和革兰氏阴性菌的鞭毛蛋白。TLR-5 介导的信号转导可以激活 NF-κB、诱导 TNF-α 和 IL-8[54]。在 DC 中，鞭毛蛋白可诱导 CD83、CD80、CD86、MHC II 类分子和淋巴结归巢趋化因子受体 CCR7 的表面表达增加[53]。

TLR-6

与 TLR-1 一样，TLR-6 是 TLR-2 的协同受体。TLR-2/TLR-6 异源二聚体识别肽聚糖和双酰化支原体脂蛋白。支原体脂蛋白与 TLR-2 和 TLR-6 结合后可诱导 NF-κB 的活化，后者在一定程度上由髓样分化蛋白 88（myeloid differentiation protein 88，MyD88）和 Fas 相关死亡结构域蛋白（Fas-associated death domain protein，FADD）介导，也可通过促分裂素原活化蛋白激酶（mitogen activated protein kinase，MAPK）p38 亚族、MyD88 和 FADD 来调节细胞凋亡[55]。

TLR-7 和 TLR-8

TLR-7 和 TLR-8 与 TLR-9 相关，与 TLR-(1~6) 相比，它们的分子质量更大。TLR-7 和 TLR-8 的自然配体尚不明确。然而，对 TLR-7 缺陷小鼠的研究显示 TLR-7 能够识别咪唑喹啉复合物，后者是一种合成的抗病毒小分子。TLR-7 的活化可导致炎性细胞因子释放。TLR-8 也能与咪唑喹啉复合物发生反应[56]。

TLR-9

TLR-9 位于细胞内部，参与识别特异性的非甲基化 CpG 寡脱氧核苷酸序列[57]。这些寡脱氧核苷酸基序的非甲基化形式可以区分细菌 DNA 和哺乳动物 DNA，因此符合典型 PAMP 的特征。活化的 TLR-9 参与启动 NF-κB 移位的细胞内途径。

中间免疫程序

作为填补人体防御缺口的重要的中间免疫程序，既具有固有免疫程序的一些特性，也具有适应性免疫程序的一些特性。如同经典的适应性免疫程序，中间免疫程序也有 T 细胞和 B 细胞的参与。然而，它可利用的受体有限，并且如同固有免疫系统的 PRR 一样，这些受体是由胚系基因编码的。在 B 细胞中，这些受体是由胚系免疫球蛋白 V 基因编码，其中很多可形成能够与细菌表面分子相互作用的受体[58]。在中间免疫程序中，B 细胞活化和向浆母细胞分化不需要 T 细胞的辅助，也不需要经历耗时的亲和力成熟的过程。因此，该系统的抗体应答并不理想，但是反应迅速。最后，中间免疫程序的 B 细胞和 T 细胞能够被迅速募集到感染可被快速检测到的解剖部位。

中间免疫程序中 B 细胞的作用

B 细胞亚群具有两种主要的表型。第一种是分布于腹膜和其他体腔的 B1 细胞，它们具有自我更新的能力，并可表达未突变的、数量有限的传统 B 细胞受体（B cell receptor，BCR），这些受体以一种非依赖 T 细胞的方式对细菌抗原作出应答。第二种表型的 B 细胞群分布于脾脏的滤泡边缘区（marginal zone，MZ），此处是它们抵御血源性病原体的理想位置。与 B1 细胞类似，它们的数量有限，且激活过程不依赖 T 细胞。激活这些 MZ B 细胞的是来自骨髓的 DC，而不是来自淋巴且参与激活传统滤泡 B 细胞的 DC。另外，LPS 能够显著加快 MZ B 细胞向 IgM 分泌型浆细胞的分化。与 B1 细胞一样，这些快速活化的非依赖 T 细胞的 B 细胞群被置于最关键的位置，在此处，血源性细菌抗原被循环中未成熟的 DC 捕获，完成它们与中间或适应性免疫系统的第一次接触。

中间免疫程序中肠道 T 细胞的作用

具有特定功能和受体种类有限的淋巴细胞群不仅仅局限于 B 细胞，肠道中的 T 细胞群也有类似的特性[59]。小鼠 GALT 中含有的 T 细胞数量相当于整个中枢免疫系统中的 T 细胞数量，其中有一半都不是来源于胸腺的。该系统的细胞中至少有一部分来源于一个被称为隐窝小结的肠道相关结构，该结构将在本章后面详述。由于单个隐窝小结所含的这种细胞数量非常少，使得发现和分析此类细胞非常困难，因此对这种细胞的分析不尽如人意。Rocha[60] 介绍了如何利用单细胞 PCR 方法分析这些 T 细胞系可能携带的标记，以及如何通过细胞分选和进一步的功能分析（过继性转移试验）对该细胞系进行分离。如同 B1 和 MZ B 细胞，这些 T 细胞分布于重要的黏膜表面，以便抵御细菌的攻击。与中间系统的 B 细胞相似，它们表达有限的受体。现在可以对这些肠道相关 T 细胞进行详细的研究。

适应性免疫应答

适应性黏膜免疫系统可以适时地调动淋巴组织，启动针对潜在病原体的特异性应答。MALT 分布于解剖学定义上的腔室。MALT 在肠道称为 GALT，而在鼻咽部称为鼻相关淋巴组织（nasal-associated lymphoid tissue，NALT）。GALT 被认为是最主要的 MALT，因为它的数量庞大，抗原负载于它暴露的位置，并且影响免疫系统。GALT 在功能上分为诱导部位和效应部位。PP 结和阑尾是肠道诱导部位的代表，而扁桃体和腺样体则在 NALT 中发挥相似的作用。在小鼠中还分离出具有诱导部位特性的淋巴滤泡[61,62]。GALT 的效应部位包括黏膜固有层和肠道上皮（图 3.2）。

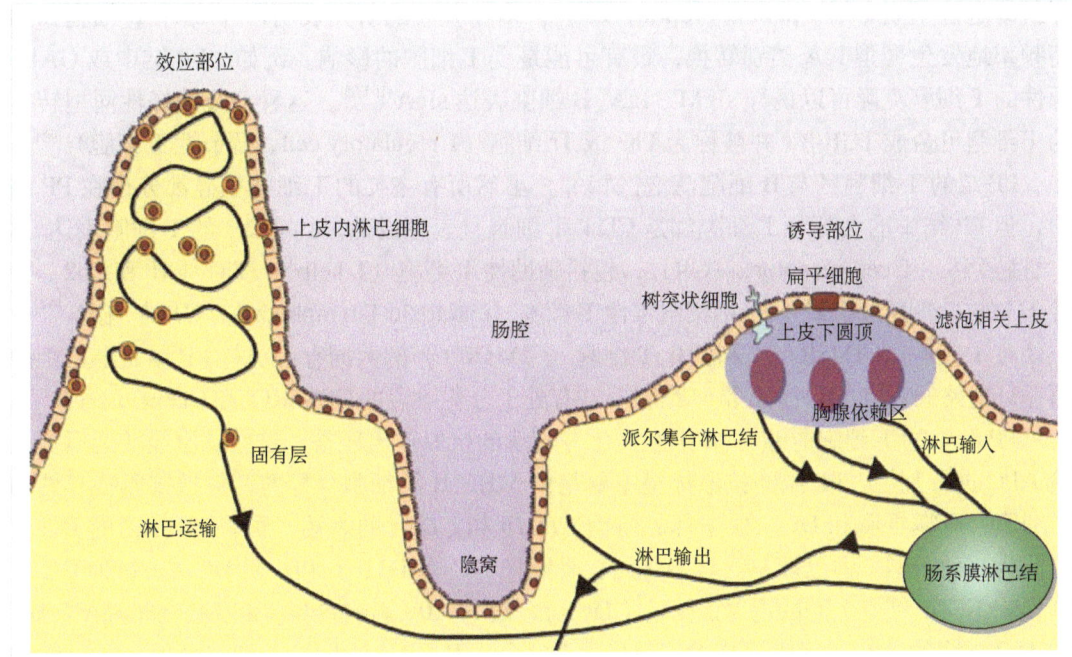

图 3.2 GALT 包括诱导部位和效应部位。PP 结的上皮下圆顶（subepithelial dome，SED）中含有 B 细胞滤泡和胸腺依赖区（thymus-dependent area，TDA）。抗原通过 M 细胞或 DC 穿越上皮，这些细胞将突起通过上皮紧密连接延伸至肠腔。效应部位的分布不规则，存在于 GALT 的整个固有层和上皮中。这些效应部位中有很多上皮内淋巴细胞（IEL），它们通过传入淋巴管补给肠系膜淋巴结（mesenteric lymph node，MLN）。

胃肠道诱导部位

派尔集合淋巴结

派尔集合淋巴结（Peyer's patch，PP 结）由肠道黏膜的淋巴组织有序集合而成，它含有滤泡中心和明确界定的细胞区。PP 结表面覆盖有滤泡相关上皮，后者是一种独特的上皮层，与邻近的柱状上皮的区别是它呈立方形且不含分泌成分。而滤泡相关上皮含有一种被称为 M 细胞（microfold cell）的特殊细胞，它具有抗原摄取功能。M 细胞形状不规则，以微皱褶替代微绒毛。与吸收性上皮细胞相比，M 细胞的刷状缘发育不良，酶活性也降低。M 细胞在基底膜形成腔室，聚集着 T 细胞、B 细胞和 DC。M 细胞能够从肠腔摄取抗原，内化之后转运给 APC。可溶性抗原和完整的细菌都可以被 M 细胞内化[63]。这些结果提示 M 细胞能调控抗原从肠腔转运至 PP 结，这是免疫监视的一部分，并最终发展成为适应性免疫应答。

PP 结中的大部分 B 细胞用于合成 IgA，而毗邻 M 细胞的 B 细胞与具有记忆表型的生发中心 B 细胞相似[36]。位于 PP 结圆顶下的生发中心含有处于分化阶段的正在经历亲和力成熟的 B 细胞，并发生 IgA 类别转换。最终合成的 IgA 在黏膜表面提供适应性免疫保护，这一内容将在下文中讨论。当 PP 结受到抗原刺激后，IgA⁺ 淋巴母细胞通过淋巴和血液循环最终定位于固有层（lamina propria，LP）。多项独立的研究表明，PP 结中 B 细胞如此高频率地发生同型 IgA 类别转换，很有可能是受 T 细胞的影响。例如，PP 结中或 GALT 源性的 T 细胞克隆可以诱导 sIgM$^+$ sIgA$^-$ B 细胞表达 sIgA^{+}[64,65]。这种涉及选择性同型转换的 T 细胞可合成 TGF-β，并被称为 Th3 或 Tr 细胞（T regulatory cell，调节性 T 细胞）[66]。

PP 结的 T 细胞区与 B 细胞滤泡区相邻。虽然所有主要的 T 细胞亚群都分布在 PP 结中，但 PP 结中的大部分 T 细胞都是 CD4$^+$ T 细胞且表型成熟。约有 2/3 的 T 细胞表达 αβ T 细胞受体（T cell receptor，TCR），包括辅助性 T 细胞（T helper，Th）Th1 和 Th2。另外 1/3 的 T 细胞为 CD8$^+$，包括细胞毒性 T 细胞（cytotoxic T lymphocyte，CTL）前体[67]。小幼稚 T 细胞（CD45RA$^+$）和活化 T 细胞（CD45RO$^-$）的共同存在支持 PP 结是淋巴细胞再循环通路的观点。另外，紧邻 M 细胞下方有处于分化阶段的 CD45RO$^+$ 和 CD69$^+$ T 细胞[68]。

PP 结中的 T 细胞能够对 M 细胞内化并转运的抗原作出应答。这些抗原经转运后提呈给 APC 进行加工。PP 结的抗原提呈主要是由 MHC II 类细胞介导的，包括抗原特异性的 B 细胞、巨噬细胞和 DC。根据标志基因 *CD11b* 和 *CD8α* 的表达，可将 PP 结内的 DC 至少分为三种亚型：淋巴样 DC（CD8α）、骨髓样 DC（CD11b）和双阴 DC[69]。每种 DC 亚型影响不同 T 细胞亚群的诱导。骨髓样 DC 可合成 IL-10，影响参与体液免疫（如 IgA 合成）的 Th2 细胞的分化，而淋巴样 DC 和双阴 DC 合成 IL-12，诱导 Th1 细胞分化，并最终诱导细胞介导的免疫应答[70]。骨髓样 DC 合成的 IL-10 和 TGF-β 也会影响 Th3 和 Tr 细胞的分化，后者参与口服抗原的无应答，即口服耐受[66]。

隐窝小结

隐窝小结代表了最近提出的一级淋巴器官（又称中枢淋巴器官），由淋巴细胞前体的多个小集群组成。这些淋巴细胞表达 c-kit$^+$、CD3$^-$、TCR$^-$ 和 RAG$^-$ 的 IL-7 受体。小鼠含有这些细胞集群，而人类肠道没有。将隐窝小结中的 c-kit$^+$ 淋巴细胞从无胸腺的裸鼠移植到被严重照射且免疫缺陷（severe combined immunodeficiency，SCID）的小鼠后，发现这些淋巴细胞具有增殖能力[61]。

胃肠道效应部位

抗原启动的 B 细胞和 T 细胞通过肠系膜淋巴结、胸导管和血流从黏膜诱导部位（GALT 或 PP 结）向黏膜效应部位迁移。这些淋巴细胞进入黏膜效应部位后（如固有层和上皮）进一步分化，如 sIgA$^+$ B 细胞分化为 IgA 浆细胞。Th1 和 Th2 合成的细胞因子能够促进这种分化的发生，如 Th1 合成的 IL-2 及 Th2 合成的 IL-5、IL-6 和 IL-10。

固有层

LP 是位于滤泡相关上皮下方并环绕淋巴样滤泡的基底膜层，它位于上皮和黏膜肌层之间，含有平滑肌细胞、成纤维细胞和造血源性细胞。除了淋巴细胞之外，在这些造血细胞中，固有层还含有大量巨噬细胞和 DC，它们负责加工穿越上皮的抗原，并将处理后的抗原肽提呈给 CD4$^+$ T 细胞。固有层中的 CD4$^+$ T 细胞大部分是 αβ TCR$^+$，更少数量的 CD8$^+$ T 细胞表达 αEβ7 整合素，提示它们会前往上皮[62]。固有层内的 T 细胞表达典型的活化 T 细胞相关的标志物。这些标志物是 α4β7$^+$、CD45RO$^+$、CD25$^+$ 和人类白细胞抗原（human leukocyte antigen，HLA）-DR$^{+[71]}$。与外周淋巴细胞相比，正常的、未激活的固有层淋巴细胞凋亡的水平升高，可能是因为它们能够表达 Fas 和 FasL[72]。这些固有层 T 细胞还能增加对 IgA 的最终合成发挥重要作用的细胞因子的合成。

B 细胞之所以能定位于固有层，是因为它们表达的 α4β7 整合素能够与黏膜上皮细胞表达的黏膜黏附素细胞黏附分子（mucosal addressin cell adhesion molecule-1，MADCAM-1）相互作用。IgA$^+$ 浆细胞前体的募集很可能是受到固有层细胞或肠道上皮细胞分泌的特异性趋化因子与 B 细胞受体之间的相互作用的介导。有趣的是，近期的一项研究显示胸腺表达的趋化因子（thymus-expressed chemokine，TECK）CCL25 是对 IgA 分泌细胞有效的选择性化学引诱物[73]。除胸腺外，肠道上皮细胞也能表达这种趋化因子，其趋化效应是由 IgA$^+$ 浆细胞前体表达的 CC 趋化因子受体 9（CC chemokine receptor 9，CCR9）介导的[73]。固有层 T 细胞合成的细胞因子 IL-2、IL-4 和 IL-5 可促进 IgA 浆细胞的生成。类别转换和 IgA$^+$ 浆细胞分化还可以以一种非依赖 T 细胞的方式进行，是由 LPS 和基质细胞分泌的 TGF-β、IL-10 和 IL-6 介导发生的[74]。IgA$^+$ 浆细胞约占固有层中单核细胞的 1/3，这些 IgA 浆细胞可主动地合成 IgA 二聚体和多聚体。在胃肠道黏膜中，超过一半的 IgA 浆细胞合成 IgA2，而在淋巴结和扁桃体中合成的 IgA 的主要形式是 IgA1[75]，这些抗体的特性将在本章后面详述。

肠道上皮

肠道上皮是另一个淋巴样效应部位，如前所述，它可能发挥重要的免疫调节作用。在肠道上皮中，位于基底膜上方上皮细胞之间的淋巴细胞群被称为上皮细胞间淋巴细胞（intraepithelial lymphocyte，IEL）。IEL 的特性与固有层和全身的淋巴细胞不同，IEL 含有 αβT 细胞和 γδ T 细胞。IEL 中 αβ TCR 和 γδ TCR 的比率在不同物种中存在差异。小鼠中 γδ TCR IEL 占优势，而人类中 αβ TCR IEL 则更常见[76]。大多数的人 IEL 为 CD8$^+$，并且表达能够与上皮的 E- 钙黏蛋白结合的 GI 整合素 αEβ7[77]。IEL 还表达活化 T 细胞的标志物，如 CD45RO$^{+[78]}$。每 4～9 个小肠上皮细胞之间就有一个 IEL。从免疫组织学的角度来讲，IEL 几乎占到所有淋巴样器官中 T 细胞总数的一半[79]。

与外周相比，拥有 γδ TCR 的 T 细胞主要存在于肠道中，尤其是感染之后，然而，它们的功能重要性还未完全阐明。研究表明，γδ T 细胞不需要抗原提呈就可以针对细菌抗原作出应答，可能是固有免疫应答机制的一部分[80]。有些 γδ T 细胞直接与人 MHC I 类分子样 MIC 分子结合，这种分子不携带抗原肽，并且可诱导性表达。在应激状态下或发生上皮肿瘤时，肠上皮细胞的 MIC 表达增加，并可被 γδ IEL 识别[81,82]。因此，γδ TCR IEL 可能负责应激细胞的识别。

另一种独特的 IEL 群是表达 CD8αα 同源二聚体的 T 细胞，这种细胞在肠道上皮之外的组织很少见。这些 T 细胞能利用不变的 FcεRIγ 链作为其 CD3 复合物的一部分。这些 IEL 在其 TCR 库中是寡克隆的[59]。多项研究表明 CD8αα IEL 具有自身反应性，属于胸腺外 T 细胞系。例如，由于缺失的原因，表达 *Mls-1*^{a} 等位基因的小鼠中缺乏传统的表达 Vβ6、Vβ8.1 和 Vβ11TCR 的 T 细胞，而后者能够与内源性逆转录病毒 Mtv-7 超抗原结合。相反，CD8αα TCR αβ IEL 的出现频率甚至比未缺失株还高[79]。为了确定 CD8αα TCR αβ

IEL 的发育是否需要 MHC I 类分子，4 种分别缺失 TAP、CD1、典型的 MHC I 类分子和 β2 微球蛋白的小鼠均经过了测试，结果显示除了 β2 微球蛋白之外，其他 3 种敲除小鼠都有胸腺外 CD8αααβ IEL[83]。这些结果表明这些细胞的发育只需要 MHC Ib 类分子。多项研究结果显示 CD8αα 不是作为 MHC I 类分子的辅助受体发挥作用，实际上这些 IEL 可能是通过辅助受体非依赖性的途径被选择的。

CTL 主要负责清除被细胞内病原体感染的细胞，如病毒感染的细胞。大部分 CTL 是 $CD8^+$ T 细胞，它们识别 MHC I 类分子结合的病毒肽。由于每 4~9 个肠上皮细胞之间就有一个 IEL，而且 2/3 的 IEL 又是 $CD8^+$ T 细胞，所以它们是抵御细胞内肠道病原体的第一道重要屏障。因为 IEL 具有组成性溶细胞活性[84]，所以它们被认为在清除细胞内病原体方面发挥作用。支持该观点的研究表明 $CD8^+$ TCR αβ 能够溶解单核细胞增生性李斯特菌感染的细胞，并且将其过继转移给 SCID 小鼠后，能够清除 RV 感染[84]。

IgA

哺乳动物分泌的 IgA 比其他所有类别抗体的总和还多，至少 80% 的浆细胞位于肠道固有层[85,86]，而且大多数 IgA 分泌入肠腔，以上这些发现引出了一些问题，即这种适应性免疫防御功能如何抵御肠道细菌和病毒的攻击。现在，人们已经对这些问题及相关问题进行了研究，包括 IgA 浆细胞的诱导部位、抗体前体的迁移方式、IgA 类别转换的关键元素及针对特定人类病原体的 IgA 应答。有趣的是，据估计，胃肠道上皮每天分泌 3g IgA[87]（图 3.3）。

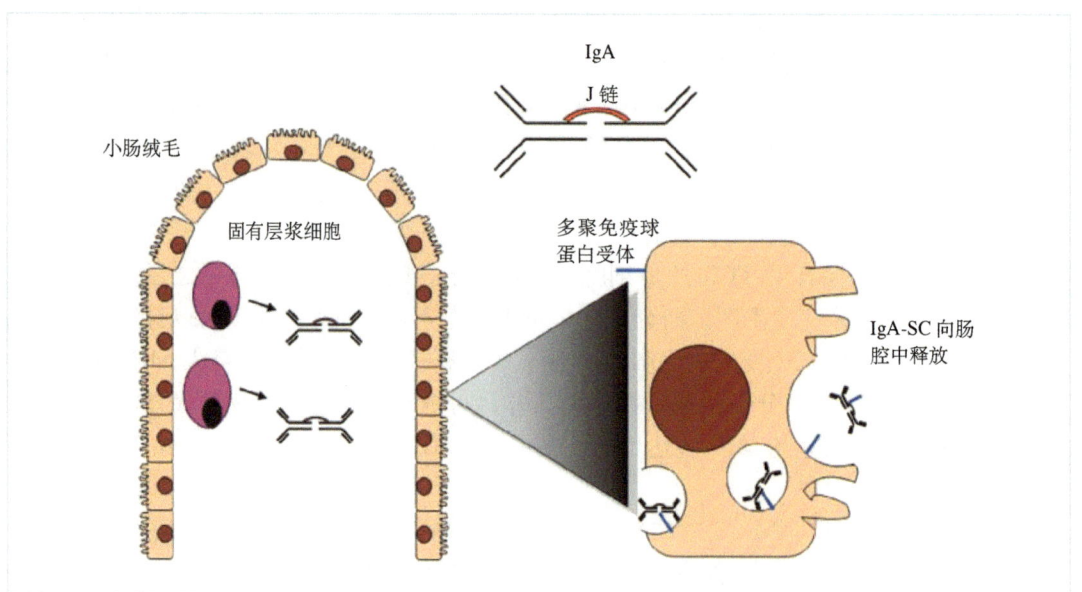

图 3.3　浆细胞分泌的多聚 IgA（pIgA）与黏膜上皮细胞底外侧表面的多聚免疫球蛋白受体（polymeric Ig receptor，pIgR）结合。IgA-pIgR 复合物被胞吞后转运至细胞顶端表面。在此过程中，IgA 与 pIgR 间形成二硫键。在细胞的顶端表面，pIgR 跨膜区和胞浆区之间的连接被酶切断，IgA-分泌成分复合物（IgA-SC）释放至外分泌液。

IgA1

虽然血清中有少量 IgA，但大部分都以分泌型 IgA（secretory IgA，sIgA）的形式存在。实际上，人类可合成两种类型的 IgA。IgA1 是 IgA 子类的其中一种，它以单体的形式存在于血清中[88]。尽管血清中 IgA 的含量要比 IgG 或 IgM 少，但人们现在正在研究它的功能。在嗜酸性粒细胞、中性粒细胞、单核细胞和巨噬细胞的细胞表面有一种 IgA1 受体，即 FcαR1/CD89，能够诱导细胞吞噬作用、抗体依赖细胞介导的细胞毒作用（antibody-dependent cellular cytotoxicity，ADCC）和炎性分子的分泌[89~92]。对转入人类 CD89 分子的转基因小鼠的研究表明，在炎性介质存在的情况下，IgA 包被的细菌能够被 Kupffer 细胞吞噬[93]。在没有局部调理作用时，病原体可以逃逸黏膜免疫系统，此时血清 IgA 可能起到备用防御的作用。

IgA2

IgA2 是由两个 IgA 分子的 α 链通过 J 链相连形成的二聚体。固有层中的浆细胞释放 sIgA，它与黏膜上皮细胞结合后，通过内吞和转运作用由细胞顶端释放。结合 sIgA 的跨膜细胞受体是多聚免疫球蛋白受体（polymeric Ig Recpotor，pIgR）。sIgA 和 pIgR 在上皮屏障的底外侧表面通过共价键结合形成受体-配体复合物。受体-配体复合物被细胞内吞后，在细胞内发生转运，经蛋白质水解后将仍然带有 pIgR N 端的 IgA 分泌至肠腔[88]，这段 pIgR 片段被称为分泌成分。有趣的是，pIgR-IgA 复合物在发生上皮细胞内转运前及转运过程中，都能够结合抗原。这样有很多好处：首先，渗入黏膜屏障的抗原能够重新回到肠腔；其次，无法通过其他方法进入肠腔的 IgG 和 IgM 可以通过上皮层的转运到达肠腔[94]；最后，研究表明，IgA 在细胞内转运的过程中能够结合并中和复制中的病毒[95]。

IgA 进入肠腔的次要途径

除了跨上皮细胞的胞吞作用外，IgA 还可通过其他两种方式进入肠腔。IgA 也可通过胆管和胆囊的胆道上皮分泌入胆汁，然后经肝胰管壶腹的十二指肠入口进入肠道[96,97]。IgA 进入肠道的另外一种途径是通过婴儿的母乳喂养。在研究母乳 IgA 对新生儿发育中的免疫系统的作用时发现，母乳 IgA 与共生菌群结合并限制它在肠道中完全定植[98]。另外，母乳喂养的婴幼儿肠道中的正常菌群组成与奶粉喂养的有所不同[99]。对具有不同免疫能力的小鼠进行研究发现，由母乳中获得的适应性免疫力非常重要。例如，人的母乳中含有针对致病菌的抗体[88]。

IgA 诱导

GALT 是黏膜免疫系统最重要的功能区，包括 PP 结和孤立淋巴滤泡（isolated lymphoid follicle，ILF）中的诱导部位及效应部位，含有 IgA⁺ 浆细胞前体。在这些免疫中心部位，B 细胞、携带抗原的 DC 和局部 CD4⁺ T 细胞之间能够发生相互作用。然而，值得注意的是，PP 结并不是 IgA 分泌型 B 细胞存在于肠道的充分条件[100]。肠道微环境持续暴露并受到外界抗原刺激的特点有利于 B 细胞增殖、IgA 类别转换和体细胞高突变的发生。另外，最近的研究结果显示 GALT 中的 B2 细胞分泌 IgA 需要两个有趣的条件，一是与辅助性 T 细胞相互作用，二是依赖与共生菌群的相互作用[101]。但是，B1 细胞合成 IgA 并不依赖于 T 细胞（B2 细胞是骨髓来源的 B 细胞，IgM 染色深而 IgD 染色浅；B1 细胞是胸腹膜来源的，IgM 染色浅而 IgD 染色深）。B1 细胞合成 IgA 依赖 T 细胞的这种特性表明它所合成的 IgA 分子在抵御肠道细菌全身侵袭的前线中发挥重要的作用。支持这一观点的证据如下：①与 B2 细胞合成的 IgA 相比，共生菌群更多的是与 B1 细胞合成的 IgA 相结合；②能够合成共生菌群特异性肠道 IgA（B1 细胞合成的）的正常小鼠血清中没有共生菌群特异性 IgG 或 IgA。相反地，IgA 缺陷小鼠的血清中存在肠道细菌特异性 IgG[102]。

IgA 归巢

IgA$^+$B 细胞从 PP 结的诱导部位迁移到肠系膜引流淋巴结，进一步增殖后，分化成浆细胞。这些细胞通过胸导管和血液归巢回到它们在肠道固有层中的优先靶位置[103]。淋巴细胞受体和上皮细胞配体之间的特异性相互作用导致浆细胞归巢至肠道效应部位。但至今仍有一个问题困惑着研究者，即为什么 IgG 和 IgM 浆细胞不能归巢至肠道固有层。只有 IgA 合成细胞采用这种迁移方式的事实表明局部肠道细胞合成一种特异性的趋化因子。对这种假说的研究发现了小鼠体内存在一种由胸腺表达的 IgA$^+$ B 细胞特异性的趋化因子 TECK/CCL25[73]，它由胸腺和小肠上皮合成。除了该趋化因子，胃肠道中某些特定细胞是 B 细胞归巢所必需的。具体来说，固有层间质细胞对 B 细胞能够存在于肠道固有层十分关键。进一步研究发现，这是由于 B 细胞归巢依赖于固有层间质细胞上的淋巴毒素-β 受体（lymphotoxin-β receptor，LTβR）[100,104]。但是，B 细胞归巢利用 LTβR 作为转导信号的机制尚不清楚。

IgA 类别转换

为了解决 B 细胞如何进行 IgA 表型类别转换的问题，人们对 B 细胞进行了体外培养。由于细胞因子已被证实能够促进和影响 B 细胞类别转换的特异性，因此在 B 细胞培养时加入了非特异性刺激物 LPS 和一系列细胞因子。结果表明，TGF-β 和 IL-4 能促进 IgM 向 IgA 转换，而且 IL-10 能够和 TGF-β 发挥协同作用[74,105,106]。IL-2 能增强这种活性，但它不是必不可少的。另外，细胞发生 IgA 转换后，IL-5 和 IL-6 能够增强抗体的分泌[107,108]。由于这些细胞因子缺陷的小鼠表现为慢性炎症，这就增加了模型分析的难度，所以目前对于这些细胞因子在 IgA 转换中重要作用的体内评价还是个难题。

感染中 IgA 的功能

IgA 在抵御肠源性感染中的作用是一个最重要的问题。先前的关于口服脊髓灰质炎疫苗研发的大量研究结果及关于轮状病毒（rotavirus，RV）与黏膜免疫系统相互作用的研究结果均支持 IgA 对黏膜免疫系统的重要性。研究表明，脊髓灰质炎减毒活疫苗通过黏膜接种产生的 sIgA 比通过注射途径接种产生的多，这一发现是揭示 sIgA 在肠道病原体免疫中发挥重要作用的关键一步。轮状病毒也被广泛地用作肠道 IgA 应答的诱导物。小鼠模型被用来研究 RV 感染，这使得研究者对病毒的清除和免疫机制有了深刻的认识。已发表的研究结果清楚地阐明了 RV 的清除、对再次感染的保护和黏膜 IgA 合成之间的关系。RV 研究的一个重要发现是：IgA 保护作用的重要性不依赖于 T 细胞的辅助作用。具体来说，这种现象是在裸鼠和 T 细胞受体敲除的动物中观察到的。在这些情况下，病毒清除与 T 细胞非依赖性的 IgA 合成有关，这也加强了前面所提到的 B1 细胞的重要性。

虽然这些研究结果明显地证明了 IgA 在防御肠道病原体中的免疫重要性，但是其他关于 IgA 缺陷的研究结果却比较复杂，有时甚至相互矛盾。一方面，选择性 IgA 缺陷的个体经常发生胃肠道感染，并且进展为结节性滤泡增生，这被认为是针对局部抗原的局部免疫应答的结果。另一方面，黏膜免疫系统的过度反应，如 IgA 缺陷时 IgG 和 IgM 的过量合成，增加了充分评价 IgA 对人类免疫中的整体作用的难度。缺陷动物模型只是增加了这种评价的不确定性，因为 IgA、J 链或 pIgR 阴性小鼠并没有发病的征象。

A. Lanzavecchia 在研究中发现，细菌产物与经典的适应性免疫系统的细胞直接接触后，最终会产生记忆性 B 细胞。IgM 记忆细胞与 B1 细胞、PP 结边缘区 B 细胞不同，它有一种突变的免疫球蛋白，是适应性 B 细胞应答的特点。在 IL-2 或 IL-15 的辅助下，IgM 记忆 B 细胞针对微生物的 PAMP CpG 的应答方式是细胞增生并分泌 IgM。相反，幼稚 B 细胞需要表面免疫球蛋白的参与。因此，微生物产物甚至是通过持续的多克隆激活来维持 B 细胞的长效记忆是必不可少的。这是有必要的，因为即使长寿命浆细胞的半衰期可长达数月，也无法解释为什么人类 B 细胞的记忆效应可以维持数年。

TCR 也能够作为超抗原的异型 PRR。多株金黄色葡萄球菌基因组测序结果显示，人们远远低估了超抗原及超抗原样序列的数量。超抗原可以连接 MHC II 类分子和 TCR 亚群，因此它可以作为非常有效的 T 细胞有丝分裂原，然而，这不是超抗原的唯一功能。在所有分析过的每一种金黄色葡萄球菌株中均存在着一种数量庞大且多样化的超抗原家族——*set* 簇。晶体分析结果显示 *Set* 蛋白中的普通超抗原结构是非常保守的，但它们不能激活 T 细胞，因此从定义上来说它们不属于超抗原[109]。所以，今后还需要进一步阐明这组新型的潜在毒力因子的功能。

多方面的数据显示经典的 B 细胞和 T 细胞应答是抵抗微生物攻击的最后的也一定是最有效的方式。然而，位于黏膜表面和一些关键位点（如脾或胃肠道）的其他类型的细胞，包括上皮细胞及中间免疫系统的 B 细胞和 T 细胞等，在病原体防御上有着比以前所认为的更为重要的作用。人们期望能够加速对该系统的更全面的认识，因为它将直接影响人们对病原体的防治策略。

胃肠道的常见感染及免疫应答

胃

胃黏膜将其下面的组织与胃腔中的抗原世界分隔开；胃中的极端 pH 可低至 1，在辅助食物消化、激活酶及将离子形式的铁转化为易吸收形式的铁等方面非常重要。盐酸还能阻止细菌在胃上皮的定植或感染，但是有一种重要的人类病原体例外，即幽门螺杆菌（*Helicobacter pylori*）。幽门螺杆菌具有在胃的恶劣环境中生存的方式，能有效地穿越黏膜层，黏附于上皮，逃逸免疫应答并长期在胃上皮定居。

流行病学

世界上约有 50% 的人口感染过幽门螺杆菌。它的传播途径很明确，即粪 - 口途径，最常见的是儿童早期发生的家庭内部传播。感染率与社会经济状况直接相关；由于发展中国家的水质和卫生条件较差，所以幽门螺杆菌的感染率也较高，在南美的某些地区接近100%。

发病机理

每一个幽门螺杆菌感染者均会表现为胃上皮炎症（慢性浅表性胃炎），其中部分个体发展为溃疡或胃癌等重症疾病。超过80%的胃十二指肠溃疡是由幽门螺杆菌引起的。另外，由于幽门螺杆菌与MALT淋巴瘤和胃癌有极强的相关性，所以将其列为与石棉和吸烟同等级别的I类致癌物。

幽门螺杆菌基因组全长1.65×10^6bp，编码约15 000种蛋白质。临床上可分离到若干不同的菌株，且部分完成了基因组测序，结果证明幽门螺杆菌具有高度的遗传变异性。实际上，幽门螺杆菌是第一种完成基因组测序和两株不同菌株比较的细菌。该研究的一项重要发现是很多株幽门螺杆菌的基因组中都存在毒力岛。在29-基因簇（29-gene cluster）中，第一种完成测序的基因是细胞毒素相关基因A（cytotoxin-associated gene A，CagA），并用它的名字来命名这种Cag毒力岛（pathogenicity island，PAI），即Cag PAI。Cag PAI中的很多这样的基因编码一种预测性的IV型分泌系统。CagA是一种分子质量为120kDa的蛋白质，它能够插入宿主细胞并被磷酸化，然后与SHP-2磷酸酶结合。Cag^+的幽门螺杆菌菌株为I型，而Cag^-为II型。虽然幽门螺杆菌株与疾病表现之间的关系非常复杂，但是非常清楚的是，Cag^+菌株更有能力去诱导促炎性上皮细胞应答，其中IL-8的释放似乎是关键（图3.4）。

幽门螺杆菌发病机理的另一种重要因子是空泡化细胞毒素VacA。这种细菌的基因产物不是Cag PAI的一部分，但是在大多数菌株中都表达。VacA能够将其自身插入上皮细胞膜，形成一种阴离子选择性电压依赖的六聚体通道，在宿主上皮细胞中生成大的空泡。VacA还能影响线粒体膜，诱导细胞色素c的释放和细胞凋亡。

作为唯一能感染人类胃表面的细菌，幽门螺杆菌进化出一种能保护自身抵御酸性环境并在胃黏膜长期定植的机制；这种革兰氏阴性螺旋菌合成的主要蛋白质是尿素酶。幽门螺杆菌也合成大量的尿素酶，后者在所有细胞蛋白合成中的占比高达15%。部分幽门螺杆菌菌群的自溶导致其毗邻的活菌表面被游离的尿素酶包被。细菌从极低pH的胃腔向温和pH的黏膜层转移时，尿素酶催化内源性尿素分解成CO_2和氨。氨能中和盐酸，使胃腔环境接近中性，直到幽门螺杆菌能够在不是那么恶劣的黏膜环境中定植并存活下来。

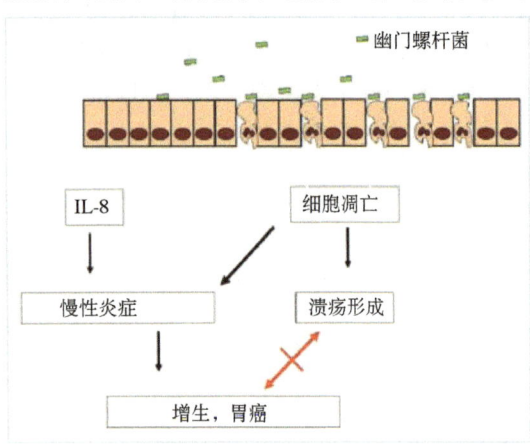

图3.4 针对幽门螺杆菌的两种关键的上皮应答是IL-8的释放和细胞凋亡。在体内外实验中都已经观察到这些现象。然而，有趣的是，临床数据显示这些结果是趋异途径的一部分，因为胃十二指肠溃疡患者发展成胃癌的概率要低得多。

幽门螺杆菌与上皮细胞的相互作用

由于这种革兰氏阴性、有鞭毛的螺旋菌采取细胞外感染的方式,所以细菌定植和发病机理都依赖于它与胃上皮细胞表面受体的结合及其相互作用。幽门螺杆菌利用多种表面蛋白与上皮细胞紧密结合。其中,最具特征性的一种 78kDa 的外膜蛋白(Hop),即黏附素 BabA,能与岩藻糖化的 Lewis B 血型抗原结合。Hop 蛋白家族的很多其他成员也介导细菌与上皮细胞的黏附。然而,上皮细胞对幽门螺杆菌结合的体内和体外应答结果表明这种结合需要宿主信号受体的参与。MHC II 类分子就是这样一种能进行信号转导的幽门螺杆菌结合的上皮表面蛋白。胃上皮是唯一能够组成性表达这种异源二聚体蛋白复合物的黏膜。另外,与幽门螺杆菌感染相关的炎症会上调 MHC II 类分子在整个胃腔的表达,这是关于该细菌如何受益于它所诱导的宿主炎症性免疫应答的重要问题的一种解释。研究表明,幽门螺杆菌尿素酶是与 MHC II 类分子结合的黏附素[110](图 3.5)。

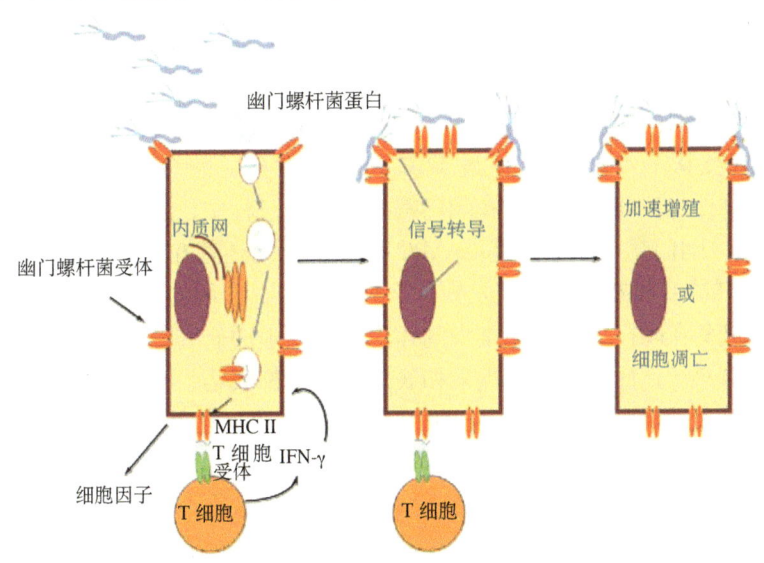

图 3.5 幽门螺杆菌受体必须表达在胃上皮的顶端,以便为这种非侵袭性细菌提供结合位点。一旦结合,就启动了促炎性信号转导。胃上皮细胞含有能通过 MHC II 类途径处理和提呈抗原的分子工具,包括 MHC II 类分子的表达。由于 MHC II 类分子在胃上皮的顶端和底外侧表面都表达,它与幽门螺杆菌结合后能将抗原提呈给固有层 T 细胞。

幽门螺杆菌诱导的局部免疫应答

由于幽门螺杆菌是细胞外感染,所以感染所诱导的局部免疫应答是由胃上皮细胞启动的。上皮细胞与幽门螺杆菌结合后释放 IL-8,后者能募集并激活中性粒细胞,中性粒细胞又能通过释放活性氧自由基(reactive oxidative species,ROS)来加重炎症反应。在抗氧化物存在的情况下,幽门螺杆菌诱导的细胞凋亡减少,因此 ROS 是幽门螺杆菌感染引起宿主细胞损伤的重要因素。这种初期炎症损伤引起 Th1 细胞因子 IFN-γ、TNF-α 和 IL-1β 的积聚。临床数据表明,高达 80% 幽门螺杆菌溃疡患者,和细菌诱导的且抗生素可以治愈的溃疡病很多病例,其上皮屏障受损。黏膜上皮层的"缺口"使幽门螺杆菌及其裂解产物能够侵入下面的组织,包括 APC、LP T 细胞和成纤维细胞。感染者中相当数量的局部 T 细胞都是幽门螺杆菌特异性的,从本质上保证了针对细菌抗原的血清阳转。

关于针对幽门螺杆菌的免疫应答的进一步研究证明它能诱导明显不同的固有免疫应答和适应性免疫应答。虽然这些防御措施与经典的外周免疫相似,但发生在胃黏膜中的固有免疫应答和适应性免疫应答具有独特的特征,这一特征反映了幽门螺杆菌感染的特殊本质。

固有免疫应答

与任何一个经典的固有免疫应答一样,在幽门螺杆菌诱导的非特异性免疫中,最重要的两个因素分别是对细菌增生的早期防御及感染信号向适应性免疫效应器的转导。

然而,至少在感染早期,由于幽门螺杆菌只存在于胃腔中,所以它与固有免疫应答因子的接触机会非常少。因此,为了了解上皮在固有免疫和适应性免疫中的作用,科学家进行了大量的研究工作。已经明确的是,胃上皮细胞合成 IL-8 及随后的中性粒细胞募集是固有免疫应答第一步中的组成部分。研究结果也证明了 IL-8 的合成需要幽门螺杆菌与上皮细胞的结合[111, 112]。这种固有免疫应答相关受体的明显候选者是 TLR 家族。

虽然对 TLR 在幽门螺杆菌感染中重要性的研究一直在进行,但在这方面几乎没有进展。当前的观点认为专职 APC 通过 TLR 和促炎性介质的合成,如 TNF-α、IL-1β 和 IL-8,对细菌产物作出应答。另外,在幽门螺杆菌感染过程中,这些细胞因子的水平升高。虽然在感染后期,幽门螺杆菌有可能与 APC 接触,但是还存在一个重要问题,即这些固有免疫应答信号转导受体在感染早期发挥什么样的作用。当前的研究集中在 TLR-2、TLR-4、TLR-5 和 TLR-9 在幽门螺杆菌感染中的作用。已发表的研究结果表明胃上皮表达 TLR-4、TLR-5 和 TLR-9[113],而且在细胞顶端和底外侧表面都表达。有趣的是,在感染过程中,TLR-5、TLR-9 的表达转移到了底外侧表面。另一研究表明虽然胃上皮细胞表达 TLR-4,但它并不用于信号转导[114]。

适应性免疫应答

虽然幽门螺杆菌诱导的固有免疫应答不足以清除感染,但它所激发的炎症反应有助于突破上皮屏障。文献报道幽门螺杆菌及其产物存在于上皮下面的固有层,这可能被解释为幽门螺杆菌具有改变顶端-连接复合体的组成和功能的能力,并最终破坏上皮屏障的功能[115]。在此处,细菌抗原被 APC 摄取和加工,启动适应性免疫应答。

大量证据表明幽门螺杆菌可以诱导特异性的细胞和体液免疫应答。在幽门螺杆菌感染过程中,CD4 T 细胞和 CD8 T 细胞均可被局部诱导。另外,从感染患者的胃窦中可以分离出幽门螺杆菌特异性的 $CD4^+$ T 细胞。关于幽门螺杆菌诱导的 CD4 T 细胞应答的进一步研究表明,从感染的动物和人中分离出的胃 T 细胞可以合成 IFN-γ 和 TNF-α,但不合成 IL-4,提示这部分 T 细胞发生了 Th1 极化[116,117]。然而,尽管 Th1 型 CD4 T 细胞占明显优势,但是针对幽门螺杆菌的抗体应答也很显著。实际上所有感染者都能产生针对多种幽门螺杆菌抗原的血清阳转,并且在外周血和胃的局部都可以检测到这些细菌特异性抗体,这些抗体包括尿素酶、鞭毛蛋白、LPS 和其他膜蛋白的特异性 IgG 及 IgA。实际上,从感染者体内分离的所有单核细胞中能合成 IgA 的比例高达 10%。

尽管大量研究向我们清楚地展示了幽门螺杆菌诱导的局部特异性免疫应答，但这种免疫应答在幽门螺杆菌介导的疾病状态形成中的作用尚缺乏了解。人们推测不同的临床结果是由不同的 T 细胞应答介导的，研究者最近发现从不同疾病状态的感染者体内分离出的 T 细胞具有不同的抗原特异性。例如，在消化性溃疡患者中，CagA 似乎是优势免疫抗原[118]。此外，细菌性溃疡患者似乎不会患 MALT 淋巴瘤和腺癌。另外，在蠕虫感染高发的国家中，幽门螺杆菌感染者发展成溃疡的概率更低，提示寄生虫可以诱导 Th2 应答水平升高，可以平衡 Th1 诱导的炎症和溃疡的长期和自我破坏性循环。然而，近期研究结果表明 T 细胞转向发生 Th2 极化后会促进幽门螺杆菌感染者中肿瘤细胞的生长，但是这些研究至今还未能很好地重复出来。

虽然还有很多尚未解决的问题，但是有一点是明确的，即黏膜免疫应答不足以清除幽门螺杆菌感染，却在影响细菌介导的疾病病程中发挥关键的作用。幽门螺杆菌患者无法清除细菌使得人们猜测幽门螺杆菌可能会干扰宿主的免疫应答。抗原的加工和提呈是产生适应性免疫应答的关键步骤，而幽门螺杆菌的空泡毒素能破坏这一过程[119]。为了根除这种胃黏膜病原体，首先需要考虑的就是有必要阐明宿主 T 细胞应答变化的机制及细菌逃逸黏膜免疫的机制。

肠道

在大肠和小肠定植的致病菌每年可导致数百万人死亡。各种各样的微生物，大多数为革兰氏阴性菌，能够进化出逃逸宿主防御的方式，有时还能将这些防御机制转化成对自身有利的条件。人类宿主和这些致病菌的共同进化对宿主和入侵的细菌来说都导致一种负担；所有潜在有害的肠道细菌都必须克服物理、化学和免疫学防御屏障才能完成定植或感染。相反，宿主黏膜免疫系统也必须建立丰富的防御系统以抵抗各种细菌复杂的入侵策略。

从一出生开始，具有适当功能的肠道黏膜免疫系统就开始发挥作用。虽然子宫内是无菌的，但在分娩后数小时内，肠道黏膜就有共生菌群定植，3～4 周后 400 多种菌群就会发育成熟。这些共生菌群的建立对于致病菌的固有防御十分重要，如果它们无法正常定植或发生功能失调，则可能是多种肠道疾病的主要原因，包括溃疡性结肠炎和克罗恩病。因此，除了与致病菌发生竞争之外，共生菌群还在宿主形成防御致病菌的局部免疫系统方面发挥着关键作用。

因此，在自己和非己的动态环境中，肠道黏膜免疫系统会对入侵的细菌作出应答；在分散存在于大小肠的免疫组织里，固有免疫和适应性免疫变化多样的"军火库"可用来抵御有害细菌的定居和繁殖。

流行病学

肠道的革兰氏阴性致病菌每年可导致超过 300 万人死亡。这些疾病中绝大多数在本质上都是腹泻/痢疾。虽然多种生物体都可以引起以血性腹泻为指征的痢疾，但是其中志贺氏菌（*Shigella dysenteriae*）最重要。痢疾志贺氏菌 1 型（Sd1）是志贺氏菌的 4 个血清型中毒力最强的，它是流行性痢疾的唯一病因。志贺氏菌是发展中国家面临的主要问题，每年可造成超过 1.5 亿病例及 100 万人死亡。沙门氏菌（*Salmonella*）虽然不像志贺氏菌那样容易危及生命，但也会给健康和经济带来重大的影响。美国疾病预防控制中心（Center for Disease Control and Prevention，CDC）每年都会接到 40 000 例沙门氏菌病例报告。据有关部门估计，美国有 140 万人感染沙门氏菌，但是每年只有 1000 人死于沙门氏菌病。老年人、婴幼儿和慢性疾病患者的症状最为严重。目前，已知的肠致泻性大肠杆菌（统称为 EEC 群）有四类。与沙门氏菌一样，肠致泻性大肠杆菌的很多菌株都可以导致水样和血性腹泻。肠出血性大肠杆菌（enterohemorrhagic *E. coli*，EHEC）O157:H7 是与出血性结肠炎相关的最常见的血清型。小肠结肠炎耶尔森氏菌（*Yersinia enterocolitica*）是肠道耶尔森氏菌病的病原体，可导致小肠结肠炎。

发病机理

肠道病原体采用相对保守的一组分子工具来逃避和抑制宿主黏膜免疫系统，以引起肠道大量的病理改变。对特定致病菌种的相似性分析及基因组研究进展发现了一些病原体具有共同的进化祖先，如大肠杆菌和肠道沙门氏菌。实际上，不同菌种在基因型和表型水平的相似性是显著的，为研究它们之间的关系和共享的策略提供了线索。相反，致病微生物的基因组必须保留一定程度的可塑性才能持续感染状态，抵抗宿主的免疫防御及发挥它们具有快速繁殖周期的优势。对致病菌几十年的研究结果显示它们的基因组中一些毒力最强的成分也是最易变和最易遗传的。这些基因组致病工具包括质粒、噬菌体和毒力岛。毒力岛在某些致病菌基因组中是散在的基因座，而在其不致病的亲本株中则没有。这些基因组叠加具有很高比例的插入序列，并且编码毒力因子，包括噬菌体受体 [120]。

很多毒力岛携带的一种这样的毒力因子是编码大分子分泌系统的蛋白质家族。革兰氏阴性菌必须将分子运进和运出双层膜系统，包括感染中重要的致病毒素。这种选择压力导致至少进化出了 5 种从简单到复杂的分泌系统。

I 型分泌系统

I 型分泌系统是由三种分泌性蛋白复合物构成的：内膜转运三磷酸腺苷酶（adenosine triphosphatase，ATPase）（由于是 ATP 结合盒而被称为 ABC 蛋白）为蛋白质分泌提供能量；外膜蛋白通过 sec 通路运出；膜融合蛋白锚定在内膜上并横跨胞质空间。

II 型分泌系统

II 型分泌系统由 12～14 种蛋白质构成，能使细胞质空间中完全折叠的蛋白质通过外膜转运 [121]。霍乱弧菌（*Vibrio cholerae*）利用 II 型分泌系统转出主要毒力因子——霍乱毒素（cholera toxin，CT）。这种毒素通过刺激肠道细胞分泌氯化物，导致大量液体分泌入肠腔，继而使宿主发生腹泻疾病。

III 型分泌系统

某些肠道致病菌利用该分泌系统，如沙门氏菌、志贺氏菌和肠致病性大肠杆菌。目前，引起腹泻疾病的大肠杆菌可分为 5 类（毒力型）：肠产毒性大肠杆菌（enterotoxigenic *E. coli*，ETEC）、肠侵袭性大肠杆菌（enteroinvasive *E. coli*，EIEC）、肠出血性大肠杆菌（enterohemorrhagic *E. coli*，EHEC）、肠致病性大肠杆菌（enteropathogenic *E. coli*，EPEC）和肠聚集性大肠杆菌（enteroaggregative *E. coli*，EAggEC）。每一类分属于一个血清亚组，具有不同的发病机理。该分泌系统至少由 20 种基因编码，能将毒素通过细菌双层膜运出[122~124]。另外，一种注射器样的大分子突起能够将细菌蛋白直接注入宿主细胞内。与霍乱弧菌（一种非侵袭性病原体）使用的不那么复杂的 II 型分泌系统不同，沙门氏菌、志贺氏菌和 EPEC 利用 III 型分泌系统进入非吞噬细胞。虽然 EPEC 利用 III 型分泌系统进入细胞，但是耶尔森氏菌却能利用这种分泌系统来逃避被吞噬细胞摄取。它是通过将一种被称为耶尔森氏菌外膜蛋白（Yersinia outer protein，Yop）的毒素注入宿主细胞，阻止细菌摄取所必须发生的骨架改变而实现的[125]。Yop 及分别由沙门氏菌和志贺氏菌合成的 SipB 和 IpaB 可以诱导巨噬细胞凋亡[126,127]。

IV 型分泌系统

III 型分泌系统由鞭毛的基本组分构成，与 III 型分泌系统不同，IV 型分泌系统利用细菌的结合蛋白。到目前为止，已发现该分泌系统能将三类物质注入宿主细胞：DNA 结合中间体、百日咳毒素（pertussis toxin，PT）和单体蛋白质，如幽门螺杆菌的 CagA 蛋白[128]。

V 型分泌系统

V 型分泌系统通过自身编码的 β 桶状区装配形成的跨膜孔将蛋白质跨越外膜运送。该分泌系统是革兰氏阴性菌中最大的蛋白质转运外膜孔蛋白家族[129]。

上皮细胞与肠道病原体的相互作用

志贺氏菌

志贺氏菌最早在结肠滤泡相关上皮（follicle-associated epithelium，FAE）的 M 细胞处突破黏膜上皮[130]。细菌从这里进入上皮细胞的底外侧表面，这是细胞最容易被侵入的部位。然而，在细菌侵入上皮细胞前后，上皮细胞通过合成大量的 IL-8 及募集中性粒细胞对志贺氏菌作出应答，而这种应答破坏了上皮之间的紧密连接，使志贺氏菌能直接进入上皮表面下[131]。除了细菌的直接入侵之外，还有两个因素能够诱导上皮细胞分泌这种炎性细胞因子。第一种因素是在早期感染过程中 LPS 与上皮细胞顶端表面的接触。第二种因素是志贺氏菌诱导巨噬细胞分泌大量的 IL-1b，并诱导巨噬细胞凋亡[132]。被感染巨噬细胞大量分泌 IL-1b 的应答是炎症进程引发临床疾病的关键。因此，细菌以宿主的上皮细胞应答为工具，通过诱导大量的上皮细胞因子释放和黏膜屏障的物理改变来增加细胞感染的概率。

沙门氏菌

与志贺氏菌一样，沙门氏菌也能将宿主上皮细胞的骨架蛋白转化为对自身有利的条件。与上皮细胞接触后，沙门氏菌能导致上皮细胞微绒毛退化[51]。然后在细菌黏附部位发生上皮细胞膜褶皱。膜褶皱又伴随着大量的巨胞饮作用，使细菌进入细胞。一旦进入宿主上皮，沙门氏菌就会定居在膜结合囊泡中，细胞形态恢复至正常状态。

沙门氏菌侵入宿主上皮细胞机制依赖于至少两种细菌毒力因子编码基因簇。一种是毒力岛 SPI1（salmonella pathogenicity island 1，SPI 1），它编码的 III 型分泌系统可将毒力蛋白注入上皮细胞。另一种是编码毒力因子 SopE1 和 SopE2 的噬菌体基因组，这些因子通过分泌系统注入细胞后，显著增加肌动蛋白的核化，这是诱导上皮细胞褶皱和巨胞饮作用，从而有助于细菌侵入细胞的重要过程。值得注意的是，在这些膜改变蛋白进入上皮细胞的同时，SPI1 中的毒力蛋白 SptP 也进入了宿主细胞质。SptP 通过拮抗 SopE 来关闭被 SopE 激活的 G 蛋白，因此有利于上皮细胞膜恢复最初形态[133]。

肠致病性大肠杆菌

虽然志贺氏菌和沙门氏菌能通过宿主细胞浆膜来分泌蛋白，直接介导细胞入侵，但是肠致病性大肠杆菌(EPEC)则诱导微绒毛的破坏和基架的形成，被称为黏附与脱落(attaching and effacing，A/E)。这一过程需要利用 III 型分泌系统将一种被称为转位紧密黏附素受体（translocated intimin receptor，Tir）的蛋白质转运至宿主细胞。该分泌系统和构建 A/E 需要的所有蛋白质都位于一个被称为肠上皮细胞脱落位点（locus of enterocyte effacement，LEE）的毒力岛。Tir 与细菌的外膜黏附和紧密黏附素密切相关，从而使 EPEC 与宿主发生黏附。因此，EPEC 不需要寻找真核生物的受体，它本身携带了受体[134]。

肠道病原体诱导的局部免疫应答

固有免疫应答

如前所述，宿主利用预存防御或从头装配的防御来抵御强毒性肠道细菌是躲避严重疾病的关键。肠道的固有免疫系统由抵御细菌入侵和增殖的结构、化学、大分子物质和细胞屏障构成。

与胃一样，肠道固有免疫系统结构部分最关键的组分是上皮衬液。上皮为抵御致病性肠道菌提供了物理屏障，也负责向潜在病原体入侵的局部免疫系统的其他部位发送首次警报信号。这种信号最常见的是以释放细胞因子和趋化因子的形式完成的。在肠道细菌固有应答调节有关因子中，研究最集中的是 IL-8、MCP-1、TNF-α、GM-CSF 和 IL-6。这些分子"哨兵"的释放通常始于前文中讨论的跨膜模式识别受体（PRR）。由于 TLR 能在病原体有机会入侵细胞前识别其特有的各种模式并作出应答，因此它是固有免疫系统的基石。有趣的是，近期的研究结果表明肠道上皮细胞含有内在的模式识别受体（PRR），这是细胞外 TLR 受体的一个补充。这样的细胞内受体有两种：NOD1 和 NOD2，它们是哺乳动物的核苷酸结合位点（nucleotide binding site，NBS）- 富含亮氨酸重复（leucine-rich repeat，LRR）蛋白超家族的成员。在人类中，NOD1 的表达普遍存在。这种蛋白质识别革兰氏阴性菌来源的肽多糖末端的两个氨基酸。NOD2 主要存在于髓系细胞，与 NOD1 相似，能识别革兰氏阳性菌和革兰氏阴性菌肽多糖的不同部位。NOD1 和 NOD2 与细菌产物配体结合后的功能包括激活 NF-κB 和增强细胞凋亡。另外，最近的研究发现 NOD2 参与杀灭肠道上皮细胞内的沙门氏菌。NOD1 和 NOD2 介导的信号转导的重要性及 TLR 诱导的信号转导对这种反应的协同作用仍在研究中[135]。

宿主针对这些肠道病原体的固有免疫应答的关键要素是位于皮下组织中的常驻细胞和新募集细胞的吞噬作用。这些细胞包括巨噬细胞、DC 和中性粒细胞，它们能够完全杀灭细菌、限制细菌复制并释放细胞因子和趋化因子介质以募集和活化另外的免疫细胞。细菌（如沙门氏菌）一旦进入吞噬体就会对宿主细胞产生的化学性防御敏感。还原型烟酰胺腺嘌呤二核苷酸磷酸（nicotinamide adenine dinucleotide phosphate，NADPH）氧化酶是一种能够催化氧分子还原的多组分酶，它与诱导型一氧化氮合酶（inducible nitric oxide synthase，iNOS）联合后能够发挥直接和长效的杀菌作用。另外，NO 衍生物除了协同氧自由基杀灭沙门氏菌外，还能表现出长期的氧化酶非依赖性的抑菌效应[136]。

适应性免疫应答

黏膜固有免疫系统作为第一道防线，能够抵御或减慢感染性肠道微生物的扩散，这是维持宿主健康的关键。然而，MALT"前线"细胞另一个同等重要的作用是将感染类型和位置向适应性免疫系统发出警告和通知。病原体诱导肠道细胞（如上皮细胞和局部巨噬细胞）合成的细胞因子和趋化因子可以启动在适应性免疫应答中十分关键的激活级联反应，包括 DC 成熟、Th1/Th2 极化和效应细胞趋化。这些反应和适应性免疫系统的体液因子联合后，极大地影响着入侵病原体的长期命运，从而为宿主将来的免疫记忆打下基础。

严重沙门氏菌感染的清除及随后获得性防御能力（免疫记忆）是组合性适应性免疫应答在抵御黏膜病原体中发挥重要作用的经典案例。具体来说，证据表明清除这种病原体需要 CD28 依赖的 T 细胞活化及特异性抗体应答[136]，而志贺氏菌诱导的适应性免疫应答偏重于体液效应。LPS 和 IpaA-D 特异性血清 IgG 及肠道 sIgA 是对志贺氏菌最重要免疫应答的特征。虽然有报道称，志贺氏菌抗原在体内能够启动 CD4$^+$ T 细胞，但是人们仍怀疑这些细胞在细菌清除方面是否发挥着重要作用，因为志贺氏菌几乎全部存在于细胞质内（MHC II 类通路的溶酶体之外）或者细胞外。相反，MHC I 类分子介导的 CD8$^+$ T 细胞应答最早被认为是对志贺氏菌的重要防御。然而，目前尚没有研究发现针对该菌的明显的细胞毒性 T 细胞启动。同样地，针对弧菌（*Vibrio*）的免疫应答在很大程度上依赖于抗体。具体来说，因为弧菌感染是非侵袭性的，所以建立在 sIgA 基础上的保护性免疫力对抵御弧菌是成功的，而不是依赖于局部免疫系统中的吞噬或细胞毒性效应因子。

胃肠道的显性免疫应答

黏膜免疫系统是抵御外源性抗原的第一道防线，包括微生物和食源性抗原。在正常情况下，黏膜免疫系统利用由独特位点构成的、严格调控的动态黏膜内信号转导来诱导宿主和黏膜环境之间适当的免疫动态平衡。共同黏膜免疫系统（common mucosal immune system，CMIS）的特性已经非常明确，它在诱导组织（如 PP 结）和效应组织（如肠道 LP）之间发挥相互作用，诱导 IgA 应答。近期的研究数据为 CMIS 非依赖性 IgA 诱导通路的存在提供了强有力的证据。黏膜 IgA 分泌性 B 细胞可分为两个不同的亚群——B1 和 B2，这在前文中已经介绍过，它们分别与 CMIS 依赖性和 CMIS 非依赖性的级联反应相关。在某些情况下，这种严格调控的黏膜免疫系统的破坏会引起针对不同肠道环境抗原的病理反应。结果导致胃肠道紊乱，如过敏性胃肠病和炎性肠病（inflammatory bowel disease，IBD）。

食物过敏的发病机制

对摄入的食源性抗原的不恰当免疫应答会造成对食物的不良反应。食物过敏必须与食物耐受不良区别开来，食物的不良反应与异常免疫应答无关。相反，真正的食物过敏是只发生在过敏个体身上的针对特定食源性抗原的免疫介导过程。胃肠道在保护宿主防止发生过敏反应方面发挥着重要作用。有两种主要的机制看起来很重要，它们是限制外源性抗原通过消化上皮吸收及调控针对这些抗原的全身性免疫应答。消化道的每一部分在这一过程中都发挥作用，肠道被认为是关键部位。当然，胃屏障的作用也已得到了认可，该屏障有一个双层物理结构，由覆盖黏液层的上皮细胞构成。细胞间紧密连接维持的上皮细胞层的连续性[137,138]、上皮细胞膜的完整性，以及黏液层的厚度和组成保证了该屏障的完整性。在正常情况下，胃屏障构成了接近完整的离子反扩散（H^+进入胃壁，Na^+进入胃腔）屏障。物理损伤及化学或细菌性物质在任何时候都有可能破坏这种屏障，可导致通过该屏障的各种分子（抗原）增加。

胃上皮还形成一个能防止细菌性、病毒性和食源性抗原侵入小肠的重要屏障。已有研究表明胃酸缺乏可能与肠道中革兰氏阳性菌加速繁殖、胃肠道感染率升高及对大分子抗原的超敏反应都有关系[139]。此外，将重碳酸盐和蛋白质混合物喂养动物后，肠道中大分子的转运增加，提示蛋白质水解可能会影响蛋白质的抗原特性或蛋白质抗原的吸收量。

多种证据表明肠道和胃都是变应性启动作用的潜在靶点。肠道含有大量发达的免疫（淋巴细胞）系统，被认为是经典的食物过敏反应的中心器官。然而，也有研究表明胃上皮与小肠上皮一样，能够吸收少量的大分子，这种抗原吸收可能会诱导IgE介导的针对这些抗原的过敏反应[140]。

临床观察和流行病学研究强烈支持遗传背景在过敏性疾病包括食物过敏中的作用，这些观察和研究表明遗传在食源性抗原启动反应的发生中发挥着重要作用，并且这些疾病在双胞胎[141, 142]和父母患有过敏性疾病的儿童中的发生率高于对照人群。关于双胞胎的其他研究发现一些与过敏性疾病相关的可量化的特征，如血清总IgE水平与皮肤试验结果表明组内相关系数在同卵双生的孩子中要比在异卵双生的孩子中高两倍。人们认为最少存在两个独立且相互分离的疾病易感基因与环境因素协同作用才能导致在特定组织中发生过敏性炎症。目前，遗传研究认为人类和鼠基因组的多个区域存在公认的遗传性过敏症基因[143]。例如，花生过敏的易感性可能取决于HLA II类遗传多态性。虽然还不知道为什么特异性抗原能导致异常的免疫应答，但是环境因素（如细菌性和病毒性刺激）也可能发挥作用。这些因素可能改变了肠道对食源性抗原的通透性或激活了局部APC表面的共刺激分子，因此有利于免疫应答的发生，而不是正常的抑制反应，后者是口服耐受的基础。

病原体和食物过敏

在调控口服耐受的环境因素中，细菌性肠道微生物群是重要的一种。肠道微生物在调节对肠腔抗原的免疫应答效应上存在互相矛盾的数据。虽然共生菌群对口服耐受的充分诱导和维持是必要的[144]，包括IgE合成系统[145]，但当抗原遇到GALT及能刺激抗原提呈的微生物时，会发生强烈的针对口服抗原的免疫应答[144]。最近有两个事实解释了这一现象：一是肠道黏膜的DC在诱导口服耐受中发挥着重要作用[146]，二是通过DC提呈对可溶性抗原的肠道反应进行调控，这依赖于炎性信号存在与否。在体外直接影响人上皮细胞生长的肠道非致病菌能明显减弱促炎性效应分子的分泌，如多种促炎性刺激物（包括致病菌诱导合成的 NF-κB）。抑制效应的机制包括：抑制性 κ-β-α 降解的阻断，活化的 NF-κB 二聚体核转运的阻止，以及炎性细胞因子基因的转录。

炎性肠病

黏膜免疫系统面临着与肠道中大量共生菌群共同生存的棘手任务（每克结肠粪便中含有 10^{12} 个细菌，大约有 1000 种，以厌氧菌居多）。然而，对于侵袭性肠道病原体，保护性免疫应答也是必需的。任何共生生物在一定环境下都有可能打破平衡成为病原体，这种平衡作用的大小体现在无害的共生大肠杆菌蛋白和它的致病性衍生物（或志贺氏菌属）之间的相似性上。无害菌和有害菌的本质区别在于毒素的合成、黏附或侵入肠道上皮细胞层的数量。

多项研究观察均支持 IBD 是由肠腔菌群或其产物的刺激诱导的免疫应答和炎症反应所导致的观点。在关键黏膜功能上发生的遗传决定性变异（包括原型细菌分子模式诱导的细胞活化）可以导致对这些功能失调发展的易感性差异，可能反映了固有免疫应答和适应性免疫应答之间发生的相互关联活化。炎症的持续和扩大很可能反映了强效刺激物的持续存在及由多种细胞因子介导的选择性 T 辅助细胞亚型、巨噬细胞和其他 APC 的复杂的自我增强活化。这些细胞因子包括 IL-2、IL-12 和 IL-18、IFN 和巨噬细胞迁移抑制因子。其他的大量促炎性细胞因子的合成，最显著的是 TNF、IL-1 和 IL-6，增强了相关炎症过程，并最终导致多种 IBD 临床症状的发生。炎症过程的整体严重程度反映了白细胞募集与黏膜修复过程下调之间的平衡。

在过去两年里，对基因改造的啮齿类动物的研究结果为了解易患肠道炎症的情况做出了巨大的贡献。缺失大量不同的免疫基因的功能，包括 IL-2、IL-10 或 αT 细胞受体的缺失，或插入 HLA-B27，其中单独一种情况都可使动物易患自发性肠道炎症，而这类动物通常在无特定病原体（specific pathogen free，SPF）或无菌环境下饲养才有可能减弱或避免炎症的发生。虽然与人类 IBD 关联的基因位点已经报道过，但是对于这些基因本身的寻找还在继续，所以许多动物的基因异常可能有些人为的因素。然而，在一定的条件下，它们确实可以支持下面的观点：黏膜免疫系统、上皮细胞层和共生菌群之间微妙平衡的破坏会导致慢性肠道炎症的发生。

Duchmann 等 [147] 研究了 IBD 肠道黏膜来源的 T 细胞克隆对共生细菌的反应性。明确的是，活动性克罗恩病患者的黏膜中活性 T 细胞的比例增加，T 细胞克隆通常被证明是一种强有力的免疫工具，因为它只需要单一的短肽表位（9～15 个氨基酸）特异性受体就可以进行 T 细胞培养。在这些克隆中，人们已经阐明了在病毒和细菌感染中辅助 T 细胞和 CTL 识别的主要抗原决定簇。这些团队在以前就提供数据说明了从对照受试者肠道黏膜分离的 T 细胞在体外增殖时能对从另一受试者的肠道（异源的）菌群中分离的细菌的相对粗提物作出应答，而对从自身菌群中分离的细菌不会作出应答。有趣的是，克罗恩病患者的肠道 T 细胞能对它们自身的菌群（自体的）作出应答。因此，克罗恩病可以被解释成对共生菌群黏膜耐受的失败，该观点与动物模型中的数据一致，也与粪便分流的临床疗效一致。虽然人类肠道微生物群具有多样性，但相关物种蛋白和多个物种不同个体的共同结构之间具有显著的同源性,所以正常个体对异源菌群反应的差异尚不清楚。

由于很难从肠道黏膜中获得在抗原刺激后增殖状况良好的T细胞,所以为了获得单一的细胞克隆,必须用非特异性的植物凝集素进行刺激,然后在经射线照射的同种异体的培养细胞上扩增(经典方式)。虽然目的是为了获得代表性的克隆,但是对细菌超声波处理产物的应答并不能反映原始T细胞的抗原特异性。在这种情况下,可能有三种主要的T细胞应答。第一种是$CD4^+$克隆对肠道厌氧菌(二裂菌和类杆菌)和需氧肠道细菌存在显著的交叉应答。第二种是IBD患者体内存在对自身菌群粗提物作出应答的细胞(T细胞克隆)。第三种是研究者分析了在异源混合分离物中哪一种菌株能够刺激溃疡性结肠炎患者的T细胞克隆,发现主要负责的是需氧的肠道细菌,而且奇怪的是,同一菌种(如大肠杆菌)的某些菌落能刺激该克隆,而另一些菌落则不能。

数据表明,IBD患者的T细胞克隆增殖应答在不同菌种间可能有交叉反应。多种共生的需氧菌种也可对异源菌群作出应答。但仍然需要解决的问题是在T细胞水平上,对自身菌群的"耐受"何时建立或崩溃。T细胞克隆具有的优势是:首先在细菌蛋白纯化出来之后,就能确定单个蛋白质分子(或其他结构性细菌组分)的特异性,这样就可以解决交叉反应的分子基础。不幸的是,由于人类MHC II类分子(将抗原肽提呈给$CD4^+$ T细胞)的多样性,导致每个人的情况都可能不同。因此,除了对共生菌群决定簇作出应答的LP $CD4^+$ T细胞存在与否之外,还有很多其他水平的调节,包括无反应性T细胞及合成下调性细胞因子而不增殖的T细胞。对于这些机制在健康人群中的相对作用,以及它们的缺陷在IBD患者中的相对作用仍在研究中。

总结

我们对人类胃肠道黏膜免疫系统的研究现状进行了综述。从上皮黏膜的屏障防御及其模式识别受体(PRR)到抗微生物肽的分子防御,局部固有免疫系统是肠道黏膜免疫系统的一个关键组成部分。局部淋巴细胞提供的病原体特异性免疫力完成了对肠道病原体的免疫应答,并且通常利用记忆细胞提供长期的免疫力。我们还讨论了在黏膜免疫系统的成熟中发挥关键作用的共生菌群,以及其如何通过与致病菌株的竞争提供固有防御。这些益生菌的重要性不仅在于它们可以起到防御作用,而且一旦它们诱导不适宜应答会产生有害作用。另外,阐述了当对微生物的免疫和耐受的微妙平衡遭到破坏时,在胃肠道发生的不良反应。

实际上,人类黏膜免疫系统和肠道致病菌之间的相互作用是一种极其动态的共进化模型。人类胃肠道免疫系统的复杂性和多层性特征是不断地受到任何一种特定肠道病原体的相对有限的致病作用的挑战。然而,细菌能够通过一个小基因组编码一组不相关联的"分子武器"来适应和抵消宿主的防御机制。这是通过细菌的快速生命周期和多种能够水平或垂直运输毒力因子的遗传工具来完成的。另外,一些致病菌不仅能逃避真核生物免疫细胞及其防御性化学产物,它们通常还将这些免疫细胞作为它们致病的原始聚集区。实际上,对宿主防御机制的最清晰认识有时是从对细菌攻击策略的阐明获得的。那么,是什么阻止了有适应能力的微生物击垮宿主呢?最确定的答案在于人类免疫系统的重重保护。胃肠道黏膜中的固有免疫和适应性免疫效应因子共同提供了结构和功能有序排列的多层防御系统。当然,黏膜免疫系统成功起作用的证据在于它克服细菌致病策略的惊人的可塑性。

致谢

作者向各方面给予的支持表示感谢。David A. Bland 得到了 McLaughlin Fellowship Fund 的资助及免疫学和黏膜防御培训项目(T32AI007626)的支持。这项工作还得到了 NIH 基金(DK050669)(V.E.R.)和得克萨斯墨西哥湾消化性疾病中心基金(DK056338)的资助。

参 考 文 献

[1] Youakim A, Ahdieh M. Interferon-gamma decreases barrier function in T84 cells by reducing ZO-1 levels and disrupting apical actin. Am J Physiol 1999;276(5 pt 1):G1279–G1288.

[2] Kucharzik T, Walsh SV, Chen J, Parkos CA, Nusrat A. Neutrophil transmigration in inflammatory bowel disease is associated with differential expression of epithelial intercellular junction proteins. Am J Pathol 2001;159(6):2001–2009.

[3] Dignass A, Lynch-Devaney K, Kindon H, Thim L, Podolsky DK. Trefoil peptides promote epithelial migration through a transforming growth factor beta-independent pathway. J Clin Invest 1994;94(1):376–383.

[4] Dignass AU, Podolsky DK. Cytokine modulation of intestinal epithelial cell restitution: central role of transforming growth factor beta. Gastroenterology 1993;105(5):1323–1332.

[5] Eckmann L, Kagnoff MF, Fierer J. Epithelial cells secrete the chemokine interleukin-8 in response to bacterial entry. Infect Immun 1993;61(11):4569–4574.

[6] Yang SK, Eckmann L, Panja A, Kagnoff MF. Differential and regulated expression of C-X-C, C-C, and C-chemokines by human colon epithelial cells. Gastroenterology 1997;113(4):1214–1223.

[7] Reinecker HC, Loh EY, Ringler DJ, Mehta A, Rombeau JL, MacDermott RP. Monocyte-chemoattractant protein 1 gene expression in intestinal epithelial cells and inflammatory bowel disease mucosa. Gastroenterology 1995;108(1):40–50.

[8] Izadpanah A, Dwinell MB, Eckmann L, Varki NM, Kagnoff MF. Regulated MIP-3alpha/CCL20 production by human intestinal epithelium: mechanism for modulating mucosal immunity. Am J Physiol Gastrointest Liver Physiol 2001;280(4):G710–G719.

[9] Dwinell MB, Lugering N, Eckmann L, Kagnoff MF. Regulated production of interferon-inducible T-cell chemoattractants by human intestinal epithelial cells. Gastroenterology 2001;120(1):49–59.

[10] Shibahara T, Wilcox JN, Couse T, Madara JL. Characterization of epithelial chemoattractants for human intestinal intraepithelial lymphocytes. Gastroenterology 2001;120(1):60–70.

[11] Kunkel EJ, Campbell JJ, Haraldsen G, et al. Lymphocyte CC chemokine receptor 9 and epithelial thymusexpressed chemokine (TECK) expression distinguish the small intestinal immune compartment: epithelial expression of tissue-specific chemokines as an organizing principle in regional immunity. J Exp Med 2000; 192(5):761–768.

[12] Wurbel MA, Philippe JM, Nguyen C, et al. The chemokine TECK is expressed by thymic and intestinal epithelial cells and attracts double- and singlepositive thymocytes expressing the TECK receptor CCR9.

Eur J Immunol 2000;30(1):262–271.

[13] Pan J, Kunkel EJ, Gosslar U, et al. A novel chemokine ligand for CCR10 and CCR3 expressed by epithelial cells in mucosal tissues. J Immunol 2000;165(6): 2943–2949.

[14] Wang W, Soto H, Oldham ER, et al. Identification of a novel chemokine(CCL28),which binds CCR10(GPR2). J Biol Chem 2000;275(29):22313–22323.

[15] Jung HC, Eckmann L, Yang SK, et al. A distinct array of proinflammatory cytokines is expressed in human colon epithelial cells in response to bacterial invasion. J Clin Invest 1995;95(1):55–65.

[16] Reinecker HC, MacDermott RP, Mirau S, Dignass A, Podolsky DK. Intestinal epithelial cells both express and respond to interleukin 15. Gastroenterology 1996;111(6):1706–1713.

[17] Maaser C, Schoeppner S, Kucharzik T, et al. Colonic epithelial cells induce endothelial cell expression of ICAM-1 and VCAM-1 by a NF-kappaB-dependent mechanism. Clin Exp Immunol 2001;124(2):208–213.

[18] Maaser C, Eckmann L, Paesold G, Kim HS, Kagnoff MF. Ubiquitous production of macrophage migration inhibitory factor by human gastric and intestinal epithelium. Gastroenterology 2002;122(3):667–680.

[19] Jordan NJ, Kolios G, Abbot SE, et al. Expression of functional CXCR4 chemokine receptors on human colonic epithelial cells. J Clin Invest 1999;104(8): 1061–1069.

[20] Colgan SP, Hershberg RM, Furuta GT, Blumberg RS. Ligation of intestinal epithelial CD1d induces bio- active IL-10: critical role of the cytoplasmic tail in autocrine signaling. Proc Natl Acad Sci USA 1999;96(24):13938–13943.

[21] Barrera C, Ye G, Espejo R, et al. Expression of cathepsins B, L, S, and D by gastric epithelial cells implicates them as antigen presenting cells in local immune responses. Hum Immunol 2001;62(10):1081–1091.

[22] Li Y,Yio XY,Mayer L.Human intestinal epithelial cellinduced $CD8^+$ T cell activation is mediated through CD8 and the activation of $CD8^-$associated p56lck. J Exp Med 1995;182(4):1079–1088.

[23] Toy LS, Yio XY, Lin A, Honig S, Mayer L. Defective expression of gp180, a novel CD8 ligand on intestinal epithelial cells, in inflammatory bowel disease. J Clin Invest 1997;100(8):2062–2071.

[24] Nakazawa A, Dotan I, Brimnes J, et al. The expression and function of costimulatory molecules B7H and B7- H1 on colonic epithelial cells. Gastroenterology 2004;126(5):1347–1357.

[25] Dwinell MB, Eckmann L, Leopard JD, Varki NM, Kagnoff MF. Chemokine receptor expression by human intestinal epithelial cells. Gastroenterology 1999;117(2):359–367.

[26] Brumell JH, Steele-Mortimer O, Finlay BB. Bacterial invasion: force feeding by Salmonella. Curr Biol 1999; 9(8):R277–R280.

[27] Galan JE. Salmonella interactions with host cells: type III secretion at work. Annu Rev Cell Dev Biol 2001;17:53–86.

[28] Kaisho T, Akira S. Critical roles of Toll-like receptors in host defense. Crit Rev Immunol 2000;20(5):393–405.

[29] Kelly CP, O'Keane JC, Orellana J, et al. Human colon cancer cells express ICAM-1 in vivo and support LFA- 1-dependent lymphocyte adhesion in vitro. Am J Physiol 1992;263(6 pt 1):G864–G870.

[30] Cario E, Rosenberg IM, Brandwein SL, Beck PL, Reinecker HC, Podolsky DK. Lipopolysaccharide activates distinct signaling pathways in intestinal epithelial cell lines expressing Toll-like receptors. J Immunol 2000;164(2):966–972.

[31] Gewirtz AT, Navas TA, Lyons S, Godowski PJ, Madara JL. Cutting edge: bacterial flagellin activates basolaterally expressed TLR5 to induce epithelial proinflammatory gene expression. J Immunol 2001; 167(4):1882–1885.

[32] Dogan A, Wang ZD, Spencer J. E-cadherin expression in intestinal epithelium. J Clin Pathol 1995;48(2): 143–146.

[33] Yio XY, Mayer L. Characterization of a 180-kDa intestinal epithelial cell membrane glycoprotein, gp180. A candidate molecule mediating t cell-epithelial cell interactions. J Biol Chem 1997;272(19):12786–12792.

[34] Huang GT, Eckmann L, Savidge TC, Kagnoff MF. Infection of human intestinal epithelial cells with invasive bacteria upregulates apical intercellular adhesion molecule-1 (ICAM-1) expression and neutrophil adhesion. J Clin Invest 1996;98(2):572–583.

[35] Parkos CA, Colgan SP, Diamond MS, et al. Expression and polarization of intercellular adhesion molecule-1 on human intestinal epithelia: consequences for CD11b/CD18-mediated interactions with neutrophils. Mol Med 1996;2(4):489–505.

[36] Yamanaka T, Straumfors A, Morton H, Fausa O, Brandtzaeg P, Farstad I. M cell pockets of human Peyer's patches are specialized extensions of germinal centers. Eur J Immunol 2001;31(1):107–117.

[37] Meijer LK, Schesser K, Wolf-Watz H, Sassone-Corsi P, Pettersson S. The bacterial protein YopJ abrogates multiple signal transduction pathways that converge on the transcription factor CREB. Cell Microbiol 2000;2(3):231–238.

[38] Schesser K, Spiik AK, Dukuzumuremyi JM, Neurath MF, Pettersson S, Wolf-Watz H. The yopJ locus is required for Yersinia-mediated inhibition of NFkappaB activation and cytokine expression: YopJ contains a eukaryotic SH2-like domain that is essential for its repressive activity. Mol Microbiol 1998;28(6):1067–1079.

[39] Lehrer RI, Ganz T. Antimicrobial peptides in mammalian and insect host defence. Curr Opin Immunol 1999;11(1):23–27.

[40] Agerberth B, Charo J, Werr J, et al. The human antimicrobial and chemotactic peptides LL-37 and alphadefensins are expressed by specific lymphocyte and monocyte populations. Blood 2000;96(9):3086–3093.

[41] Ouellette AJ, Bevins CL. Paneth cell defensins and innate immunity of the small bowel. Inflamm Bowel Dis 2001;7(1):43–50.

[42] Lehrer RI, Ganz T. Defensins of vertebrate animals. Curr Opin Immunol 2002;14(1):96–102.

[43] Durr M, Peschel A. Chemokines meet defensins: the merging concepts of chemoattractants and antimicrobial peptides in host defense. Infect Immun 2002; 70(12):6515–6517.

[44] Masson PL, Heremans JF. Lactoferrin in milk from different species. Comp Biochem Physiol B 1971;39(1): 119–129.

[45] Vorland LH. Lactoferrin: a multifunctional glycoprotein. APMIS 1999;107(11):971–981.

[46] Ellison RT, III, Giehl TJ, LaForce FM. Damage of the outer membrane of enteric gram-negative bacteria by lactoferrin and transferrin. Infect Immun 1988;56(11): 2774–2781.

[47] Tomita M, Bellamy W, Takase M, Yamauchi K, Wakabayashi H, Kawase K. Potent antibacterial peptides generated by pepsin digestion of bovine lactoferrin. J Dairy Sci 1991;74(12):4137–4142.

[48] Olson KA, Verselis SJ, Fett JW. Angiogenin is regulated in vivo as an acute phase protein. Biochem Biophys Res Commun 1998;242(3):480–483.

[49] Strydom DJ. The angiogenins. Cell Mol Life Sci 1998; 54(8):811–824.

[50] Hooper LV, Stappenbeck TS, Hong CV, Gordon JI. Angiogenins: a new class of microbicidal proteins involved in innate immunity. Nat Immunol 2003; 4(3):269–273.

[51] Takeuchi A. Electron microscope studies of experimental Salmonella infection. I. Penetration into the

intestinal epithelium by Salmonella typhimurium.Am J Pathol 1967;50(1):109–136.

[52] Alexopoulou L, Holt AC, Medzhitov R, Flavell RA. Recognition of double-stranded RNA and activation of NF-kappaB by Toll-like receptor 3. Nature 2001;413(6857):732–738.

[53] Means TK, Hayashi F, Smith KD, Aderem A, Luster AD. The Toll-like receptor 5 stimulus bacterial flagellin induces maturation and chemokine production in human dendritic cells. J Immunol 2003;170(10): 5165–5175.

[54] Zhou X, Giron JA, Torres AG, et al. Flagellin of enteropathogenic Escherichia coli stimulates interleukin-8 production in T84 cells. Infect Immun 2003;71(4):2120–2129.

[55] Into T, Kiura K,Yasuda M, et al. Stimulation of human Toll-like receptor(TLR) 2 and TLR6 with membrane lipoproteins of Mycoplasma fermentans induces apoptotic cell death after NF-kappa B activation. Cell Microbiol 2004;6(2):187–199.

[56] Jurk M, Heil F, Vollmer J, et al. Human TLR7 or TLR8 independently confer responsiveness to the antiviral compound R-848. Nat Immunol 2002;3(6):499.

[57] Hemmi H, Takeuchi O, Kawai T, et al.A Toll-like receptor recognizes bacterial DNA. Nature 2000;408(6813): 740–745.

[58] Goodyear CS, Narita M, Silverman GJ. In vivo VLtargeted activation-induced apoptotic supraclonal deletion by a microbial B cell toxin. J Immunol 2004; 172(5):2870–2877.

[59] Regnault A, Cumano A, Vassalli P, Guy-Grand D, Kourilsky P. Oligoclonal repertoire of the CD8 alpha alpha and the CD8 alpha beta TCR-alpha/beta murine intestinal intraepithelial T lymphocytes: evidence for the random emergence of T cells. J Exp Med 1994; 180(4):1345–1358.

[60] Rocha B. Characterization of V beta-bearing cells in athymic(nu/nu) mice suggests an extrathymic pathway for T cell differentiation. Eur J Immunol 1990;20(4):919–925.

[61] Saito H, Kanamori Y, Takemori T, et al. Generation of intestinal T cells from progenitors residing in gut cryptopatches. Science 1998;280(5361):275–278.

[62] Farstad IN, Halstensen TS, Lien B, et al. Distribution of beta 7 integrins in human intestinal mucosa and organized gut-associated lymphoid tissue. Immunology 1996;89(2):227–237.

[63] Jones BD, Ghori N, Falkow S. Salmonella typhimurium initiates murine infection by penetrating and destroying the specialized epithelial M cells of the Peyer's patches. J Exp Med 1994;180(1):15–23.

[64] Kawanishi H, Saltzman L, Strober W.Mechanisms regulating IgA class-specific immunoglobulin production in murine gut-associated lymphoid tissues. II. Terminal differentiation of postswitch sIgA-bearing Peyer's patch B cells. J Exp Med 1983;158(3):649–669.

[65] Kawanishi H, Saltzman LE, Strober W. Mechanisms regulating IgA class-specific immunoglobulin production in murine gut-associated lymphoid tissues. I. T cells derived from Peyer's patches that switch sIgM B cells to sIgA B cells in vitro. J Exp Med 1983; 157(2):433–450.

[66] Fukaura H, Kent SC, Pietrusewicz MJ, Khoury SJ, Weiner HL,Hafler DA. Induction of circulating myelin basic protein and proteolipid protein-specific transforming growth factor-beta1-secreting Th3 T cells by oral administration of myelin in multiple sclerosis patients. J Clin Invest 1996;98(1):70–77.

[67] London SD, Rubin DH, Cebra JJ. Gut mucosal immunization with reovirus serotype 1/L stimulates virusspecific cytotoxic T cell precursors as well as IgA memory cells in Peyer's patches. J Exp Med 1987; 165(3):830–847.

[68] Farstad IN, Halstensen TS, Fausa O, Brandtzaeg P. Heterogeneity of M-cell-associated B and T cells in human Peyer's patches. Immunology 1994;83(3):457–464.

[69] Iwasaki A, Kelsall BL. Localization of distinct Peyer's patch dendritic cell subsets and their recruitment

by chemokines macrophage inflammatory protein(MIP)- 3alpha, MIP-3beta, and secondary lymphoid organ chemokine. J Exp Med 2000;191(8):1381–1394.

[70] Iwasaki A, Kelsall BL. Unique functions of CD11b+, CD8 alpha+, and double-negative Peyer's patch dendritic cells. J Immunol 2001;166(8):4884–4890.

[71] Schieferdecker HL, Ullrich R, Hirseland H, Zeitz M. T cell differentiation antigens on lymphocytes in the human intestinal lamina propria. J Immunol 1992;149(8):2816–2822.

[72] De Maria R, Boirivant M, Cifone MG, et al. Functional expression of Fas and Fas ligand on human gut lamina propria T lymphocytes. A potential role for the acidic sphingomyelinase pathway in normal immunoregulation. J Clin Invest 1996;97(2):316–322.

[73] Bowman EP, Kuklin NA, Youngman KR, et al. The intestinal chemokine thymus-expressed chemokine (CCL25) attracts IgA antibody-secreting cells. J Exp Med 2002;195(2):269–275.

[74] Coffman RL, Lebman DA, Shrader B. Transforming growth factor beta specifically enhances IgA production by lipopolysaccharide-stimulated murine B lymphocytes. J Exp Med 1989;170(3):1039–1044.

[75] Crago SS, Kutteh WH, Moro I, et al. Distribution of IgA1-, IgA2-, and J chain-containing cells in human tissues. J Immunol 1984;132(1):16–18.

[76] Faure F, Jitsukawa S, Triebel F, Hercend T. Characterization of human peripheral lymphocytes expressing the CD3-gamma/delta complex with anti-receptor monoclonal antibodies. J Immunol 1988;141(10): 3357–3360.

[77] Cepek KL, Shaw SK, Parker CM, et al. Adhesion between epithelial cells and T lymphocytes mediated by E-cadherin and the alpha E beta 7 integrin. Nature 1994;372(6502):190–193.

[78] Brandtzaeg P, Farstad IN, Helgeland L. Phenotypes of T cells in the gut. Chem Immunol 1998;71:1–26.

[79] Rocha B, Vassalli P, Guy-Grand D. The V beta repertoire of mouse gut homodimeric alpha CD8+ intraepithelial T cell receptor alpha/beta + lymphocytes reveals a major extrathymic pathway of T cell differentiation. J Exp Med 1991;173(2):483–486.

[80] Williams N. T cells on the mucosal frontline. Science 1998;280(5361):198–200.

[81] Groh V, Steinle A, Bauer S, Spies T. Recognition of stress-induced MHC molecules by intestinal epithelial gammadelta T cells. Science 1998;279(5357):1737–1740.

[82] Wu J, Groh V, Spies T. T cell antigen receptor engagement and specificity in the recognition of stressinducible MHC class I-related chains by human epithelial gamma delta T cells. J Immunol 2002;169(3): 1236–1240.

[83] Gapin L, Cheroutre H, Kronenberg M. Cutting edge: TCR alpha beta+ CD8 alpha alpha+ T cells are found in intestinal intraepithelial lymphocytes of mice that lack classical MHC class I molecules. J Immunol 1999; 163(8):4100–4104.

[84] Franco MA, Greenberg HB. Role of B cells and cytotoxic T lymphocytes in clearance of and immunity to rotavirus infection in mice. J Virol 1995;69(12):7800–7806.

[85] Brandtzaeg P, Farstad IN, Haraldsen G. Regional specialization in the mucosal immune system: primed cells do not always home along the same track. Immunol Today 1999;20(6):267–277.

[86] van Egmond M, Damen CA, van Spriel AB, Vidarsson G, van Garderen E, van de Winkel JG. IgA and the IgA Fc receptor. Trends Immunol 2001;22(4):205–211.

[87] Conley ME, Delacroix DL. Intravascular and mucosal immunoglobulin A: two separate but related systems of immune defense? Ann Intern Med 1987;106(6):892–899.

[88] Macpherson AJ, Hunziker L, McCoy K, Lamarre A. IgA responses in the intestinal mucosa against pathogenic and non-pathogenic microorganisms. Microbes Infect 2001;3(12):1021–1035.

[89] Weisbart RH, Kacena A, Schuh A, Golde DW. GM-CSF induces human neutrophil IgA-mediated phagocytosis by an IgA Fc receptor activation mechanism. Nature 1988;332(6165):647–648.

[90] Monteiro RC, Kubagawa H, Cooper MD. Cellular distribution, regulation, and biochemical nature of an Fc alpha receptor in humans. J Exp Med 1990;171(3):597–613.

[91] Deo YM, Sundarapandiyan K, Keler T, Wallace PK, Graziano RF. Bispecific molecules directed to the Fc receptor for IgA (Fc alpha RI, CD89) and tumor antigens efficiently promote cell-mediated cytotoxicity of tumor targets in whole blood. J Immunol 1998; 160(4):1677–1686.

[92] Patry C, Herbelin A, Lehuen A, Bach JF, Monteiro RC. Fc alpha receptors mediate release of tumour necrosis factor-alpha and interleukin-6 by human monocytes following receptor aggregation. Immunology 1995; 86(1):1–5.

[93] van Egmond M, van Garderen E, van Spriel AB, et al. FcalphaRI-positive liver Kupffer cells: reappraisal of the function of immunoglobulin A in immunity. Nat Med 2000;6(6):680–685.

[94] Kaetzel CS, Robinson JK, Lamm ME. Epithelial transcytosis of monomeric IgA and IgG cross-linked through antigen to polymeric IgA. A role for monomeric antibodies in the mucosal immune system. J Immunol 1994;152(1):72–76.

[95] Kaetzel CS, Robinson JK, Chintalacharuvu KR, Vaerman JP, Lamm ME. The polymeric immunoglobulin receptor (secretory component) mediates transport of immune complexes across epithelial cells: a local defense function for IgA. Proc Natl Acad Sci U S A 1991;88(19):8796–8800.

[96] Orlans E, Peppard J, Reynolds J, Hall J. Rapid active transport of immunoglobulin A from blood to bile. J Exp Med 1978;147(2):588–592.

[97] Jackson GD, Lemaitre-Coelho I, Vaerman JP, Bazin H, Beckers A. Rapid disappearance from serum of intravenously injected rat myeloma IgA and its secretion into bile. Eur J Immunol 1978;8(2):123–126.

[98] Kramer DR, Cebra JJ. Early appearance of "natural" mucosal IgA responses and germinal centers in suckling mice developing in the absence of maternal antibodies. J Immunol 1995;154(5):2051–2062.

[99] Mackie RI, Sghir A, Gaskins HR. Developmental microbial ecology of the neonatal gastrointestinal tract. Am J Clin Nutr 1999;69(5):1035S–1045S.

[100] Kang HS, Chin RK, Wang Y, et al. Signaling via LTbetaR on the lamina propria stromal cells of the gut is required for IgA production. Nat Immunol 2002;3(6): 576–582.

[101] Macpherson AJ, Gatto D, Sainsbury E, Harriman GR, Hengartner H, Zinkernagel RM. A primitive T cellindependent mechanism of intestinal mucosal IgA responses to commensal bacteria. Science 2000; 288(5474):2222–2226.

[102] Fagarasan S, Honjo T. Intestinal IgA synthesis: regulation of front-line body defences. Nat Rev Immunol 2003;3(1):63–72.

[103] McWilliams M, Phillips-Quagliata JM, Lamm ME. Mesenteric lymph node B lymphoblasts which home to the small intestine are precommitted to IgA synthesis. J Exp Med 1977;145(4):866–875.

[104] Newberry RD, McDonough JS, McDonald KG, Lorenz RG. Postgestational lymphotoxin/lymphotoxin beta receptor interactions are essential for the presence of intestinal B lymphocytes. J Immunol 2002;168(10): 4988–4997.

[105] Kunimoto DY, Harriman GR, Strober W. Regulation of IgA differentiation in CH12LX B cells by lymphokines. IL-4 induces membrane IgM-positive CH12LX cells to express membrane IgA and IL-5 induces membrane IgA-positive CH12LX cells to secrete IgA. J Immunol 1988;141(3):713–720.

[106] Defrance T, Vanbervliet B, Briere F, Durand I, Rousset F, Banchereau J. Interleukin 10 and transforming growth factor beta cooperate to induce anti-CD40- activated naive human B cells to secrete

immunoglobulin A. J Exp Med 1992;175(3):671–682.

[107] Beagley KW, Eldridge JH, Kiyono H, et al. Recombinant murine IL-5 induces high rate IgA synthesis in cycling IgA-positive Peyer's patch B cells. J Immunol 1988;141(6):2035–2042.

[108] Kunimoto DY, Nordan RP, Strober W. IL-6 is a potent cofactor of IL-1 in IgM synthesis and of IL-5 in IgA synthesis. J Immunol 1989;143(7):2230–2235.

[109] Arcus VL, Langley R, Proft T, Fraser JD, Baker EN. The Three-dimensional structure of a superantigen-like protein, SET3, from a pathogenicity island of the Staphylococcus aureus genome. J Biol Chem 2002; 277(35):32274–32281.

[110] Fan X, Gunasena H, Cheng Z, et al. Helicobacter pylori urease binds to class II MHC on gastric epithelial cells and induces their apoptosis. J Immunol 2000;165(4): 1918–1924.

[111] Crabtree JE, Farmery SM, Lindley IJ, Figura N, Peichl P, Tompkins DS. CagA/cytotoxic strains of Helicobacter pylori and interleukin-8 in gastric epithelial cell lines. J Clin Pathol 1994;47(10):945–950.

[112] Crowe SE, Alvarez L, Dytoc M, et al. Expression of interleukin 8 and CD54 by human gastric epithelium after Helicobacter pylori infection in vitro. Gastroenterology 1995;108(1):65–74.

[113] Schmausser B, Andrulis M, Endrich S, et al. Expression and subcellular distribution of toll-like receptors TLR4, TLR5 and TLR9 on the gastric epithelium in Helicobacter pylori infection. Clin Exp Immunol 2004;136(3):521–526.

[114] Backhed F, Rokbi B, Torstensson E, et al. Gastric mucosal recognition of Helicobacter pylori is independent of Toll-like receptor 4. J Infect Dis 2003;187(5):829–836.

[115] Amieva MR, Vogelmann R, Covacci A, Tompkins LS, Nelson WJ, Falkow S. Disruption of the epithelial apical-junctional complex by Helicobacter pylori CagA. Science 2003;300(5624):1430–1434.

[116] Bamford KB, Fan X, Crowe SE, et al. Lymphocytes in the human gastric mucosa during Helicobacter pylori have a T helper cell 1 phenotype. Gastroenterology 1998;114(3):482–492.

[117] Karttunen R, Karttunen T, Ekre HP, MacDonald TT. Interferon gamma and interleukin 4 secreting cells in the gastric antrum in Helicobacter pylori positive and negative gastritis. Gut 1995;36(3):341–345.

[118] D'Elios MM, Manghetti M, Almerigogna F, et al. Different cytokine profile and antigen-specificity repertoire in Helicobacter pylori-specific T cell clones from the antrum of chronic gastritis patients with or without peptic ulcer. Eur J Immunol 1997;27(7): 1751–1755.

[119] Molinari M, Salio M, Galli C, et al. Selective inhibition of Ii-dependent antigen presentation by Helicobacter pylori toxin VacA. J Exp Med 1998;187(1):135–140.

[120] Perna NT, Mayhew GF, Posfai G, et al. Molecular evolution of a pathogenicity island from enterohemorrhagic Escherichia coli O157 : H7. Infect Immun 1998;66(8):3810–3817.

[121] Russel M. Macromolecular assembly and secretion across the bacterial cell envelope: type II protein secretion systems. J Mol Biol 1998;279(3):485–499.

[122] Kubori T, Matsushima Y, Nakamura D, et al. Supramolecular structure of the Salmonella typhimurium type III protein secretion system. Science 1998;280(5363): 602–605.

[123] Blocker A, Gounon P, Larquet E, et al. The tripartite type III secreton of Shigella flexneri inserts IpaB and IpaC into host membranes. J Cell Biol 1999;147(3): 683–693.

[124] Knutton S, Rosenshine I, Pallen MJ, et al. A novel EspAassociated surface organelle of enteropathogenic Escherichia coli involved in protein translocation into epithelial cells. EMBO J 1998;17(8):2166–2176.

[125] Donnenberg MS. Pathogenic strategies of enteric bacteria. Nature 2000;406(6797):768–774.

[126] Hersh D, Monack DM, Smith MR, Ghori N, Falkow S, Zychlinsky A. The Salmonella invasin SipB induces macrophage apoptosis by binding to caspase-1. Proc Natl Acad Sci U S A 1999;96(5):2396–2401.

[127] Hilbi H, Moss JE, Hersh D, et al. Shigella-induced apoptosis is dependent on caspase-1 which binds to IpaB. J Biol Chem 1998;273(49):32895–32900.

[128] Christie PJ, Vogel JP. Bacterial type IV secretion: conjugation systems adapted to deliver effector molecules to host cells. Trends Microbiol 2000;8(8):354–360.

[129] Yen MR, Peabody CR, Partovi SM, Zhai Y, Tseng YH, Saier MH. Protein-translocating outer membrane porins of gram-negative bacteria. Biochim Biophys Acta 2002;1562(1–2):6–31.

[130] Sansonetti PJ, Arondel J, Cantey JR, Prevost MC, Huerre M. Infection of rabbit Peyer's patches by Shigella flexneri: effect of adhesive or invasive bacterial phenotypes on follicle-associated epithelium. Infect Immun 1996;64(7):2752–2764.

[131] Perdomo JJ, Gounon P, Sansonetti PJ. Polymorphonuclear leukocyte transmigration promotes invasion of colonic epithelial monolayer by Shigella flexneri. J Clin Invest 1994;93(2):633–643.

[132] Zychlinsky A, Fitting C, Cavaillon JM, Sansonetti PJ. Interleukin 1 is released by murine macrophages during apoptosis induced by Shigella flexneri. J Clin Invest 1994;94(3):1328–1332.

[133] Stebbins CE, Galan JE. Modulation of host signaling by a bacterial mimic: structure of the Salmonella effector SptP bound to Rac1. Mol Cell 2000;6(6):1449–1460.

[134] Celli J, Deng W, Finlay BB. Enteropathogenic Escherichia coli (EPEC) attachment to epithelial cells: exploiting the host cell cytoskeleton from the outside. Cell Microbiol 2000;2(1):1–9.

[135] Hisamatsu T, Suzuki M, Reinecker HC, Nadeau WJ, McCormick BA, Podolsky DK. CARD15/NOD2 functions as an antibacterial factor in human intestinal epithelial cells. Gastroenterology 2003;124(4):993–1000.

[136] Mastroeni P. Immunity to systemic Salmonella infections. Curr Mol Med 2002;2(4):393–406.

[137] Karczewski J, Groot J. Molecular physiology and pathophysiology of tight junctions III. Tight junction regulation by intracellular messengers: differences in response within and between epithelia. Am J Physiol Gastrointest Liver Physiol 2000;279(4):G660–G665.

[138] Gasbarrini G, Montalto M. Structure and function of tight junctions. Role in intestinal barrier. Ital J Gastroenterol Hepatol 1999;31(6):481–488.

[139] Sarker SA, Gyr K. Non-immunological defence mechanisms of the gut. Gut 1992;33(7):987–993.

[140] Sampson HA. Food allergy: immunology of the GI mucosa towards classification and understanding of GI hypersensitivities. Pediatr Allergy Immunol 2001;12(Suppl 14):7–9.

[141] Bardella MT, Fredella C, Prampolini L, Marino R, Conte D, Giunta AM. Gluten sensitivity in monozygous twins: a long-term follow-up of five pairs. Am J Gastroenterol 2000;95(6):1503–1505.

[142] Sicherer SH, Furlong TJ, Maes HH, Desnick RJ, Sampson HA, Gelb BD. Genetics of peanut allergy: a twin study. J Allergy Clin Immunol 2000;106(1 pt 1):53–56.

[143] Pietrzyk JJ. [Genetic background of atopy]. Pediatr Pol 1996;71(1):7–10.

[144] Par A. Gastrointestinal tract as a part of immune defence. Acta Physiol Hung 2000;87(4):291–304.

[145] Sudo N, Sawamura S, Tanaka K, Aiba Y, Kubo C, Koga Y. The requirement of intestinal bacterial flora for the development of an IgE production system fully susceptible to oral tolerance induction. J Immunol 1997;159(4):1739–1745.

[146] Mowat AM, Donachie AM, Parker LA, et al. The role of dendritic cells in regulating mucosal immunity and tolerance. Novartis Found Symp 2003;252:291–302.

[147] Duchmann R, Neurath MF, Meyer zum Buschenfelde KH. Responses to self and non-self intestinal microflora in health and inflammatory bowel disease. Res Immunol 1997;148(8–9):589–594.

第4章
胃肠道病毒学

Richard L. Ward, Xi Jiang, Tibor Farkas, and Dorsey M. Bass

胃肠道病毒

胃肠道（gastrointestinal tract，GI）是最常见的病原体入侵门户之一，且病毒常通过粪口途径传播。脊髓灰质炎病毒是已知的历史上第一种能引起广泛发病和死亡的肠道病毒。脊髓灰质炎病毒疫苗是第一种针对肠道病毒感染开发的疫苗，它包括非经肠道施用的灭活疫苗和口服减毒活疫苗。脊髓灰质炎病毒疫苗非常有效，自1989年以来，西半球就再也没有野生型病毒感染病例的报道。虽然脊髓灰质炎病毒通过胃肠道进入宿主体内，但脊髓灰质炎病毒疫苗通过诱导血清中和抗体阻止肠道外的病毒扩散来防御系统性麻痹。然而，对于那些发病率和病死率仅与肠内复制有关的肠道病毒感染来说，血清中和抗体几乎不起保护作用。因此，针对这些病毒的有效疫苗的开发面临着新的挑战，因为需要以黏膜免疫为基础，而非系统性免疫。

至少从20世纪40年代开始，人们就认识到病毒可能是重症胃肠炎的病原体，因为当时人们发现从胃肠炎暴发样本中得到的无菌粪便滤液可将胃肠道疾病成功地传染给志愿者[1~5]。在60年代，人们利用电镜在患有胃肠炎的小鼠和小牛的肠内容物[6,7]及健康猴子的直肠拭子中[8]观察到车轮状外观的病毒颗粒，后来被确认为轮状病毒（rotavirus，RV）的特征。尽管如此，直到1972年在流行性病毒性胃肠炎患儿的粪便中发现诺瓦克病毒[9]和1973年在重症胃肠炎患儿的呕吐物内分离出RV[10]之后，人类胃肠道疾病与特定病毒的相关性才得以确定。虽然其他病毒也与胃肠道疾病相关，但目前已确定的作为最常见的重症胃肠道疾病病因的三个肠道病毒群分别是轮状病毒、杯状病毒和星形病毒。本章节将重点介绍每一种病毒的主要结构特点、复制周期、发病机制和免疫力。就像40多年前的脊髓灰质炎病毒那样，阻止上述病毒引发疾病的唯一可靠的预防策略就是疫苗接种，但还没有获得许可的疫苗用于这些GI病毒。然而，两种候选RV疫苗最近进行了大规模的III期临床试验，因此，用于全世界婴幼儿常规免疫的RV疫苗有望很快产生。

轮状病毒

轮状病毒（RV）是引起全世界婴幼儿重症胃肠炎的唯一的最重要病原体。仅在美国，RV 每年导致超过 5 万幼儿住院，大约 40 人因此死亡[11]。进一步估计，每年 RV 腹泻导致约 60 万的门诊或急诊病例。RV 疾病每年在美国造成至少 5 亿美元的直接医疗费用及 10 亿美元的非医疗支出[12]。全世界范围内，RV 每年导致超过 60 万人死亡（U. D. Parashar，2004，个人通信）。因为以上原因，RV 疫苗成为优先发展的目标。

RV 通过粪口途径传播，这为其普遍暴露提供了高效机制。在发达国家和发展中国家中，大约 90% 的儿童在 3 岁以前都感染过 RV[13]。RV 疾病的典型症状是腹泻和呕吐，伴随发热、恶心、食欲减退、腹部绞痛、萎靡不振，这些症状可以是轻微的并持续较短时间，或可导致严重的脱水。重症疾病主要发生于幼儿，以 6~24 月龄儿童最常见。RV 感染通常对后续的重症疾病提供短期的保护和免疫力，而不能提供终生免疫力；此外，还有大量再次感染病例的报道。新生儿同样可以感染 RV，但是这种感染是在某些环境下作为地方病发生，并且通常无症状[14~17]。据报道，此类新生儿感染可以降低日后 RV 感染的发病率[15,16]。成人及老年人也可出现 RV 疾病，与其他的继发性 RV 感染一样，症状通常较为轻微。然而，日本近期的研究表明，RV 可导致成人住院[18]，青少年发病率显著上升[19]。

考虑到 RV 感染的普遍性及再次感染后疾病严重程度通常降低的现象，RV 疫苗的现实目标是预防严重病例的发生。人们已经研发了多种候选疫苗，并在婴幼儿评价中获得了有前景的结果。如果发达国家将有效的 RV 疫苗列入婴幼儿免疫规划，将可减少 40%~60% 的幼儿腹泻住院率及 10%~20% 的总体腹泻病死率[20]。在有效的 RV 疫苗可以使用之前，对 RV 疾病的控制局限于非特异性方法，主要是补液疗法。

轮状病毒历史

1963 年，在小鼠和猴子的肠组织和直肠拭子中，人们首次通过电镜观察到一种后来认为其形态学特征与 RV 有关的病毒[6,8]。这些病毒分别被称为幼鼠流行性腹泻病毒和猴病毒 11，均为 70nm 大小、车轮状外观的病毒颗粒。因此，人们后来以车轮的拉丁语 "rota" 命名了该病毒[13]。1969 年，Mebus 及其同事[7]在腹泻小牛的粪便中发现了这些病毒颗粒，说明这些病毒与家畜的腹泻疾病有关。1973 年，Bishop 及其同事[10]利用电镜对急性胃肠炎患儿的十二指肠黏膜进行活检，第一次报道了这些病毒与人类腹泻疾病的相关性。在这项重要的研究中，研究者鉴定出了之前在动物粪便中发现的车轮状外观的病毒颗粒。不久之后，他们及其他研究者证实了粪便中存在的 RV 与急性胃肠炎之间的相关性。现在，这些人类及动物 RV 被分类为呼肠孤病毒科轮状病毒属的成员。

轮状病毒颗粒的性质

利用冷冻电镜技术(cryoelectron microscopy, cryo-EM)获得的 RV 颗粒的计算机成像(图 4.1)表明其直径约为 100nm，衣壳由三个同心的蛋白质层组成[21,22]。外层由 VP7 糖蛋白（780 个分子/病毒粒子）和 60 个 VP4 蛋白二聚体组成，后者形成的刺突样突起延伸出 VP7 层之外 11~12nm[21~24]。VP4 蛋白锚定在由 780 个 VP6 蛋白分子组成的颗粒中间层。最内层含有 120 个 VP2 蛋白分子，与 12 个病毒转录酶（VP1）和鸟苷酸转移酶（VP3）分子及双链 RNA 基因组的 11 个节段相互作用。这些基因组节段编码 6 个结构蛋白和 6 个非结构蛋白 NSP1~6（表 4.1）。除了第 11 节段是双顺反子之外[25]，其他每个节段编码一种已知的病毒蛋白，这些蛋白质的功能已被研究，但仍不是十分清楚。这些基因组节段的长度为 660~3300bp，其编码蛋白的分子质量为 12~125kDa。

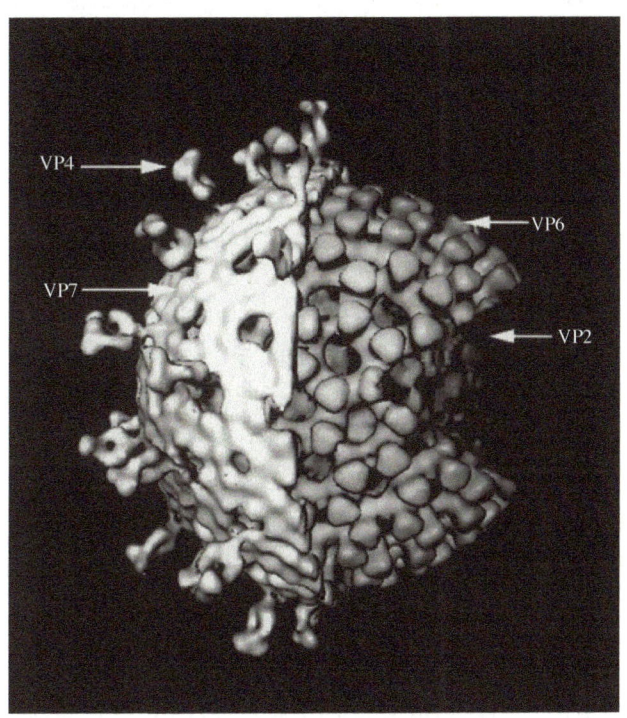

图 4.1　利用冷冻电镜技术获得的三层 RV 颗粒的计算机成像。剖图显示外壳由 VP4 刺突和 VP7 衣壳组成，中间层为 VP6，内层为 VP2 围绕着由 11 个双链 RNA 节段与 VP1 和 VP3 组成的核心（Source: Courtesy of B.V.V. Prasad，Baylor College of Medicine，Houston，Texas）。

表 4.1　RV 基因节段的大小和编码蛋白的特性

RNA 节段	碱基对数量	编码蛋白	蛋白质相对分子质量（×10^{-4}）	蛋白质的性质
1	3300	VP1	12.5	内层核心蛋白，RNA 结合，RNA 转录酶
2	2700	VP2	10.2	内层衣壳蛋白，RNA 结合
3	2600	VP3	9.8	内层核心蛋白，鸟苷酸转移酶
4	2360	VP4	8.7	外层衣壳蛋白，HA，NP，受体结合，促融合蛋白
5	1600	NSP1	5.9	非结构蛋白，RNA 结合，含有锌指结构，宿主范围决定簇（？）
6	1360	VP6	4.5	中间层衣壳蛋白，组和亚组抗原
7	1100	NSP3	3.5	非结构蛋白，RNA 结合，翻译调控

续表

RNA 节段	碱基对数量	编码蛋白	蛋白质相对分子质量（×10⁻⁴）	蛋白质的性质
8	1060	NSP2	3.7	非结构蛋白，RNA 和 NSP5 结合，NTPase
9	1060	VP7	3.7	外层衣壳糖蛋白，NP
10	750	NSP4	2.0	非结构糖蛋白，跨膜蛋白，肠毒素
11	660	NSP5	2.2	非结构蛋白，磷酸化，O-糖基化，与 NSP2 相互作用，病毒体
		NSP6	1.2	非结构蛋白，与 NSP5 相互作用

HA：血凝素；NP：中和蛋白；NTPase：三磷酸核苷水解酶

轮状病毒分类

轮状病毒组

除了具有独特的形态，RV 共用一种组抗原[13]，后来被确认是保守的、构成中间层衣壳的 VP6 蛋白。1980 年，在猪体内发现了一种与已知的 RV 在形态学上无差别，但缺少共同组抗原的病毒颗粒[26,27]。随后，基于共同组抗原鉴定出了归属于其他 6 个组的 RV（B~G），而最初的 RV 株归为 A 组。只有 A~C 组与人类疾病有关，且绝大多数由 A 组病毒引起。然而，B 组与中国尤其是中国成人的大流行有关[28,29]，C 组与世界范围内尤其是日本的许多小流行有关[30]，预示着这些非 A 组病毒在未来将有可能成为主要的病原体。大量血清流行病学研究显示 C 组 RV 抗体在不同国家存在高流行，这也支持了上面的预示。

轮状病毒的电泳型和基因型

根据流行病学研究的目的，利用不同的分类方案对 RV 进行特征描述。然而，每一种方案都与基因组分节段病毒的独特特性分不开，即重配的能力。在病毒复制周期中病毒装配的最初阶段，最后包装于病毒颗粒中的新合成的正链 RNA 在形成复制中间体之前是可以自由结合的[31]。子代病毒的装配就是从这些基因组前体中选择合适的节段数量和组合进行的。超过一种病毒共感染细胞可引起来自于不同亲代的正链 RNA 的重配。如果是病毒的不同毒株共感染，信使 RNA（mRNA）重配产生的子代是共感染毒株的遗传嵌合体。这些新毒株或重配株的鉴别依据其特殊的基因节段排列，通常是根据它们在聚丙烯酰胺凝胶电泳（polyacryamide gel electrophoresis，PAGE）中的迁移率（如电泳分型）。新病毒株的性质取决于哪些基因节段从哪种亲代毒株遗传得到，以及每一种特定的节段组合及其蛋白质产物的功能行为。

RV 在细胞培养及实验动物共感染中极易发生重配，这至少是自然界中存在各种各样 RV 株的部分原因。然而，RV 株之间重配的形成并不是普遍现象。例如，没有证据表明不同组的 RV 株会发生重配[32]。即使在 A 组 RV 内，可形成稳定重配株的毒株组合也有严格的限制，这种限制似乎与毒株之间的遗传变异度直接相关[33]。RV 株之间形成限制性重配的一个结果是遗传家族或遗传组概念的产生[34]。遗传组是由基因节段能够形成毒株间 RNA-RNA 杂交链的 RV 株组成的，这种 RNA-RNA 杂交链足够稳定并在 PAGE 中迁移形成清晰的条带[34]。因此，同一个遗传组的成员具有高度的遗传相关性，且与其他遗传组成员的遗传同源性明显降低。由于 RV 遗传组似乎具有种属特异性[34,35]，所以其种属间传播可通过遗传组的分析来进行检测。几乎所有的人类 RV 属于 Wa 或 DS-1 组[36,37]，因此这些毒株被定义为原型株。遗传组的概念已经广泛用于确定引起人类感染和疾病的 RV 的来源，尤其是用于检测含有动物来源的基因节段的病毒或重配株。

轮状病毒的血清型

RV 的两种外层衣壳蛋白 VP4 和 VP7 都含有中和表位，因此都可以用于血清分型的确定。最初的血清分型只依据 VP7 蛋白的差异，因为 RV 超免疫动物产生的中和抗体大多数是针对 VP7 蛋白的。对于这些超免疫血清的交叉中和研究可以很容易地将这些毒株分成不同的 VP7 血清型[38,39]。后来，研究者发现 VP4 在某些情况下也能成为优势中和蛋白[40~43]，因此需要一种双重血清分型方案。虽然 VP7 血清型可以比较容易地通过交叉中和试验来确定，但是 VP4 血清分型更加困难。因此，两种数字系统被设计用来对 RV 株的 VP4 蛋白进行分类：一种基于比较核酸杂交和序列分析（基因型），其类别在括号中标出；第二种以抗血清进行中和试验为基础（血清型），这些抗血清是针对杆状病毒表达的 VP4 蛋白[44]或含有特异性 VP4 基因的重配毒株的[45]。

根据 VP4 和 VP7 RV 被分为 P 型和 G 型，来分别揭示这两种蛋白质的蛋白酶敏感性和糖基化结构[46]。到目前为止人们已经鉴定出 15 个 G 血清型和 22 个 P 基因型[47,48]。然而，Liprandi 等[49]在 2003 年描述了一株猪 A 组 RV（A34），根据该病毒 VP4 基因的 VP8 区部分序列（13~250 位氨基酸）的分析，推测该毒株可能属于新的 P 基因型，并暂定为 P[23]。另外，基于 VP4 基因全序列的对比，一株名为 TUCH 的猕猴 RV 被鉴定为新的 P 基因型[50]。根据 A34 株全序列的分析，可将其归类为 P[23]或者 P[24]。

已经分离出 10 个 G 血清型的人 RV（human rotavirus，HRV），但是到目前为止绝大多数的 HRV 经鉴定为 G1、G2、G3 或 G4 型[13]。事实上这 4 种血清型病毒均能引起疾病，而且这些疾病的严重程度几乎没有差别[51~53]。同时也发现了 10 个 P 基因型的 HRV，但是几乎所有的疾病都跟 P 基因型 4、P 基因型 6 和 P 基因型 8 有关[13]。当然，在某些情况下，也经常能分离出其他的 G 型和 P 型，尤其是 G9 株分布于世界范围内，有时还在所有分离株中占很大比例。

轮状病毒基因节段之间的联系

如果 HRV 的 G 型和 P 型在重配形成时可以自由结合，那么理论上预测有关蛋白质类型的组合就可能随机发生。然而，事实并非如此。例如，G1P[8]和 G2P[4]分别与其原型株 Wa 和 DS-1 株相似，它们经常被分离到，由于分属于 HRV 的两个不同的遗传组[34]，因此，它们应该极少形成稳定的重配，这一推断已经通过对大量病毒株的分析所证明。基因节段的其他关联性也已经被发现。根据蛋白质本身抗原性的差异，VP6 蛋白或组抗原可以分为 4 个亚组（Ⅰ、Ⅱ、Ⅰ/Ⅱ和非Ⅰ/Ⅱ）[54,55]。几乎所有的 G2 和 G8 型 HRV 都属于Ⅰ亚组，而 G1、G3、G4 和 G9 型 HRV 仅属于Ⅱ亚组。G3 型也是动物毒株的一个常见血清型，但是与 HRV G3 株相反，几乎所有的 G3 型动物 RV 属于Ⅰ亚组。另外，人Ⅰ亚组毒株表现为典型的电泳短型,并且第10和第11节段的迁移顺序反转,而动物Ⅰ亚组毒株无此现象[56]。因此,可以通过血清型、基因型、亚型、电泳型分析及遗传组测定发现独特的遗传连锁。

轮状病毒的复制

细胞附着

RV在体内的组织嗜性非常特异,它们通常只通过小肠绒毛顶端感染肠上皮细胞。虽然在体外RV可以与多种类型的细胞结合,但是只能有效地感染肾和小肠来源的细胞系,这就意味着结合前与结合后的选择过程调节着RV的复制。细胞结合的条件在毒株之间存在差异。某些病毒株,尤其是动物毒株在最初附着时需要唾液酸（sialic acid,SA）,但这种需要也不是必需的,因为不需要唾液酸的变异株也已经被分离到[57,58]。此外,许多动物RV和绝大多数HRV都不需要这种受体。对于这些病毒株而言,有多种细胞表面蛋白充当最初的附着分子,包括神经节苷脂GM1和GM3及整合素α2β1[59~62]。一些RV VP4蛋白的VP5*区（308~310位氨基酸）含有α2β1配体序列DGE[60,63],因此提示病毒通过VP4分子中的部分序列与细胞之间发生最初的相互作用。然而,有报道称VP4蛋白的VP8*区的第155位和第188~190位氨基酸在该蛋白质的唾液酸结合活性中发挥着不可或缺的作用[64]。在进入细胞之前,RV首先与初级受体接触,继而与一个或更多的次级受体结合（图4.2）。这些次级受体包括但绝不限于热激蛋白hsc 70[65]及整合素αXβ2、α4β1和αVβ3[60,63,66]。与整合素的结合似乎是通过与VP7而不是与VP4蛋白的相互作用完成的[60,65]。研究发现,VP7蛋白也能调节某些VP4介导的表型,包括受体结合[67,68]。

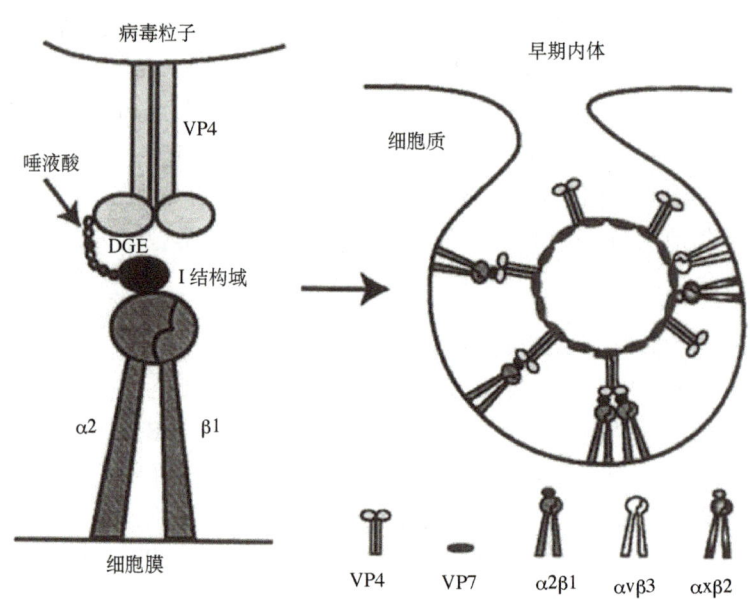

图4.2 参与RV与细胞膜附着及通过内含体摄取病毒颗粒进入细胞的整合素模型（Source：Graham et al.[60],with permission of the American Society for Microbiology）。

脂类的亲和力差异导致了细胞膜上存在着鞘脂和胆固醇富集的脂微区或脂筏[69,70]。对于特定去污剂具有耐受性的脂筏不仅可以选择性结合 RV，而且还可富集 RV 受体，如神经节苷脂 GM1、整合素亚单位 α2 和 β3 及 hsc 70[71]。这一结果提示去污剂耐受性微区可能为促进 RV 受体与病毒颗粒的有效相互作用提供了一个平台。

进入细胞和转录激活

胰蛋白酶将 VP4 蛋白裂解为 VP5* 和 VP8* 亚单位的病毒活化过程是病毒结合后发生产毒性感染所必需的。目前已经提出了两种病毒颗粒内化的机制。基于电镜观察的早期研究表明病毒通过胞吞作用进入细胞，内体中的病毒颗粒被迅速地转运至溶酶体，发生脱壳和转录激活[72,73]，这种机制通常与其他 RNA 病毒的雷同。后来，有报道称这种途径可能被非胰蛋白酶活化的 RV 所采用，病毒半衰期为 30~50min，并且在细胞表面消失后导致顿挫型感染[74,75]。相反，活化的病毒半衰期为 3~5min，并以直接侵入的方式进入细胞。亲溶酶体药剂几乎不影响病毒复制，这一结果进一步证明了 RV 不在溶酶体内活化[74~77]。

最近有新的证据表明 RV 结合后的吸收在内体完成，这正如最初假设的一样[78,79]（图 4.2）。然而，病毒的外层衣壳蛋白在低 Ca^{2+} 浓度的内体中发生脱衣壳，而不是进入溶酶体。从这一点来说，内体膜具有渗透性，并且使具有转录活性的双层 RV 颗粒被释放到细胞质中[78]。在进入过程中，细胞膜可能通过与结合病毒的 VP5* 亚单位蛋白相互作用而暂时变得可渗透[80]，因此导致了放射性铬的释放及诸如 α-次黄嘌呤等毒素的内化[75,81,82]。虽然根据现有的数据能够提出了其他的进入和转录激活机制，但是以上表述是对已有观察结果的最合理综合解释。

转录和复制

具有转录活性的病毒颗粒释放入细胞质后立即合成 11 条病毒正链 RNA，这些 RNA 是通过病毒颗粒顶部的 VP2 和 VP6 蛋白层通道从病毒核心进入细胞质的[83,84]。每个颗粒包括 12 个 VP1 和 VP3 分子，而且每个蛋白质的每一分子与每一基因组节段都有关，由 VP1 转录并通过 VP3 酶活性加帽。这些最初的转录子必须作为 mRNA 合成病毒蛋白。翻译效率取决于 RV NSP3 的合成，后者可与病毒 mRNA 的 3′ 端和真核起始因子 eIF4G 有效结合[85]。这种细胞蛋白可以作为"脚手架"募集其他的翻译起始蛋白并通过促进 mRNA 环化进行有效的翻译。由于 NSP3 与 eIF4G 有高亲和力，所以 NSP3 可以通过阻止细胞 mRNA 的环化来抑制细胞蛋白质的合成[86,87]。

在病毒复制周期的早期，其他两种非结构蛋白 NSP2 和 NSP5 一旦合成，就会形成细胞质电子致密颗粒结构，被称为病毒体，病毒 RNA 的包装和复制及双层病毒颗粒的装配都被认为是在这里完成的[88~90]。病毒颗粒的装配可能起始于病毒质中由 11 个基因节段转录出的正链 RNA，以及 VP1、VP3 和 RNA 结合的非结构蛋白 NSP2、NSP5 和 NSP6 所组成的复合物的形成[91,92]。虽然机制仍不清楚，但是病毒忠实地在每一个前体病毒复合物中装配和包装一个拷贝的每一条正链 RNA。该复合物最后丢掉非结构蛋白，并在相继加入 VP2 和 VP6 之后形成双层病毒颗粒，其单链 RNA 也转化成双链基因组节段。由于两个共感染的病毒基因组可非常高效地发生重配，并且正链 RNA 可以在病毒进入胞液后从病毒质中释放[84]，所以来源于共感染 RV 的具有转录活性的双层颗粒可以进入共享的病毒质，在这里完成正链 RNA 的合成和重配，并最终包装入病毒颗粒，这就解释了反向遗传系统并不适于 RV 的原因[84]。

病毒成熟和释放

在感染细胞的胞液内合成的 5 种 RV 蛋白似乎在双层病毒颗粒的装配中并不发挥作用，也似乎没有被转运入病毒质。一种是 NSP3，它在病毒 mRNA 翻译过程中的作用前文中已经描述。另一种是非必需的 NSP1 蛋白[93]，据报道它可与干扰素调节因子 3（interferon regulatory factor 3，IRF-3）相互作用，因此可以抑制 IRF-3 激活，减弱细胞的干扰素反应[94]。另外 3 种蛋白质（VP4、VP7 和 NSP4）在病毒成熟的最后阶段发挥特定的不可或缺的作用。VP7 和 NSP4 都是在内质网（endoplasmic reticulum，ER）结合的核糖体合成的糖蛋白，通过信号肽序列嵌入内质网膜。相反地，有报道称，VP4 蛋白定位于病毒质外缘与 ER 外表面之间的空间内[95,96]。在病毒成熟的最终阶段，病毒质中完整组装的 RV 双层颗粒似乎与 ER 外膜相关，这可能就是 VP4 的加入位点。然而，直到最近，有实验提示 VP4 的加入可能是成熟过程的最后一步[97]。有报道指出，不管 VP4 何时加入，未成熟的病毒颗粒与 VP7 和 NSP4 联合穿过 ER 而完成出芽，并获得暂时性的包膜，这个包膜会随着病毒颗粒向 ER 内部的移动而移开[79]。VP4 包含在这些病毒颗粒中，还是在随后的步骤中加入，这一问题仍然有待确定。

完全成熟的三层病毒颗粒从感染细胞中释放的机制尚未完全阐明。有数据表明，这可能是 RV 感染刺激了细胞内 Ca^{2+} 浓度增加而导致了细胞的意外死亡（坏死）[98]，也可能是这些感染引起了细胞的程序性死亡（细胞凋亡）[99]。Jourdan 等[100]曾提出，在细胞死亡之前，完全成熟的 RV 颗粒通过"非常规的小囊泡"从 ER 转运至细胞顶端表面。在更近一段时间，有研究表明成熟的 RV 颗粒在细胞内与脂筏结合并转运到细胞表面[101]。因为已经发现 VP4 与这些脂筏有关，表明这些脂筏是 VP4 加入和病毒颗粒最终成熟的场所[97]。这些脂筏的结构与那些细胞膜中富集 RV 受体的脂筏相似[71]，因此提示病毒进出细胞涉及相似的细胞膜/病毒相互作用。因为大多数 RV 的双层和三层颗粒在细胞裂解后仍与细胞碎片结合，所以 Musalem 和 Espejo 提出可能是这些病毒颗粒在细胞内就与这些结构结合[102]。

轮状病毒致病机制

人感染轮状病毒的疾病表现

RV 是儿童脱水腹泻的最常见病原体。RV 感染的主要部位是小肠绒毛膜顶端的上皮细胞，潜伏期为 2~4 天，随后突发呕吐和腹泻。疾病通常是自限性的，持续 4~8 天。如需住院治疗，住院时间通常较短，2~14 天不等，平均 4 天[103]。其他肠道 RV 感染相关的临床表现包括发热、腹部不适和轻度脱水。个别感染者出现呼吸系统症状，如咳嗽、咽炎、中耳炎和肺炎，但是这些症状与 RV 感染的关系尚不清楚，并且呼吸道分泌物中不一定都能分离到 RV。其他与 RV 感染相关的病因学或者偶发的临床表现包括脑炎和脑膜炎、川崎病、婴儿猝死综合征、肝脓肿、胰腺炎、新生儿坏死性小肠结肠炎[104]和糖尿病[105,106]。肠套叠和 RV 自然感染的关系备受关注，因为在美国有报道显示获得许可的四价 RRV 疫苗（Rotashield™, Wyeth, Philadelphia, PA）与肠套叠有关，所以在 1998 年，即上市不到一年后该疫苗被撤市[107]。多项研究调查了可能引发肠套叠的感染性病因学，大部分研究的结论是 RV 的自然感染不是主要原因[108,109]。虽然没有被证明，但是 Rotashield 接种与肠套叠之间的特殊相关性说明 RRV 具有其他 RV 毒株没有的独特的特征。

轮状病毒感染后小肠绒毛的变化

RV 经粪 - 口途径传播后，感染起始于小肠，并且通常引起一系列的组织学和生理学改变。RV 感染引起的可见病理改变绝大多数都局限于小肠，并且主要是以动物模型进行的研究。RV 感染在不同动物中引起的肠道组织学改变的范围差别显著，从很少或没有改变（如成年鼠）到广泛改变（如新生小牛和仔猪）。在小牛和仔猪中的研究表明，RV 感染使绒毛上皮细胞由柱状变为立方状，导致绒毛缩短和生长迟缓[110,111]。绒毛膜顶端的细胞裸露在外（图 4.3），而下方固有层中网状细胞的数量增加且能观察到单核细胞浸润。感染开始于小肠近端，并向远端发展，最突出的改变通常但并不总是发生在近端小肠[112]。

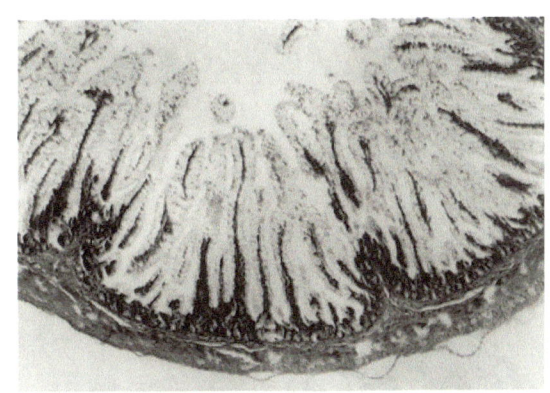 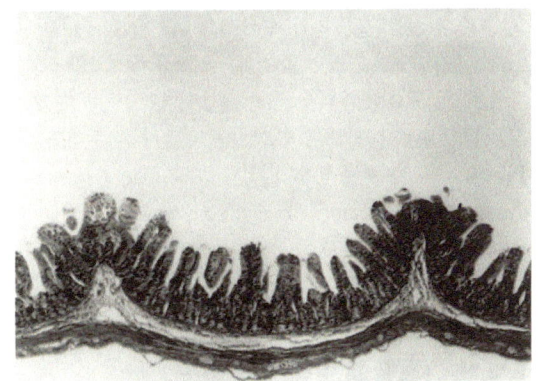

图 4.3 左图：8 日龄无菌猪回肠的正常组织形态。绒毛上覆盖着正常的成熟的具有空泡的吸收细胞。苏木精伊红（hematoxylin and eosin, HE）染色。右图：口服接种强毒性 HRV（Wa 株）的 8 日龄无菌猪的回肠。发现明显的严重绒毛萎缩和早期隐窝增生。HE 染色（Source: Courtesy of L.A. Ward, Ohio Agricultural Research and Development Center, Ohio State University, Wooster, OH）。

关于 RV 感染小鼠的病理学开展了很多研究，由于异源性病毒在鼠中的复制受限，所以很多利用异源性病毒开展的研究需要的病毒量要比鼠病毒株更大才能引起感染。然而，这些异源性毒株与小鼠 RV 感染引起的组织学改变相似。小鼠在出生两周内易患 RV 腹泻，且近期有一系列引人注目的关于新生小鼠感染鼠 RV 的明确的实验结果[113]，这些结果包括组织学改变（图 4.4）、RV 复制动力学（图 4.5）、肠绒毛缩短（图 4.6）、细胞凋亡诱导和细胞迁移动力学改变（图 4.7）。一些试验对人类小肠的病理改变进行了研究，结果发现与小牛和仔猪的相似[114,115]。

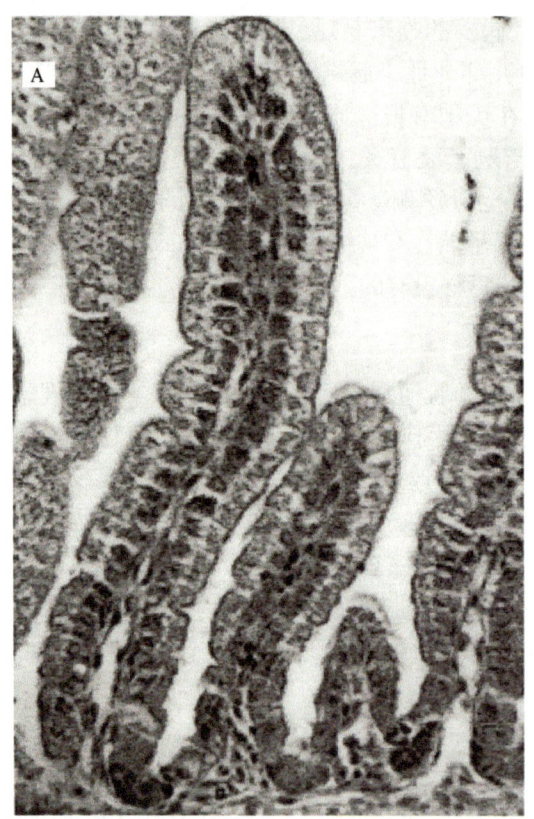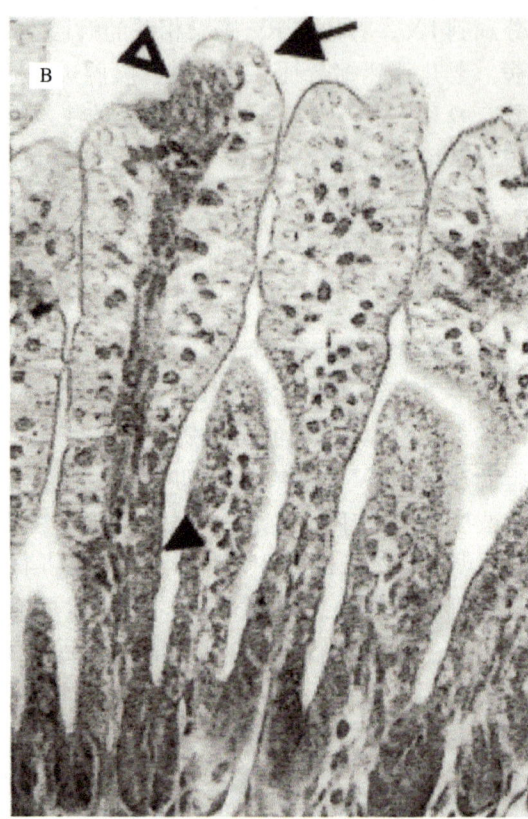

图 4.4 鼠 RV 感染 1 天后,小肠的组织病理损伤。A. 对照组动物,肠细胞两极化,其细胞核位于基底部。B. 感染小鼠,肠细胞有许多空泡,绒毛顶端肿胀(箭头),细胞基底部缩小,细胞核不规则地位于细胞内(实箭头)。在许多绒毛中,病变位于顶端(空心箭头)(Source: Boshuizen et al.[113], with permission of the American Society for Microbiology)。

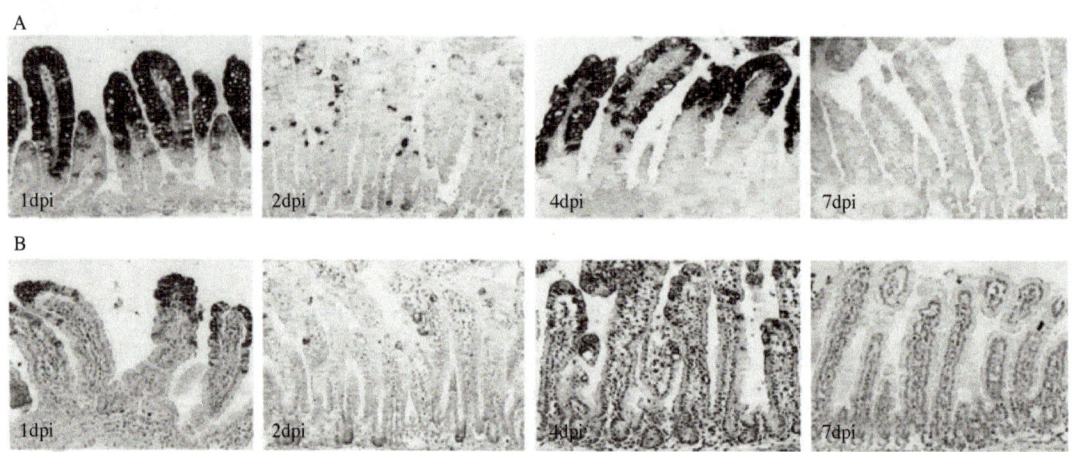

图 4.5 小鼠小肠中 RV 复制的动力学。在小鼠 RV 感染后的各天(dpi),分别用原位杂交和免疫组化测定空肠中 NSP4 信使核糖核酸(mRNA)(A)和蛋白质(B)表达的水平(Source: Boshuizen et al.[113], with permission of the American Society for Microbiology)。

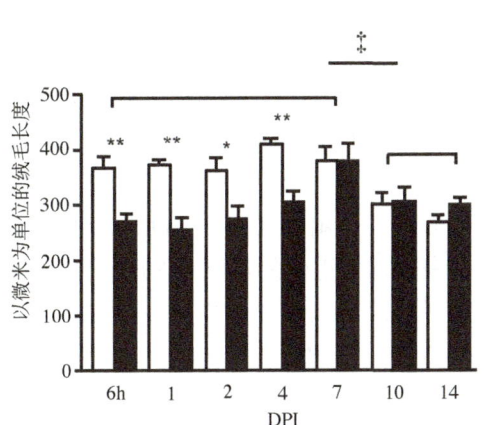

图 4.6 感染后各天（dpi）中，对照小鼠（白色）和鼠 RV 感染的小鼠（黑色）的空肠绒毛长度。数据表示 3~5 个动物的平均绒毛长度和平均值的标准差（SEM）（误差线）。*$P< 0.05$；**$P< 0.01$（t 检验）。对对照组在 6dpi 和 7dpi 同 10dpi 和 14dpi 的绒毛长度进行方差分析，随后进行了非配对 t 检验（‡ $P< 0.05$）(Source: Boshuizen et al.[113], with permission of the American Society for Microbiology)。

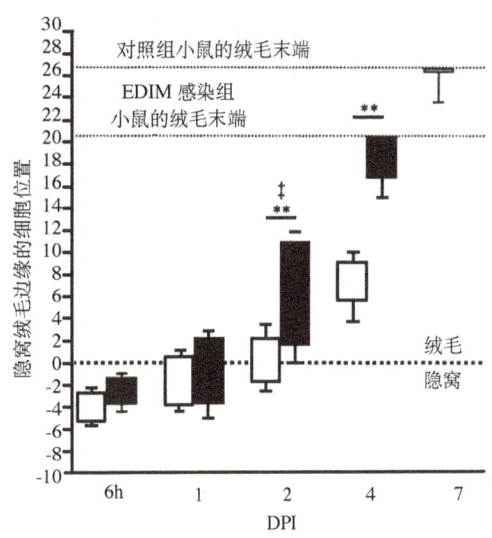

图 4.7 RV 感染后（dpi）小鼠小肠（回肠）的细胞迁移。最上面和最下面的标记细胞位置表示隐窝-绒毛边缘的细胞数量。对照组动物用白色表示，感染组动物用黑色表示。感染后 2~7 天，与对照组相比，感染组的标记细胞明显向绒毛上方迁移（**$P<0.01$）。在感染后第 2 天，细胞数量也有所增加（‡ $P<0.05$）。EDIM，幼鼠流行性腹泻病毒（Source: Boshuizen et al.[113], with permission of the American Society for Microbiology）。

腹泻的机制

虽然 RV 引起包括人在内的多种动物严重腹泻，但其致病机制尚未确定，可能是由多因素共同作用所致。在早期的幼猪体内研究表明，对照组和感染组体内的钠离子和氯离子流量无差别，但是葡萄糖介导的钠离子吸收却因病毒感染而减少[116]。根据此结果和其他的生理学改变，作者推断，非感染肠细胞分化迟缓，病毒感染之后细胞从隐窝处加速移行，导致吸收异常。另外，根据小猪的研究推论，绒毛膜上皮细胞的破坏导致碳水化合物吸收不良和渗透性腹泻[117]。据报道，小鼠不像小猪那样存在碳水化合物吸收不良，因此，隐窝细胞分泌可能导致液体丢失[118]。在人和动物的进一步研究显示有关 RV 感染后跨越肠表面的大分子吸收改变不是通常模式。一些分子的摄取增加，如辣根过氧化物酶和 2-鼠李糖；一些分子的摄取减少，如乳果糖和 D-木糖。因此，病毒感染导致的肠黏膜的吸收性和腹泻的关系仍不清楚。

在幼鼠和大鼠腹腔内接种 RV 的 NSP4 或者来源于这种蛋白质的 22-氨基酸肽，都会引起腹泻[119,120]。根据观察表明，外源性加入这种蛋白质或者多肽，可以导致昆虫细胞内 Ca^{2+} 浓度增加[121]。在随后的试验中证明，NSP4 蛋白及其多肽可以通过激活钙依赖性信号转导途径动员 Ca^{2+}[122] 从内质网流出以增加其浓度[121,123]。进一步研究显示，NSP4 能够破坏胞膜的稳定性[124, 125]，可能是由于细胞膜内 Ca^{2+} 浓度增加，导致细胞骨架解体和细胞死亡[98,126~128]。因此，NSP4 从感染细胞中释放出来之后，与肠上皮结合，改变离子转运引起腹泻。分泌的 NSP4 的另外一个可能的靶点是肠神经系统，它位于绒毛上皮下方。有报道称，RV 感染可以激活小鼠体内的这个系统，阻断神经活性的药物在体外减弱 RV 引起的液体分泌，在体内则可以减轻腹泻[129]。RV 感染后 NSP4 是否是引起腹泻的主要因素还有待确定。一些关于小鼠的更多研究支持 NSP4 作为引起腹泻的原因[130,131]，但另一些研究表明，无论在人体内还是小鼠体内，NSP4 的突变并不会引起 RV 的毒力减弱[132~134]，因此，它对于引起自然界中的腹泻的重要性仍是个疑问。

根据其引起腹泻的能力来定义 RV 致病性的分子基础，目前尚未确定。Offit 及其同事们[135]报道了异源性病毒产生的重配株的毒力，并在表达毒力更强的毒株的 VP4 蛋白的小鼠模型上对重组毒株的毒力做了测试。研究所用的病毒株（猴和牛的毒株）在小鼠体内均不高效复制，提示该观察也许限制了病毒的适应性。对鼠/猴 RV 重配株的一项最新研究显示 VP4 蛋白和毒力之间没有联系[136]，但研究中却发现毒力与基因产物之间关系最密切的是非结构蛋白 NSP1。毒力和具体基因节段的关系也在小猪中进行了检测。仅 VP4 基因变异的毒力突变株从一头受感染的猪的粪便中分离得到[137]。用有毒力的猪 RV 和减毒的 HRV 的重配株对小猪进行另一研究，发现了猪 RV 表达的 VP3、VP4、VP7 和 NSP4 全部与它对小猪的毒力有关[138]。这些观察是否有广泛适用性或仅针对根据蛋白质之间的特异相互作用 RV 限定的组合，尚未被确定。

轮状病毒流行病学

轮状病毒的年龄依赖易感性

虽然 RV 感染到以前未感染过 RV 的动物或人中没有严格的年龄限制，但 RV 腹泻在所有物种中都有严格的年龄限制。小鼠在出生两周内易感 RV 引起腹泻[139]。同样，小猪和小牛在出生后的前几天或数星期内最易感染 RV 引起腹泻[140,141]，甚至非人类灵长类动物在出生后的前几天也易感引起腹泻[50]。人在 6 个月和 24 个月年龄最容易发生严重的 RV 腹泻（图 4.8），但是轻微的病症可终生发生。人们已经着重调查出现年龄限制性的可能原因，特别在人身上。肠道内随着年龄的不同会发生非免疫性变化，包括与幼鼠相比，成年鼠体内的病毒特异性受体也减少，这可能就导致了随着年龄的增长腹泻的严重性降低[142]。人们对小牛也提出了相似的意见[143]。这也许部分地解释了为什么小孩子比大孩子和成人更易受感染。

新生儿与较大婴儿相比，他们的小肠分泌物中可以裂解 VP4 的蛋白酶浓度减少，这一因素有助于解释为何新生儿对于 RV 有较高的抵抗力[144]。然而，对婴儿在其生命之初的几个月内能够抵抗严重 RV 疾病的更好解释是其存在通过胎盘获得母传抗体。有报道称，

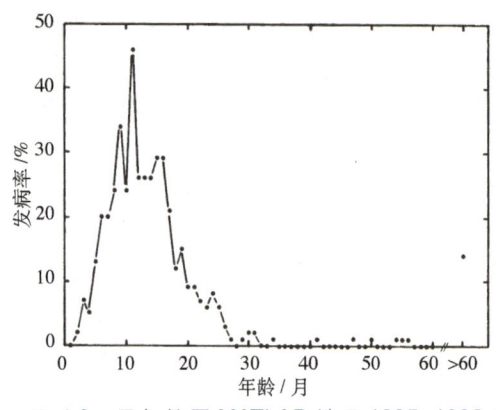

图 4.8 孟加拉国 MATLAB 地区 1985~1986 年的居民与年龄有关的 RV 发病率[190]

婴儿 RV 疾病初发时间与母传抗体滴度下降时间相同 [145]。此外，观察结果显示对 RV 活疫苗的反应与经胎盘传播的疫苗株中和抗体滴度之间存在极强相关性（R. L. Ward 等，未发表）。胎盘转移抗体保护肠感染的机制尚未明确。向人和动物的肠道中被动转移中和抗体都与保护作用有关，但是外周 RV 特异性 IgG 的保护作用很小，即使有的话，也是在动物中。也可能人母传 IgG 抗体在感染之前便被转移至肠道，从而中和病毒。

在大孩子和成人体内，疾病严重性减弱大概主要是因为先前的感染激活了免疫反应。在感染过 RV 的孩子和成人体内，对 RV 感染和疾病的保护与循环和肠道 RV 抗体滴度相关 [146~152]。这些抗体是否具有保护作用尚有待确定。

轮状病毒的跨种传播

RV 感染范围很宽，但是自然的物种间交叉感染比较罕见，特别是在动物和人之间。然而，在病毒组和序列分析中发现，很多人分离株似乎是动物毒株或动物 - 人 RV 重配株，这些毒株在疾病中的重要性也许是有限的。然而，有人提出这些毒株一旦适应了在人体内复制，可能会成为人的重要病原体 [34]。实验性动物研究显示 RV 在异种肠道中的复制通常是有限的，如果可检测到子代病毒排出，那么只能是向动物接种了高剂量的异种病毒。

宿主范围限制性的基因学基础未知，可能是由很多基因共同作用所致。给小鼠接种鼠和猴 RV 重配株，结果发现宿主限制性与编码 NSP1 的基因 5 有关 [136]。其他研究也报道了 RV 在培养的细胞 [153] 和小鼠 [154] 中共感染后，非随机地选择了基因 5，提示该基因可能与病毒生长有关。*NSP1* 基因在 11 个 RV 基因 [80] 中最易变并且不同种 RV 的基因序列差异很大 [46]，因而它可能起宿主限制作用。由于 NSP1 是病毒复制非必需的 [93]，它唯一的作用是干涉干扰素反应 [94]，它可能就是通过这个作用帮助保持种属特异性。然而，值得注意的是，在猪体内顿挫感染的牛 RV 的 NSP1 替换猪 RV 的 NSP1，新的重配株在小猪体内仍可有效复制 [155]。因此，NSP1 不是唯一的宿主限制因素。

轮状病毒流行株的季节性和起源

与其他呼吸道和肠道病毒相比，RV 具有明显的季节性。特别是在温带，RV 使冬季腹泻死亡率剧增。该季节性在热带不明显，但是仍然在干冷季节流行 [156]。引起季节性的原因是人们关注的焦点，但目前仍不清楚。由于 RV 疾病在少发季节会降低到几乎不可测的水平，所以该病毒每年大多数时间必须维持在不活跃状态。由于有物种间限制性，人类 RV 在两流行季之间不可能寄居在动物体内。因此，该病毒可能会继续在人体内低水平复制，直至出现适宜流行的条件。偶尔发生在淡季的 RV 疾病支持人体是一个病毒储蓄池的说法。也可能是病毒在终年持续暴露的环境中存活，但仅在流行季导致持续 RV 疾病。RV 在极高浓度下排出 [157]，室温下能够维持其感染性数月 [158,159]，并在环境表面易检出 [160]。因此，环境对人类 RV 来说可能是一个储蓄池，为季节性流行提供来源。

为了提供引起流行的 RV 株来源的有关线索，对循环中的病毒特征进行了广泛的研究，主要利用电泳分型和血清型。由此，RV 株在特定地点连续多个流行季既可以变化很小，也甚至可以在同一流行季就会有显著变化。此外，在流行季的任何时间，同一地区往往同时存在多种病毒株。由于 RV 共感染后普遍基因重配，在特定的地理区域内难以确定新毒株的来源。它们可能是来自外部，也可能是当地传染源，或者可能是循环株产生的基因重配株。显然，如果引起年度流行的病毒的来源可确定，就可以对 RV 流行病学有更多的了解。

轮状病毒的免疫

人们已经对预防 RV 感染的免疫效应器有了部分认识，特别是通过对动物模型的研究，但对其在人类中的机制仍然知之甚少。由于 RV 在肠上皮细胞复制，导致相关的胃肠道症状，人们普遍认为，效应器机制应该发生在肠黏膜。最明显的免疫器是分泌型免疫球蛋白 A（immunoglobin A，IgA）。小鼠感染了高剂量的异源 RV 后，其肠道固有层中大部分 IgA 分泌细胞都是 RV 特异性的[161]。此外，对口服免疫小鼠的预防 RV 感染作用与肠道（粪便）和血清 RV 特异性 IgA 滴度相关，但与血清特异性 IgG 无关[162,163]。在人类中，血清 RV 特异性 IgG 和 IgA 及肠道 IgA 滴度与自然感染后的保护作用相关。但是，自然感染或接种疫苗后任何同型的 RV 特异性抗体滴度不能始终与保护相关。因此，RV 抗体有可能仍然仅仅是一个指标，而不是保护的实际效应器。

抗体的最明显保护机制是中和病毒。人们已经在对人和动物的研究中发现中和抗体的消耗与被动保护相关。对于口服接种活 RV 或 RV 自然感染诱导的主动免疫是否是由中和抗体完成，研究结果各不相同[164~166]。例如，牛和猴 RV 最初的疫苗试验提示，在没有中和抗体的情况下，也会诱导对循环的 HRV 株的保护作用。然而，与它不一致的是，在随后的恒河猴 RV（RRV）试验中，产生的保护作用是血清型特异性的[167,168]。这些结果引领了含有 HRV 中和蛋白基因的牛和猴 RV 疫苗株的研制，它们已经或正在婴幼儿体内评估[11]。即使在这些试验中，血清中和抗体滴度与保护作用的关系也存在矛盾，而且保护大于人血清特异性中和抗体对循环 RV 株的反应[169]。

动物研究的大多数数据表明，经典的中和反应不是唯一的保护机制。最具免疫活性的蛋白是 VP6，它似乎并不刺激中和抗体反应。但有证据表明，VP6 特异性 IgA 具有保护性，但机制尚未完全明确[170,171]。接种因缺乏外衣壳蛋白而不诱导产生中和抗体的 VLP 或嵌合 VP6 蛋白均可以引起对成年小鼠的保护性免疫[172,173]。将以前感染（口服）过同源或异源 RV 株的小鼠的脾 CD8$^+$ T 细胞过继性移植给新生小鼠，可使其产生针对鼠 RV 疾病的被动保护作用[174]。同样，RV 感染的小鼠的脾 CD8$^+$ 细胞或上皮内淋巴细胞可以消除重症联合免疫缺陷病（severe combined immunodeficiency，SCID）小鼠的慢性 RV 排毒[175]。因此，细胞毒性 T 细胞至少在预防 RV 疾病和消除 RV 排毒的被动保护方面起作用。

一个成年小鼠 RV 感染模型在研究鼠针对 RV 的主动免疫中十分有用[176]。由于成年小鼠感染 RV，但不发病，这一模型将对感染的保护作为其终点。根据这一模型，经口施用的鼠轮状活病毒所产生的保护作用，与对应攻毒的血清或肠道中特异性中和抗体滴度不相关[166]。然而，它与总血清和粪便 RV 的 IgA 滴度[162,163,177]及在肠道黏膜表面高滴度的 RV 特异性 IgA 相关[178]。随后，对不能产生抗体的 B 细胞缺陷小鼠的研究结果表明，以前感染 RV 所产生的长期保护，至少部分取决于抗体[179,180]。即使在肠道外免疫，抗原提呈细胞从外周淋巴组织向肠道相关淋巴组织迁移，可能会促成黏膜 IgA 反应和保护作用[181]。虽然这种模型的保护作用典型地与 RV 的 IgA 相关，但是遗传修饰小鼠在活病毒免疫后也得到了保护作用，这可能与 RV 的 IgG 滴度升高有关[182]。研究还证明了整合素介导的小肠 B 细胞归巢对抗 RV 效果的重要性[183]。

RV 排毒消除和针对鼠 RV 继发感染的保护与 RV 特异性 CD8+ T 细胞相关。在 B 细胞缺陷的小鼠口服接种活的鼠 RV 之前去除 CD8+ T 细胞，使其缺失，会阻碍初次感染的消除[179,180]。因此，在抗体产生之前，细胞毒性 T 细胞对初期消除排毒是至关重要的。然而，完全免疫能力的小鼠体内，在有抗体的情况下，CD8+ 细胞的缺失只是延迟了排毒的消除时间。最近研究结果表明，嵌合 VP6 蛋白或 VP6 的 14 氨基酸肽加上一个有效的佐剂鼻腔内或口服接种小鼠，在攻毒后可以减少 95% 以上的排毒现象[173,184]。后来发现，引起这种保护作用唯一需要的淋巴细胞是 CD4+ T 细胞[185]。因此，B 细胞、CD8+ T 细胞和 CD4+ T 细胞都被认为是对小鼠排毒保护的效应器，它们各自的相对重要性取决于免疫原和免疫方法。在该成年小鼠模型中总结的免疫机制主要结果见表 4.2。

表 4.2 在成年鼠中得到确认的清除与保护的机制

小鼠品种	免 疫	结 果	参 考
BALB/c（常规的）	经口，少量活的同源 RV 和不同源 RV	保护与血清 RV 的 IgA 有关	163
BALB/c	经口，活 RRV，EDIM	保护与肠道 RV 的 IgA 有关	162, 178
J$_H$D（B 细胞有效的）	经口，活的鼠 RV	清除作用依赖于 CD8 T 细胞；保护主要依赖于抗体	179, 180
BALB/c	肌内，活的鼠 RV	肠外免疫后肠道 IgA 产生	181
BALB/c	经鼻，VLP 或 VP6 加佐剂	几乎对 RV 排毒完全保护	172, 173
IgA −/−	经口，活的鼠 RV	与保护有关的肠道 IgG	182
β7 −/−	免疫 B 细胞或 CD8+ T 细胞过继性移植进入慢性排毒的 Rag-2 缺陷小鼠	非 CD8+ T 细胞，而是 B 细胞需要 α4β7 归巢受体	183
J$_H$D	经鼻，VP6	保护只需要淋巴细胞中的 CD4 T 细胞	185

EDIM：幼鼠流行性腹泻病毒；IgA：免疫球蛋白 A；RRV：恒河猴 RV

轮状病毒的控制和预防

非特异性的支持疗法，如口服或静脉补液是治疗 RV 疾病的唯一方法，因此，人们正在研制疫苗以防止这些疾病。人们认为，通过诱导局部肠道免疫反应可以获得最好的保护，而且发现 RV 自然感染至少可对继发 RV 疾病产生部分保护，基于这两点，最初研发疫苗的方向是口服减毒活疫苗[11]。大多数致力于使用动物 RV 株，它们对人类来说是自然减毒株，而且能够激活异源免疫反应 [如 RIT4237（牛）、WC3（牛）和 RRV（猴）]。最近将人类 RV 基因已引入这些动物毒株产生重配病毒,以提高其与人类 RV 血清型的关联度[如 Rotashield 和 RotaTeq^{TM}（Merck，West Point，PA）]。Rotashield 是以猴 RRV 为亲本的四价重配疫苗，是在美国唯一获批的 RV 疫苗，但在 1999 年由于引起少数肠套叠而退出市场[107]。RotaTeq 疫苗是以牛 WC3 株为背景的五价重配苗，该候选疫苗最近在超过 3.5 万婴儿的Ⅲ期临床中进行了安全性评价，正在美国提出市场准入申请（P. Heaton，个人通信，2004）。

人类 RV 也已经被研发成候选疫苗，大多数是自然减毒的新生儿病毒株。然而，获得最广泛评价的 HRV 候选疫苗是 89-12 株，为 G1[P8] 型，是从有症状的儿童的粪便中分离的，并通过多次细胞培养传代使其减毒[186]。该毒株已经被葛兰素史克公司（Rixensart, Belgium）减毒，以形成新的候选疫苗，称为 Rotarix™。最近在多个国家超过 35 000 名婴儿中对其进行了 III 期临床评价（B. DeVos，个人通信，2004），并于 2004 年 7 月在墨西哥获批。这些候选疫苗的研发摘要见表 4.3。

表 4.3 Rotashield™、RotaTeq™ 和 Rotarix™ 三种候选疫苗研发中的部分重要研究

疫苗	国家	受试者人数	受试剂量	保护率[a]（全部/重症）
RIT 4237	芬兰	178	1	50/58
	芬兰	328	2	58/82
	卢旺达	145	3	0/0
	冈比亚	245	3	0/37
	秘鲁	391	3	40/75
WC3	美国（宾夕法尼亚州费城）	104	1	43/89
	美国（俄亥俄州辛辛那提）	206	1	17/41
	中非共和国	472	2	0/36
RRV	美国（纽约罗彻斯特）	176	1	0/0
	委内瑞拉	247	1	68/100
	芬兰	200	1	38/67
	委内瑞拉	320	1	64/90
	美国（纽约罗彻斯特）	223	1	66/N.D.[b]
	美国（印第安保留区）	321	1	0/N.D.
RRV 重配体				
RRV G1	芬兰	359	1	67/N.D.
RRV G2				66/N.D.
RRV G1	美国（纽约罗彻斯特）	223	1	77/N.D.
RRV G1	美国	898	3	69/73
RRV TV				
RRV G1	美国	1187	3	54/69
RRV TV				
RRV TV	芬兰	2273	3	66/91
RRV TV	委内瑞拉	2207	3	48/88
WC3 重配体				
WC3 G1	美国（纽约罗彻斯特）	325	3	64/87
WC3 TV	美国	417	3	73/73
89–12	美国	215	2	89/100

a. 免疫后第一年测得；b. N.D.：未测定

亚单位和 DNA 疫苗、各种表达载体、合成肽，以及由杆状病毒表达的 RV 衣壳蛋白产生的 VLP 也被视为替代候选疫苗。该 VLP 不可复制，具有安全性和高度免疫原性，能

诱导免疫保护[172,187~189]。鼻内或口服接种嵌合蛋白 VP6 联合黏膜佐剂也被证明在成年小鼠模型中对 RV 排毒具有保护作用[173]。

人们发现连续出现 RV 疾病，甚至是由同一血清型的 RV 引起的，并不罕见，因此很难想象任何一种口服的活疫苗能够自身激发针对所有 RV 疾病的全面而持久的保护。因此，目前候选疫苗的理性目标是要在儿童最脆弱的时期，即 6~24 个月时，消除严重的 RV 疾病。为做到这一点，该疫苗接种必须在早期，而此时母传成分如经胎盘抗体和可能的先天抗阻因子可能会限制对它的免疫反应，同时免疫系统还不成熟。为了克服可能的年龄依赖性抑制因素并促进更持久的免疫反应，人们考虑采用肠道外接种的疫苗。动物研究表明，该免疫途径可单独或配合口服免疫提供良好的保护作用。人们正在调研采用新型低创手段肠道外接种疫苗，它可能会提高这一接种途径的可行性，并有助于克服更多的儿童肠道外接种疫苗的阻力。目前的重要目标仍然是确认疫苗的保护作用。如果这一目标可以在儿童中实现，将大大简化今后新 RV 疫苗的评价工作。

杯状病毒

杯状病毒科包括一组形态学相似，但遗传性和抗原性多样化的病毒，可分为 4 个属[191]。诺如病毒（norovirus，NV）属和札如病毒（sapovirus，SV）属，根据诺瓦克病毒和札幌病毒原型的名称，先前分别被称为"诺瓦克样病毒"和"札幌样病毒"，主要引起人类急性胃肠炎，因此现在被称为人类杯状病毒（human caliciviruses，HuCV）。其他两个属——囊泡病毒和兔病毒属，没有发现在人类引起疾病，但可以引起很多动物疾病，包括呼吸道感染、流产、出血性疾病和肠胃炎。形态学上，SV 有典型的杯状病毒形态——由与许多动物杯状病毒相似的刚性表面结构组成，而 NV 是非典型杯状病毒形态——由病毒粒子的光滑表面结构组成。因其物理学特征，NV 以前被称为"小圆结构病毒"（small round structured virus，SRSV）。从遗传性角度，NV 和 SV 的亲缘关系较远，SV 与动物 CV 的基因同源性比与 NV 的更近，而且具有与兔出血症病毒相似的基因结构[192]。

HuCV 通过粪口途径传播，可造成急性胃肠炎，通常 2~3 天自愈。这些病毒可能只在胃肠道复制。因为 HuCV 感染通常不会引起强烈的免疫反应，所以感染个体可再次感染同一毒株，这使得 CV 肠胃炎成为最常见的人类疾病之一。NV 和 SV 广泛的遗传多样性是引起疾病频发的另一个原因，因为感染了某一毒株的个体仍然会对其他有抗原性差异的毒株易感。NV 有一个特别重要的意义就是引起传染性急性肠胃炎，因为这些病毒很容易通过污染的水和食物传播，其结果往往引起大暴发。这种疫情可能发生在全封闭或半封闭单位内，如学校、托儿所、餐馆、医院、养老院、游船和军事设施。由于这些暴发通常具有较高的发病率，影响所有年龄组，并能引起公众恐慌，NV 已在国立卫生研究院（National Institutes of Health，NIH）/疾病预防控制中心（Centers for Disease Control and Prevention，CDC）被列为 B 类传染病。SV 偶尔也会引起成年人暴发急性胃肠炎，但主要感染儿童。由于 SV 的诊断方法有限，其分布和重要性仍有待详细说明。本章也涵盖了 SV 已有的发现，但重点还是集中在 NV。

杯状病毒的简要历史

半个世纪前，人们已开始了对 NV 的研究，当时研究者对志愿者进行调查以期发现急性胃肠炎可能的病毒病因学。这些研究表明，口服急性胃肠炎患者粪便的滤过液可将疾病传染给健康的志愿者，这表明致病因子是可滤过性病毒。在 20 世纪 70 年代初期，Kapikian 等用免疫电镜（IEM）[9]，在 1968 年俄亥俄州诺瓦克某小学暴发的急性胃肠炎患者粪便标本中第一次观察到病原体——诺瓦克病毒[193]。这一发现开始将病原体与腹泻病联系起来。发现诺瓦克病毒不久后，人们又发现了很多有相似形态且与急性胃肠炎有关的诺瓦克样病毒，其中包括夏威夷病毒、陶顿病毒、蒙哥马利病毒和雪山病毒等株[194~197]。在同一时期，人们还发现了札如病毒，是被人们发现的具有典型 CV 形态且引起幼儿急性胃肠炎的第一个 HuCV[198]。在发现了诺瓦克病毒之后，HuCV 的研究进入了第一阶段，即研究临床表现、免疫学和流行病学等基本特征的阶段。但是，HuCV 不能在细胞中培养且缺乏动物模型，不久就制约了研究的快速发展。

随后，在 20 世纪 90 年代，对诺瓦克病毒原型株[199]及随后的其他许多诺瓦克样病毒的克隆和序列分析开创了 HuCV 的分子病毒学研究领域的一个新的篇章。许多 HuCV 的基因测序[199,200]使 NV 在基因学上归类于杯状病毒科。序列信息还促进了逆转录聚合酶链反应（reverse-transcriptase polymerase chain reaction，RT-PCR）技术用于 HuCV 诊断的发展[201,202]。很多实验室用这些新方法对不同人群和国家的急性胃肠炎进行监测，积累了大量关于 HuCV 遗传变异、流行率和分布的资料。先进的分子技术还使研究病毒基因组 RNA、功能性蛋白与病毒基因组复制成为可能。用杆状病毒[203]和其他表达系统[204,205]成功表达 NV 衣壳蛋白进而自发形成 VLP[203]为研究病毒和宿主的相互作用提供了有价值的手段，包括免疫反应[206,207]和病毒受体识别[208,209]。这些重组 VLP 也为 NV 的诊断[210~216]、疫苗研发[205,217~219]和原子结构测定[220,221]提供了有价值的材料。

杯状病毒颗粒的性质

在电子显微镜下，NV 和 SV 都是小的（直径约 38nm）、圆形的病毒（图 4.9）。最初描述的诺瓦克病毒粒子的直径为 27nm。继杆状病毒表达诺瓦克病毒衣壳蛋白后，用冷冻 EM 和原子结构分析更准确地测量 VLP 的平均直径为 38nm[222]。NV 和 SV 病毒的外观截然不同。SV 具有典型 CV 形态，即与很多动物 CV 相似的"大卫之星"外观。NV 表面是光滑的，通常不会显示"大卫之星"外观。

人们通过冷冻电子显微镜法（图 4.9）和结晶学研究杆状病毒表达[220~222]原型株诺瓦克病毒重组衣壳蛋白，很大程度上阐明了 NV 衣壳的结构。杆状病毒表达的诺瓦克病毒衣壳蛋白能够自动组装成形态和抗原性类似于真实病毒颗粒的 VLP。诺瓦克病毒的衣壳由 180 个主要衣壳蛋白分子组成，该主要衣壳蛋白被称为病毒蛋白 1（VP1），由开放阅读框（open reading frame，ORF）2 编码。最近的报告表明，ORF3 编码的蛋白质（VP2）也存在于病毒粒子中，可能与病毒基因组相关。通过冷冻电镜和计算机图像处理分析重组诺瓦克 VLP，呈现出一个清晰的 T a=3 的二十面体对称结构。病毒衣壳由 90 个衣壳蛋白二聚体组成，该衣壳蛋白含有一个外壳（S）区和一个拱状突起（P）区。这些拱状结构排列在二十面体上的五重体和三重体的位置，并形成大的空洞。

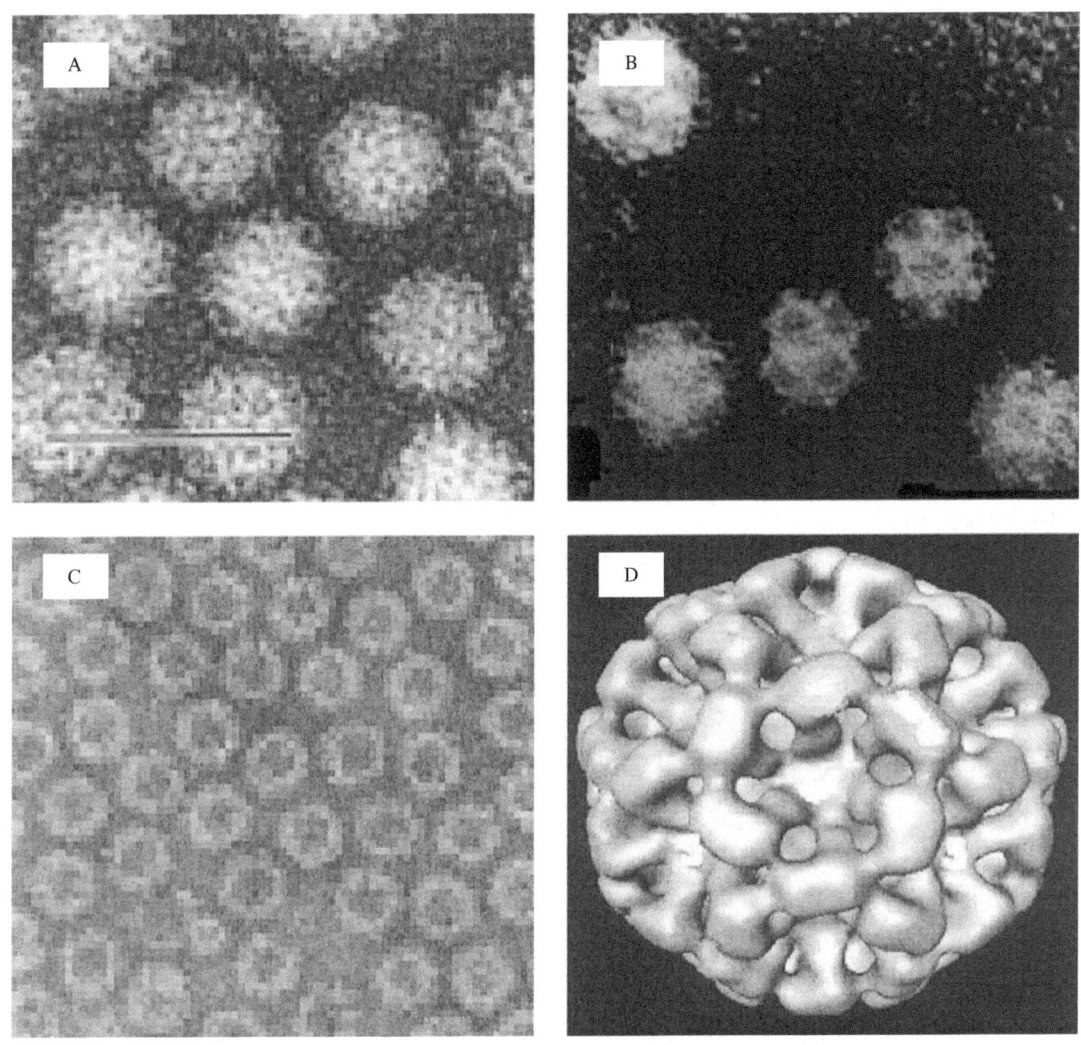

图 4.9 电子显微镜成像：诺瓦克病毒（A）、札如病毒（B）、杆状病毒表达的诺瓦克病毒重组 VLP（C），以及从冷冻电子显微镜得到的计算机生成的 VLP 三维结构（D）。标尺 =50nm（Source: Part D from Prasad et al.[308]. Reprinted with permission from Springer Science+Business Media）。

　　人们通过冷冻电镜证实重组诺瓦克 VLP 的原子结构解析[220,222]。N 端的 225 个残基构成 S 区并折叠成一个典型的 8 股反平行 β- 三明治结构。S 区负责组建二十面体外壳。S 区的表达导致了小于完整衣壳颗粒的光滑粒子的形成。其余的蛋白质构成 P 区，通过短的柔性铰链与 S 区连接，形成拱状突起。P 区由两个亚单位组成：P1 和 P2 亚单位。P2 位于衣壳表面，在不同的 NV 中其序列变异比 P1 的大，最近已被证明是病原体和宿主的相互作用的关键因素。对定点突变之后的序列同源性进行分析表明，位于 P2 的袋状结构与受体结合有关[223,224]。

杯状病毒的分类

遗传学分类

在诺瓦克病毒基因组分子克隆之前，人们根据病毒衣壳的形态和结构将其归类于 CV。人们从被感染的志愿者的粪便样本中分离出病毒蛋白，对其进行生化研究发现单个 60kDa 的病毒相关蛋白。这一特征与来自动物 CV 原型株的数据相符，动物 CV 原型株也有一个分子质量为 60~70kDa 的结构蛋白[225]。支持 NV 是 CV 的更直接的证据来自于对首个诺瓦克病毒互补 DNA（complementary DNA，cDNA）的分析，其序列与猫 CV 相似[199]。随后对诺瓦克全长基因组的描述[200]，以及获得的许多 NV 的部分和全长基因组序列证实了这些病毒都属于杯状病毒科。与动物 CV 相似，NV 含有一条约 7.7kb 的含多聚腺苷酸尾的正义、单链 RNA 基因组。诺瓦克病毒的病毒基因组包含三个主要 ORF。ORF1 编码一个可被裂解成多个非结构蛋白的多聚蛋白，ORF2 编码衣壳蛋白，ORF3 编码一个小结构蛋白[200]。

人们积累了 NV 的序列数据之后，也克隆了原型株札如病毒[226]和许多札如样病毒，如曼彻斯特、休斯敦 90、休斯敦 86、帕克维尔和伦敦 92 病毒。序列分析表明，SV 也含有一个典型的 CV 基因组，但在种族发生方面它与动物 CV 的关系比与 NV 的更密切。SV 基因组只包含两个主要的 ORF[192]。第一个 ORF 既编码非结构蛋白也编码衣壳蛋白，其衣壳蛋白与非结构多聚蛋白的 C 端融合。将 HuCV 归类于 CV 科的支持依据是在基因学上很多动物 CV 与 HuCV 的密切相关，并且 HuCV 可引起家畜腹泻[227~230]。目前尚缺乏说明 CV 胃肠炎是一种人畜共患病的证据。

即使病毒国际分类委员会（International Taxonomy Committee for Viruses，ITCV）在 2000 年出版了分类准则[191]，但 HuCV 的基因分类和命名法仍有矛盾。虽然建立一个新的基因簇或基因组需要完整的衣壳基因序列，但大多数序列数据却来源于 RNA 聚合酶区。Katayama 等[231]表明，衣壳的 N 端壳（S）结构域足以进行正确的基因分型，但最近 NV 受体和衣壳上的"连接袋"的发现表明，突出（P）结构域也应加以考虑[224]。Ando 等首次提出对 NV 的基因簇或基因型编号[232]，随后 Schuffenecker 等也为 SV 提出相似建议[233]。然而，还有一些人喜欢用病毒原型株的名称聚类代表病毒。目前这两种系统都被使用，不一致性依然存在，如不同的号码或"原型株"被应用到同一簇，即便是专家也很难分清。随着不断发现新的独特毒株和自然产生的重配株，目前亟须一种一致和公认的命名法。

抗原性分类

NV 和 SV 属均包含多个成员。在 1990 年诺瓦克病毒克隆之前，个别病毒的名字用最初它们的发现地的名字来命名，如前所述。对病毒 RNA 的生物进化分析表明两个属都存在广泛的遗传变异。根据序列的一致程度，可将目前已有的 NV 和 SV 分为不同的基因组和基因簇。虽然 Alphatron 和类似株往往被视为基因组 IV，而最近发现的小鼠 NV 被视为第 5 基因组[234]，NV 属至少包含 3 个基因组 20 个基因簇（图 4.10）[232]。人们曾认为 SV 属的变异性比 NV 的小，但最近的数据显示，它至少包含 5 个基因组 9 个基因簇（图 4.10）。

因为 HuCV 具有抗原性多样性，现有的方法并不能检测出所有类型，不同 HuCV 之间的抗原关系仍有待充分说明。NV 克隆提供了更广泛的检测方法，但在此之前，人们根据对志愿者的交叉竞争研究在几个原型株病毒中鉴别出很多血清型[197]。重组酶免疫测定

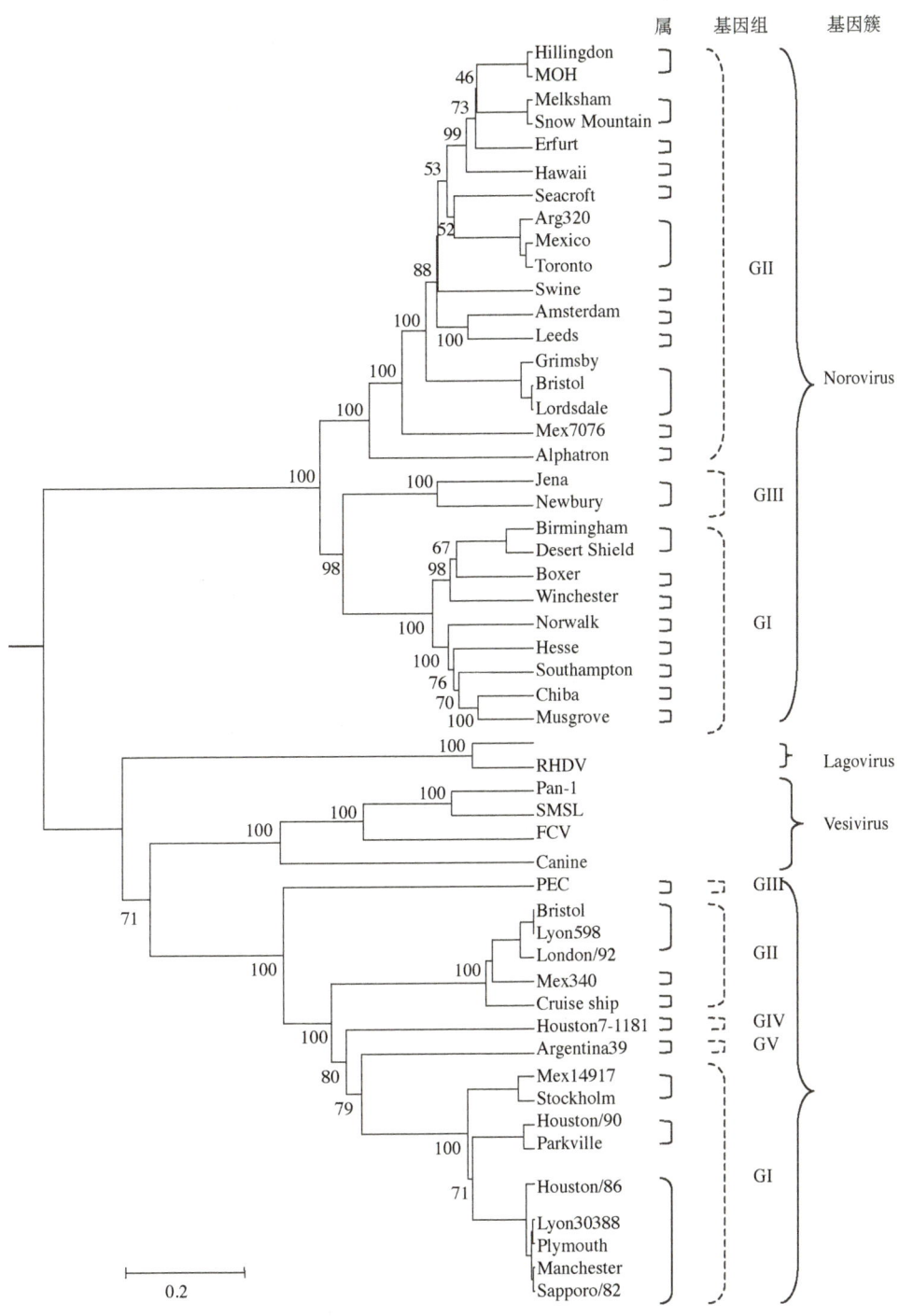

图 4.10　基于完整衣壳序列的杯状病毒科的系统树。该树通过 UPGMA 聚类分析法建立（MEGA v2.1）。125% 复制率表示显示数值。

法（enzyme immunoassay，EIA）发展后，人们研究了若干 HuCV 株的抗原关系[235]。一般情况下，抗原类型与基因类型相关[236,237]。这些结果仍是初步的，因为还需要额外的重组衣壳蛋白和高滴度抗体。此外，用于抗原分型的方法是基于抗原识别，而不是中和反应，未来还需要通过细胞培养体系或者动物模型测定其中和类型。最后，根据人类的组织血型（后面详述），发现人 NV 宿主感染特异性范围很宽。

杯状病毒的复制

杯状病毒的体外培养

尽管很多研究者做出了努力，但 HuCV 仍然很难在细胞培养中生长。一个早期的假设是，限制病毒在体外复制的因素可能是培养细胞上缺乏适当的受体以便病毒附着和进入，这一假设受到了近期研究数据的挑战。White 等以重组 VLP 为探针，研究宿主与病原体的相互作用，表明诺瓦克 VLP 可与不同来源的 13 个细胞系特异性结合[238]。分化的 Caco2 细胞属人结肠癌细胞系，明显比其他细胞系结合更多的 VLP，而且约 7%VLP 进入细胞。后来 Marionneau 等表明，这种结合是 Caco2 和胃十二指肠上皮细胞表面上的 H 型 1 和（或）H 型 3/4 组织 - 血型抗原（histo-blood group antigen，HBGA）介导的[209]。然而，Caco2 细胞即使是在分化后，也不能支持 NV 复制，表示在附着和穿入后，存在阻碍病毒复制的步骤。

最近 Duizer 等的一份报告总结了两个实验室尝试用细胞培养 NV 的结果[239]。虽然结果是阴性，但值得一提的是，他们使用了各种不同的方法。这些研究是基于一个假设，即在体外 NV 能否成功地复制取决于能否在细胞培养系统模拟肠上皮细胞分化的真实过程和最匹配的肠腔微环境。这些研究采用 20 多种人类和灵长类动物细胞系并评价不同的培养条件，包括向培养基中补充其他物质、不同的粪便样本处理制备方法、不同的细胞单层维持条件、不同的细胞接种方法和不同的病毒株。进行系列盲传，通过免疫法和 RT-PCR 法监测每一代的致细胞病变效应（cytopathic effect，CPE）和新合成的病毒产物。虽然在一定阶段会检测到阳性信号，但未发生可重复的 NV 诱导的 CPE，而且所有 RT-PCR 阳性产物继续培养后转阴。

最近报道了一个有希望的系统，用来分析 NV 在哺乳动物细胞中的复制，它是将表达诺瓦克病毒 RNA 的自然形态进行分析，该 RNA 没有来自于表达载体的外源核苷酸序列（Asanaka 等，第二届国际杯状病毒会议，法国第戎市，2004 年）。当病毒亚基因组 RNA 得到表达，就形成空病毒颗粒（VP1 和 VP2 基因）。当全长病毒基因组 RNA 得到表达，就可以检测到非结构蛋白衣壳蛋白（VP1）和亚基因组 RNA。这些结果表明基因组 RNA 能够复制，而且亚基因组 RNA 由基因组 RNA 表达并被翻译成 VP1。基因组和亚基因组 RNA 在系统中的联合表达能够产生含有基因组 RNA 的病毒颗粒，该病毒颗粒在氯化铯梯度中的密度类似于从粪便中分离纯化的真正病毒的密度。

猪 CV（PEC）的适应和培养是在体外培养肠道 CV 唯一的例子[240]。PEC/Cowden 在遗传学上属于 SV 属并会引起家猪的肠胃炎。该病毒最初适应在猪原代肾细胞中生长，然后在培养基中添加了来自于非感染的无菌猪的肠道内容物（intestinal content，IC）的条件下，它适应在传代肾细胞系（LLC-PK）中生长。PEC 在 LLC-PK 细胞中多次传代后，会引起其适应和减毒，因为它不再引起无菌猪腹泻[241,242]。对野生型和适应组织培养的 PEC/Cowden 进行序列比较，发现 RNA 聚合酶中有 2 个氨基酸改变，而且衣壳蛋白中有 1 个远端氨基酸和 3 个氨基酸簇发生变化。成簇突变发生在高变区，并导致局部更强的亲水性。PEC 的高变区对应于诺瓦克病毒衣壳蛋白的突起（P）区，该区被认为是负责抗原识别和受体结合的区域。因此，衣壳高变区的这些氨基酸突变可能与适应细胞培养和减毒相关。即使适应了在组织中培养，PEC/Cowden 的繁殖仍然需要在培养基中补充 IC。猪的不同肠道酶，如胰蛋白酶、胰酶、碱性磷酸酶、肠激酶、弹性蛋白酶和脂肪酶均不支持 PEC 复制。Chang 等的近期研究[243]表明，胆汁酸是 PEC 在组织培养中复制所必需的 IC 促进因子。人们提出 PEC 复制可能需要涉及蛋白激酶 A 细胞信号转导途径和固有免疫下调的机制。人们希望，类似的适应机制也可适用于 NV。

最近人们已经报道了鼠诺如病毒 1 型（MNV-1）能够适应在树突状细胞（dendritic cell，DC）和巨噬细胞中组织培养[244]。MNV-1 增长由干扰素 αβ 受体和 STAT-1（信号转导因子和转录激活因子）抑制，还与细胞内膜广泛重排有关。系列传代和蚀斑纯化会导致毒株的毒力减弱。虽然 MNV-1 不是一个典型的肠杯状病毒并且最初被发现于免疫缺陷小鼠，但这些发现有助于研究 HuCV 的繁殖策略。

杯状病毒的体内复制和发病机理

人们在对急性胃肠炎暴发和志愿者的研究中最早描述了 NV 相关疾病的临床表现[197,245-247]。NV 胃肠炎的潜伏期是 12~24h，疾病通常是轻微的、自限性的，症状持续 24~48h。主要临床症状包括突发性呕吐、腹泻、腹部绞痛、恶心、疲倦，有时发热。腹泻的粪便往往呈水状，没有黏液、血液或白细胞。在儿童中发生呕吐多于腹泻，而在成人中发生腹泻更为频繁。目前尚不明确该疾病是否具有种属特异性。该病毒可在粪便中排毒数天。最近用更敏感的分子诊断研究分析表明，大量的志愿者是隐性感染者，他们的排毒期（7~21 天）比以前认为的更长。这些发现对疾病暴发控制和预防非常重要，尤其当疾病暴发是通过食物从业者传播时。

荷兰和芬兰的纵向研究表明，NV 和 SV 肠胃炎临床特点相似。与学龄儿童相比，SV 更易感染婴儿和学步期儿童，而 NV 可在各年龄段儿童体内检测到[248]。它们的主要症状相似，但 NV 肠胃炎中呕吐更加常见[249,250]。

通过用诺瓦克病毒和其他 NV 对志愿者进行攻毒的研究，人们描述了 NV 相关疾病的病理，认为 NV 在近端小肠复制。可以通过对感染的志愿者进行空肠活检观察到组织病变。表现为小肠绒毛扩大和钝化，隐窝细胞增生，细胞质空泡化，固有层中性细胞和单核细胞浸润，但黏膜本身保持完整。这种病变也伴随着小肠刷状缘的酶活性下降和轻微营养成分吸收减少。盐酸、胃蛋白酶的分泌和内在因素与这些病变相关，并出现胃排空延迟。人们认为 NV 胃肠炎的恶心和呕吐是由于胃动力降低所致。

无菌猪是 CV 相关胃肠炎的一个有效动物模型，猪肠道 CV 能够诱导无菌猪产生腹泻[241,242,251]。虽然动物感染野生型 PEC/Cowden 后的整体组织病理学和病理生理学表现与感染 HuCV 后所观察到的类似[241,242,251]，但该模型还提供了更多的信息——病毒复制位点和 PEC 感染的病毒血症阶段。通过对十二指肠和空肠的黏膜压印涂片进行免疫荧光染色可检测到 PEC 感染的肠细胞。这一结果与以下病理改变一致：PEC 主要感染近端小肠的绒毛上皮细胞并诱发感染的无菌猪的十二指肠和空肠病变。人们检测结肠和肠外组织或器官，没有发现明显的病毒复制迹象。因此，小肠的上端是 PEC 复制的主要位点。

有趣的是，除了完整的病毒颗粒，人们在 NV 患者的粪便标本中还发现一种截短的衣壳蛋白。这种蛋白质浓度一定很高，因为它很容易通过蛋白质印迹（Western blot，WB）检测到。人们已经绘制了这种截短蛋白质的完整结构，它含有衣壳蛋白的整个 P 区[252]。在铰链区与 P 区的连接处有一个胰蛋白酶裂解位点，负责在体内外产生 P 蛋白[252]。人们在昆虫细胞培养表达的诺瓦克病毒衣壳蛋白中也发现了类似的截短蛋白，但由上游的糜蛋白酶消化位点负责切割[203]。由于 P 区位于衣壳表面并含有最高遗传变异区，人们认为 P 区在病毒复制和抗原性上发挥了重要作用。最近的数据表明，实际上 P 区负责识别 HBGA，至少对病毒附着和穿入非常重要[223,224]。然而，这些功能并不能解释为什么在粪便中只发现了 P 蛋白而没有 S 区。是否该截短蛋白还存在其他的功能，如在病毒复制和发病机理方面，尚不清楚。

诺如病毒宿主范围

19 世纪 70 年代初，人们在 NV 暴发的感染和免疫及对志愿者的研究中观察到一些独特的现象，随后提出假设：一种遗传因素与 NV 的宿主特异性有关。与没有抗体的志愿者相比，具有高水平的诺瓦克病毒抗体的志愿者更易感染。甚至有些没有抗体检出的个体，在受到诺瓦克病毒攻击后从不感染。一些研究表明，个体对诺瓦克病毒有短期免疫（6~14 周）[197]，但可以在 27~42 个月后被 NV 再次感染[246]。最后，大暴发时 NV 感染往往具有家庭聚集性。这些现象提示，除了宿主的获得性免疫，某种遗传因素在对 NV 易感或抵抗感染时，同样发挥作用。

人们报道了兔出血病病毒（rabbit hemorrhage disease virus，RHDV），它是一种动物 CV，与 ABH- 组织血型组家族的抗原结合，随后通过对原型株诺瓦克病毒的研究，首次提出人 HBGA 与 NV 感染的联系[253]。第一份研究表明，诺瓦克病毒能够识别肠道组织和唾液分泌器官（表达 H 抗原）中的人 HBGA，而不能识别非分泌器官的人 HBGA[209]。利用含有人 HBGA 表位的寡糖轭合物和这些寡糖表位特异性的单克隆抗体，人们发现通过 1，2- 岩藻糖 - 转移酶（1,2-fucosyl-transferase，FUT-2）加在人 HBGA 上的岩藻糖残基负责两者的结合。泌乳女性的乳汁可封闭这种结合特异性，以及诺瓦克 VLP 能结合岩藻糖－转移酶基因转染的中国仓鼠卵巢（Chinese hamster ovary，CHO）细胞，进一步证实了这种结合的特异性。用寡糖作为 HBGA 特异性试剂进行血凝试验，Hutson 等[254]也发现重组诺瓦克 VLP 和人 HBGA 之间存在特异性相互作用。

人们在临床研究中也提出了 NV 感染与 HBGA 的联系。在对受诺瓦克病毒攻击的志愿者的回顾性研究中，O 型个体受感染的风险明显高于其他血型，而 B 型个体受感染的风险最低[255]。在可能由 NV 造成的疾病暴发事件中也观察到了同样的现象[256]。随后 Lindesmith 等在对志愿者的研究中获得了支持"诺瓦克病毒识别的 H 抗原（分泌基因的产物）作为感染的受体"这一说法的直接证据[257]。在受诺瓦克病毒攻击的 77 名志愿者中，根据唾液样本的血型，22 人是 H 抗原非分泌者，其余 55 名是 H 抗原分泌者。22 名 H 抗原非分泌者中，在受到诺瓦克病毒攻击后均没有感染，并且他们的唾液不与诺瓦克 VLP

结合。此外，唾液为 B 型的个体不与诺瓦克 VLP 结合或结合很弱，而且他们受到诺瓦克病毒攻击后感染的风险很低。在 55 名 H 抗原分泌者中，根据临床症状和在粪便中检测到的病毒或抗体反应判断，34 位（62%）受感染。唾液样本中测得 sIgA 动力学在感染个体和非感染个体之间有差异，这表明获得性免疫在 NV 感染中也发挥了作用。

初步描述了诺瓦克病毒的结合模式之后，很多不同的实验室已经将研究扩展到其他 NV。通过使用相同的唾液结合实验方法和一种重组 NV 衣壳抗原结果，Huang 等[208]表明，不同 NV 识别不同的 HBGA，基于唾液捐助者的 ABO 血型、分泌型及 Lewis 血型，至少存在 4 种 NV 的受体结合模式（图 4.11）。原型株诺瓦克病毒代表了 4 种结合模式之一，它

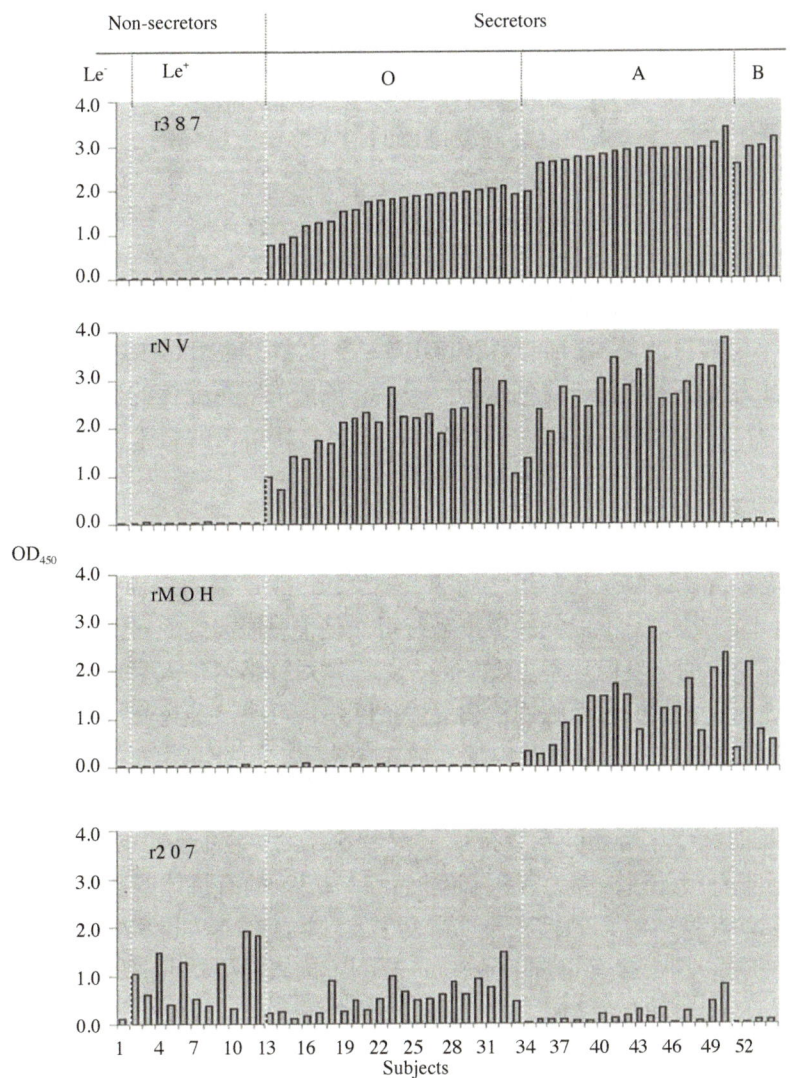

图 4.11　重组诺如病毒（NV）衣壳抗原与来自 51 名欧洲志愿者和 3 名非欧洲血统（B 型）志愿者的唾液样本的结合。唾液样本被稀释至 1∶5000 后进行了测定。个体的组织血组型显示在顶部，志愿者编号在底部。54 名受试者根据他们的组织血型分组，且根据最低到最高的光密度值（OD 值）将每组中与 VA387 株结合的唾液量分类。

识别 A 型和 O 型，而非 B 型分泌者。其他三种结合模式分别是结合 A 型、B 型和 O 型分泌者（VA387），A 型和 B 型分泌者（MOH）及 Lewis 分泌者和非分泌者（VA207）。根据人 HBGA 的生物合成途径，人们已经推导出了每个结合模式的结合靶点。因此，这项研究首次提出了存在 NV 的宿主范围变异的可能性。由于三个人类 HBGA 家族中几乎所有已知的抗原都参与 NV 的结合，因此很可能所有的人对 NV 都易感。然而，由于还没有发现能够与所有 HBGA 都结合的 NV，因此预测一种 NV 株能够感染所有人是不太可能的。

前面描述的 NV 的不同结合模式提示 NV 对于不同的个体和宿主范围所用的结合模式不同，这可能有助于解释 NV 的流行病学，虽然前面描述的 4 种结合模式中有 3 种模式的受体结合数据尚缺乏。例如，VA387 是一种 Lordsdale 样病毒株，它能够识别代表了近 80% 人群的 A 型、B 型和 O 型分泌者，这种受体结合的广谱性解释了为什么该组病毒在全世界普遍流行。预言的宿主特异性解释了为什么一些没有抗体的志愿者受 NV 攻击时不会感染。它也解释了为什么一些拥有高滴度抗体的个人比没有抗体的个人更容易受到 NV 感染[246,258]，讨论见"诺如病毒的免疫"部分。

这些结果表明，NV 受体可能对其他领域的研究产生重大影响。例如，根据对病毒衣壳的结构及其与细胞受体相互作用的认识可以合理设计抗 NV 病毒药物。了解宿主特异性可能会克服在研究这些病毒的过程中长期存在的障碍，如它们无法在细胞中培养复制或病毒的动物模型也不可靠。此外，研究 NV 和 HBGA 受体之间的相互作用可能会增加我们对病原微生物及其人类宿主共同进化的认识。最后，研究 NV 与受体的相互作用可能作为其他以 HBGA 作为其受体的病原体的一种模式。总之，在不久的将来，对 NV 受体和宿主特异性的研究是一个很有发展前景的新领域。

杯状病毒的年龄限制

虽然幼儿和老年人比这两个年龄组之间的人群更易出现严重的症状，但 NV 感染没有明确的年龄限制。对于幼儿，不成熟的免疫系统可能是主要原因。而对于老年人，健康状况不良和可能伴随老龄的免疫退化是主要原因。然而，对许多老年人疾病暴发的报道来自于养老院，其中环境因素如护理设施拥挤和卫生条件差，可能是疾病流行的主要原因。

SV 相关感染和急性胃肠炎在幼儿中比在成人中常见，可能是由于 SV 自然感染引起的保护作用比 NV 感染引起的长。因此，成年人可能在童年接触流行株时获得了后天免疫保护，虽然该长期免疫作用还缺乏直接证据。1985 年的一项研究表明，血清抗体的存在与抵御 SV 肠胃炎有相关性，因为疾病暴发时，只有 3% 的有抗体的婴幼儿发病，而有 75% 的无抗体的婴幼儿发病[259]。人们在一项研究中发现宿主的 NV 和 SV 抗体水平有差异，显示在生命之初的第一周，含有母源 Lordsdale 样 NV 抗体的婴幼儿（90%）比含有母源 London92 样 SV 抗体的婴幼儿（23%）多得多（Farkas T.，未发表）。该发现的临床解释和意义仍不清楚。

杯状病毒的动物流行病学

目前尚没有 CV 跨物种传播的直接证据。最近发现的人类 NV 识别人 HBGA 表明，NV 不可能跨物种传播，因为人类的主要 HBGA 表位与其他哺乳动物的不同。利用重组诺瓦克 VLP 作为探针，Hutson 等表明诺瓦克病毒只可以促进人类和黑猩猩红细胞凝集[254]。利用同样的重组 VLP 进行分析，猪 CV（SW918）并不与能够代表所有已知的人类 HBGA 类型的 52 位捐助者的唾液的位点结合（Farkas T.，未发表的结果）。

许多 NV 和 SV 与家畜急性胃肠炎有关，这一发现表明这些家畜可能是人类病原体的一个传染源。虽然这些动物 CV 是与人株无关的谱系（基因组或基因簇），而且全球监测报告表明它们不易跨越物种屏障感染人类，但病毒单链 RNA 基因组的高变异性和突变性，以及适应生长的要求可能很低，对物种屏障的突破可能在过去已经发生或将在未来发生。

杯状病毒的人群流行病学

人们发现诺如病毒是引起非细菌性急性胃肠炎最重要的病原，发展中国家和发达国家均存在，不分年龄，不分地域。诺如病毒通常引起在封闭或半封闭的社区及各种机构中暴发急性肠胃炎，如学校、餐馆、医院和养老院，最常见的是大型游船和战舰。虽然还可能有其他途径，NV 和 SV 主要是通过粪-口途径传播（图 4.12）。一些作者提出感染者的呕吐物产生的气溶胶也会传播 HuCV[260~262]。

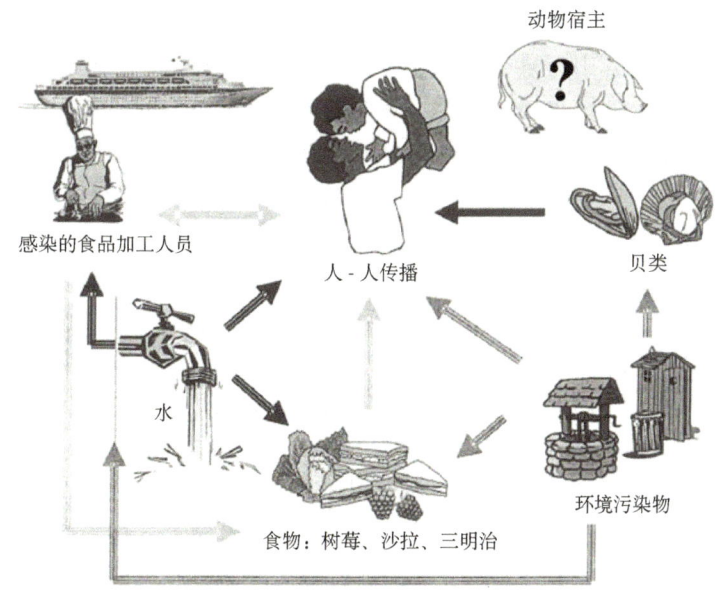

图 4.12 人类杯状病毒传播途径

人们曾记载过因社区或家庭供水系统污染引起的疾病暴发，但由于市政供水系统污染引起水源性疾病暴发的情况还很罕见。食用污染的食物如生贝类和未煮食品如沙拉火腿和三明治造成食源性暴发是常见的。NV 和 SV 全年均可感染，但呈现冬季的季节性流行优势。洗手仍是最有效的预防人与人之间传播的个人干预措施。为了在全球范围内控制 NV，人们已经建立了几个报告制度，包括疾病预防控制中心建立的 CaliciNet 邮箱（CALICINET@CDC.GOV）和欧盟建立的欧洲网络中的食源性病毒监控（WWW.EUFOODBORNEVIRUSES.CO.UK）。

20 世纪 90 年代初随着新的重组酶免疫学方法的发展，通过血清监测首次表明了 NV

为儿童急性胃肠炎的重要病因[263~268]。在很多国家的研究表明，儿童在非常年幼时就获得NV抗体，抗体水平持续上升到成年。在发展中国家抗体的阳性率比发达国家的高。人们在粪便样本中检测出了病毒同样也表明了NV作为儿童疾病病因的重要性。虽然在不同研究和不同国家的儿童中NV的检出率不同，但人们一致认为，NV胃肠炎是一种典型的儿童疾病。该看法由以下结果支持：NV在腹泻儿童中的检出率明显高于无腹泻儿童的[269]。在急性胃肠炎住院儿童（4%~53%，平均15%）[270~273]、急诊儿童（31%）[274]和门诊儿童（1.3%~16%）[275~278]中普遍检出诺如病毒，也为NV是引起儿童重症腹泻的病原体提供了证明。一般来说，虽然NV相关性腹泻的整体临床症状没有RV的严重，但HuCV被视为儿童急性胃肠炎的第二大主要病原体，仅次于RV。

在不同国家进行的NV监测观察到了重要的现象：NV相关急性胃肠炎在发展中国家和发达国家同样重要。发展中国家（如阿根廷、智利、墨西哥、中国、印度尼西亚和南非）的检出率为3%~25%，而且住院儿童中的检出率比门诊儿童的高[269,277~283]；发达国家（如英国、爱尔兰、法国、西班牙、日本和澳大利亚）的检出率为4%~30%，最高的也是住院患者[249,250,270~272,274~276,284~291]。这似乎与以下发现相矛盾：发达国家儿童的NV血清阳性率比发展中国家的低，这可能是由于不同国家使用了不同的实验室方法导致了检出率差异造成的。例如，在一些研究中，只有少数倾向选择人群接受检查，因此也就无法确定整个人群的发病率。这些研究的结果显然不能与其他选用大量受试者的研究相比。此外，由于HuCV的遗传高度多样性，不同国家的主要流行株可能不同，而且常用检测方法的敏感性也可能会有所不同。因此，关键的问题是：在不同的国家什么是真正的HuCV感染流行株？人们在一些研究中发现NV检出率较高，而且与其他肠道致病菌混合感染的比率也很高（超过50%），特别是RV，有时也可以是腺病毒或星形病毒，甚至可以观察到NV和SV的混合感染[271,284,287]。因此，在这些情况下许多疾病的病因无法确定。

与NV相比，对SV的研究就略显落后，这可能是因为SV主要感染儿童，引起的疾病比较轻微，较少有实验室研究SV，此外，SV的诊断方法仍然有限。因此，我们目前对SV流行病学的了解仍然是初步的。与粪便标本中SV的检测结果相反，抗体分布研究表明，几乎所有儿童5岁前均感染过SV，表明SV感染很普遍。SV疾病散发，大多数感染是无症状的。然而，使用高度保守的引物检测NV和SV，结果显示，在墨西哥儿童队列研究中40%的HuCV相关性腹泻与SV有关[269]。随着方法的改进和反应引物的扩展，人们将继续分离出新的SV毒株。

NV和SV具有遗传多样性，而且具有不同遗传特性的多种毒株通常在同一环境内同时流行。在NV属中，基因组Ⅱ（GⅡ）株被认为比GI株更为普遍，而且引起散发病例明显比暴发病例多[284,292]。一项研究表明，GI株常在美海军人员中检出[293]。此外，每个基因组也都有其优势群，如GⅡ/4群（Bristol/Lordsdale，包括Grimsby）是GⅡ株的优势群，而GⅡ/1（Hawaii）、GⅡ/3（Toronto/Mexico）和GⅡ/2（Snow Mountain/Melksman）株的检出率则较低。报道最多的GI株属于GI/2群（Southampton）、GI/4（Chiba）和GI/3（desert shield virus，沙漠盾牌病毒）[263,294]。报道最多的SV属于GI/1群（Sapporo/82）[285,295]。

最近的报道已经将HuCV列为能够引起免疫受损个体产生并发症的病原体。有报道称，诺如病毒能够导致干细胞移植接受者[296]发生腹泻、肠道和肝脏移植接受者发生长期的严重的分泌性腹泻[297]、HIV感染儿童发生慢性腹泻[298]。

诺如病毒的免疫

因为在志愿者中局限性观察结果和无法用一般传染病原理所能解释的疾病暴发，NV的免疫性一直是有争议的话题[197,245,246,299]。也就是在对志愿者的攻毒研究中发现具有高水平NV抗体的个体反而比具有低水平NV抗体的个体易感。最近对NV识别HBGA的发现为该现象提供了一个解释。由于HBGA识别的变异性，预计NV的宿主范围会有广谱性。因此，在对志愿者进行攻毒的研究中，因为其血型和攻毒的毒株的种类，只有部分的个体对攻击的病毒易感。此外，由于NV包含许多基因型和可能的血清型，用于酶免疫检测的NV抗体并不是特异性的中和抗体，这就是为什么一些有抗体的个体对病毒的攻击没有保护力。人们在不同的NV中发现了交叉反应抗原表位，但这些表位可能不会引起交叉反应的中和抗体。具有高滴度的NV抗体但容易受到感染的个人，有可能是他们的血型与病毒相匹配。然而，这些人也可能感染过抗原性相关但血清学上有显著差异的毒株。因此，高水平的抗体可以作为敏感性和既往感染某些毒株的指标，但其并不能代表有保护性免疫。

研究结果一再表明，如果短时间内（6~14周）再次受到相同病毒的攻击，个体可受到保护。然而，首次感染很长一段时间后再次受到病毒攻击的个体不受保护。此外，如果再次攻击的NV与首次感染的NV基因型不同，个体也不受保护。因此，NV可能只会引起针对同源毒株的短期免疫力。

人们在NV相关的急性胃肠炎暴发事件中也观察到了对同源毒株的保护性。在研究战舰里暴发的急性胃肠炎的免疫反应过程中，检测患者和无症状船员的血清中针对一系列重组衣壳抗原的抗体水平，这些抗原代表NV的不同基因群，包括在暴发中分离的毒株[300]。结果表明，个体对不同毒株有不同的抗体水平，只有暴露前体内的流行株特异性抗体滴度>1:3200的个体受到保护。毒株抗体对同一基因组（GI）内密切相关的但不在同一基因聚类的毒株不具有保护性。这项研究表明，针对NV的获得性免疫是高度特异的。

诺如病毒疫苗的发展

对HuCV疫苗的需求一直未能像RV那样明确。然而，在发达国家和发展中国家各年龄段，HuCV是引起流行性和地方性非细菌性急性胃肠炎的最重要病原体，这似乎为发展用于普通人群包括儿童的针对这些病毒有广谱保护性的疫苗提供了充足的理由。这种疫苗将对高危人群，如老人、前往流行地区的旅游者、食品行业从业人员、游船的船员和军事人员特别有用。良好的疫苗对于对抗生物恐怖主义袭击也将非常重要。

自从对NV成功地进行分子克隆后，人们一直在研发HuCV疫苗，其中一种由重组HuCV衣壳制成。选择该方法是基于以下几点：①在杆状病毒培养物中表达重组衣壳抗原高效、简单；②由杆状病毒表达的重组衣壳抗原组成的VLP在形态和抗原性上与真实的病毒颗粒相似，且用常规生化方法很容易纯化；③NV的VLP在冷冻和冻干后以及较宽的 pH 范围内是稳定的[217,301]。

大多数针对 NV 重组疫苗的研究采用原型株诺瓦克病毒 VLP 的方式。类似的方法也已通过采用其他的表达系统来研发，如转基因植物载体[302]和委内瑞拉马脑炎（Venezuelan equine encephalitis，VEE）病毒复制子[303]。转基因植物载体，如马铃薯、番茄、香蕉的主要优势是它们可以提供一个"可食用的"疫苗，从而以低成本方便重复性接种。诺瓦克病毒重组衣壳的第一种载体是马铃薯。饲喂转基因马铃薯表达的诺瓦克病毒衣壳能够成功地诱导小鼠和人类志愿者免疫应答[205,304]。在 VEE 载体产生的 NV 衣壳蛋白也形成 VLP，但因为载体源自致病性病毒，人们仍担心该疫苗的安全性。

将诺瓦克病毒重组衣壳抗原作为一种候选疫苗的研究已完成了小鼠的临床前和人类志愿者的 I 期临床评价。结果表明，小鼠通过不同途径接种杆状病毒表达的诺瓦克 VLP 是安全的和具有免疫原性的[219,305]。它也表明人类口服该疫苗也是安全的和具有免疫原性的[217~219,306]。免疫接种后抗体分泌细胞增加，表明它刺激 IgA 和 IgG 反应，它还适度诱导细胞免疫应答。人们发现这种疫苗不加佐剂接种也是有效的[218]。最近的一项研究表明，添加霍乱毒素 CT-E29H 作为佐剂被认为对肠道派尔集合淋巴结起作用，可观察到免疫效果加强[307]。

NV 疫苗发展的一个主要挑战是缺乏动物模型用于研究疫苗效力，这也阻碍了对自然感染后的发病机制和免疫机制的研究。另一个挑战是该家族中基因型和抗原型的高度变异性。诺如病毒自然感染后可以诱导保护性免疫，但这种保护很可能是同源性的[300]。因此，若想能够得到广泛使用和有效的疫苗，可能需要能够代表 HuCV 主要中和表位的多价疫苗。

杯状病毒感染的控制和预防

由于 NV 主要是通过人与人之间和污染的环境表面传播，因此，良好的个人卫生习惯是抵御 NV 感染的最重要武器，如饭前便后洗手。在家庭环境中，使用常规的家用漂白剂或其他消毒剂溶液去消毒被污染的区域是有效的。对于在社区暴发的情况，找到并消除感染源和可能的传播方式也很重要。感染病毒的食品行业从业人员是食源性暴发的最常见病源。人们发现，NV 通常导致亚临床感染，且患者的排毒期比之前确定的长，这就增加了控制由感染的食品行业从业人员引起的食源性暴发的难度。

星形病毒

星形病毒是小儿肠胃炎的一个重要病因。它们是星形病毒科的成员，并根据电镜负染测得的独特形态命名。作为有衣壳的、单链、正义 RNA 病毒，它们与细小 RNA 病毒科和杯状病毒科类似，但也与它们有些明显不同的差异因此建立该病毒科很有意义[309]。

星形病毒的历史

1975 年，Madeley 和 Cosgrove 在呕吐和腹泻婴儿的粪便中首次发现星形病毒[310]。它们的形态不同于其他小圆病毒，如先前被确定为胃肠炎病原体的诺如病毒。随后几年人们在许多物种的粪便中发现了类似的病毒。在 20 世纪 80 年代初期，通过在细胞培养基中添加胰蛋白酶可以用细胞培养繁殖星形病毒[311]。这一发现推动血清分型试剂和适用于 EIA

的单克隆抗体的发展，并最终促进星形病毒克隆和测序的发展。

星形病毒属颗粒的性质

通过电镜负染测量，星形病毒是一个直径为 27~34nm 的小颗粒（图 4.13）。可以看出，10%~15% 的病毒颗粒形态如其名呈星形，该形状可能代表了未完全降解的颗粒[312]。根据氯化铯梯度，纯化的星形病毒的浮力密度为 1.35~1.38。人类星形病毒颗粒的冷冻电镜计算机增强重建图像显示了其含有 30 个放射刺突二聚体的衣壳[313]。

通过十二烷基硫酸钠（sodium dodecyl sulfate，SDS）凝胶电泳测定，该衣壳由 2~3 种分子质量为 24~36kDa

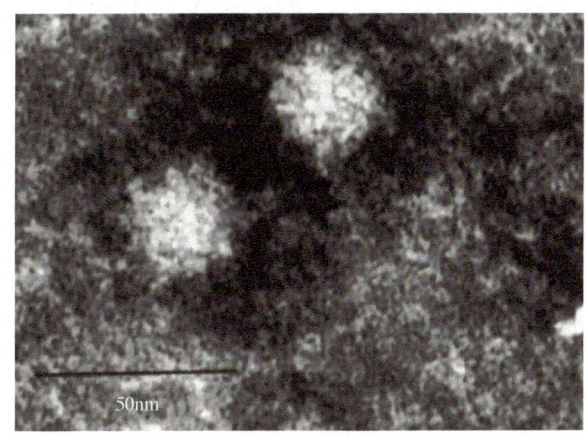

图 4.13　星形病毒的电子显微镜负染图。标尺 =50nm。

的蛋白质组成。囊壳蛋白来自于约 97kDa 的前体多肽。基因组由含有 3 个 ORF 的正义单链 RNA 组成（图 4.14）。ORF1a 包括一个蛋白酶基序、跨膜螺旋及核糖体移码和核定位信号，ORF1b 包括一个 RNA 聚合酶基序，而 ORF2 编码衣壳前体多聚蛋白。

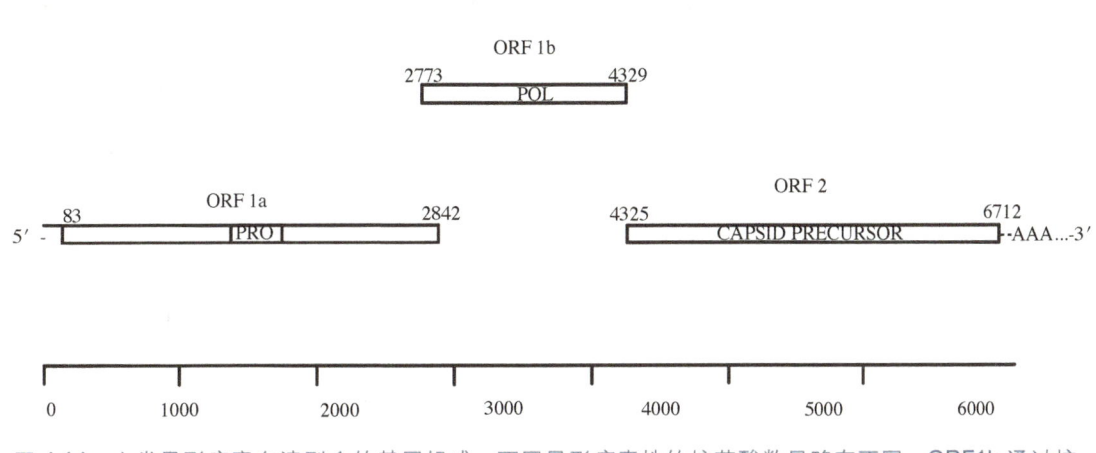

图 4.14　人类星形病毒血清型 1 的基因组成。不同星形病毒株的核苷酸数量略有不同。ORF1b 通过核糖体移码机制定位于 ORF1a 的 3′ 区起始，从而受到激活。图中描述了蛋白酶（PRO）、聚合酶（POLY）和衣壳前体区域。

星形病毒的分类

星形病毒科包括人类和动物/鸟类星形病毒属。哺乳动物星形病毒通常与本地肠道疾病相关，而鸟类的星形病毒可能与免疫缺陷[314]、间质性肾炎[315] 或肝炎[316] 相关。

从不同的物种分离出的星形病毒在血清学上互不相关，但在核苷酸序列水平上存在一定的同源性。人们通过中和实验、特异性 EIA 或 RT-PCR 分析至少可以鉴别出人星形病毒的 8 种血清型。

星形病毒的复制

尽管星形病毒复制的许多细节尚不清楚，但在最近几年已经取得了很大的进步。星形病毒基因组由正义、单链 RNA 的近 6800 个核苷酸组成。正如前面所说的，它有三个 ORF：ORF1a、ORF1b 和 ORF2。ORF1a 编码一种病毒蛋白酶，其中包括跨膜螺旋、功能性核定位信号和自我催化位点[317]。ORF1a 的体外翻译产物具有丝氨酸蛋白酶活性，关键残基突变后该活性丧失[318]。ORF1b 的第一个密码子 AUG 在 ORF1a 的 3′ 端区域内。通过核糖体移码机制激活[311,319]，ORF1b 编码病毒的 RNA 聚合酶。ORF2 编码约 87kDa 的结构前体蛋白。在感染的细胞内也可发现 ORF2 作为亚基因组 RNA，推动大量衣壳蛋白合成，从而包装子代病毒颗粒[309]。

在细胞培养中，星形病毒只在胰蛋白酶存在的情况下繁殖[311]。趋溶酶体试剂如氯化铵和丹酰戊二胺可有效抑制星形病毒复制，这表明胞吞途径对病毒进入细胞很重要[320]。电子显微镜显示星形病毒在细胞的内陷小窝被其吸收并被运至符合内含体特征的大的平滑小囊泡[320]。对星行病毒感染的细胞进行免疫荧光的研究表明，病毒感染细胞 7h 后产生抗原[321]。这些研究显示了病毒感染的小的核内荧光灶。在以后的时间点，感染细胞的电子显微图像显示子代病毒颗粒呈晶状排列聚集。

脉冲追踪实验结果表明，最初翻译为一个 87kDa 的蛋白质后，ORF2 产物在胞质内转换成 70kDa 的蛋白质，形成病毒衣壳[322]。该转换过程包括衣壳前体羧基末端的蛋白质裂解[323]。这个初步处理似乎便于形成衣壳和病毒从细胞中释放[324]，该过程可被天冬氨酸特异性半胱氨酸蛋白酶抑制剂阻断。虽然含 70kDa 蛋白衣壳的病毒颗粒可锚定到细胞，但它们感染性很小[322]。随后经胰蛋白酶处理将衣壳蛋白裂解成为约 34kDa、27kDa 和 25kDa 的小肽[322,323]。此裂解过程与病毒的感染力增强密切相关[322]。病毒依赖细胞外胰蛋白酶的这一特性可能对星形病毒向肠道上皮细胞趋化发挥作用。在细胞培养中，人星形病毒可诱导细胞凋亡[324]。

星形病毒引起的临床疾病

在哺乳动物物种中，星形病毒是引起肠胃炎的原因之一。人类星形病毒株主要与儿科疾病有关，表现为呕吐、腹泻、发热和全身乏力，典型的症状比 RV 疾病轻。在同龄的墨西哥儿童中，星形病毒腹泻是 4.3 次 / 天，而 RV 感染的是 7.1 次 / 天[325]。腹泻是水样、无血或脓。星形病毒胃肠炎的潜伏期为 1~3 天，持续 4~5 天，RT-PCR 检测排出的病毒可能持续数周[326]，免疫受损个体的症状可能会延长。许多感染，特别是在年龄较大的儿童或成人，都无症状。

对星形病毒感染的诊断最初是通过粪便样本的电镜负染[310]。近年来，敏感和特异的 EIA 已获得发展，该方法已经商品化。事实证明，RT-PCR 技术的灵敏度更高，而且可用于确定血清型[327]。

星形病毒的发病机制

由于缺乏常规的小型哺乳动物模型，限制了人们对于星形病毒发病的了解，人们仅能在人类和一些大型动物上进行一些有限的观测性研究。在早期病例报告中[328]，人们在一些患有慢性腹泻的儿童的小肠活检中观察到了星形病毒颗粒。在感染者的绒毛上皮细胞也可观察到病毒颗粒。

对成年志愿者的研究表明，尽管大多数人口服接种后出现血清转化现象，但只有极少数受试者发生胃肠炎样症状[329,330]，但在这些感染中未采集肠组织。一位长期患有星形病毒腹泻的4岁骨髓移植接受者的组织病理显示绒毛钝化，绒毛上皮细胞呈立方状，固有层炎症增加[331]。免疫荧光显示星形病毒抗原位于绒毛顶端上皮细胞，电镜显示这些细胞中的病毒颗粒呈类结晶排列。

在无菌羔羊体内，星形病毒感染与轻度绒毛萎缩、伴随病毒复制的绒毛上皮细胞隐窝增生及上皮下巨噬细胞散布有关[332~334]。在牛的感染中，病毒倾向于感染派尔集合淋巴结的圆顶上皮细胞已被阐明[335]。牛星形病毒属似乎对小牛相对无致病性，但会加重RV感染。一日龄的鸡和火鸡感染星形病毒后产生胃肠炎[336]，这与肠道二糖酶活性降低有关。鸭子感染可导致其独特的星形病毒肝炎[316]。一些鸟类星形病毒似乎是与胸腺萎缩、肠病变和免疫反应受抑制有关[337]，而另一些则与间质性肾炎和生长迟缓有关[315]。

总之，已知星形病毒感染绒毛上皮细胞，会导致伴随适度炎症改变的细胞死亡，进一步研究可探明这些变化如何引起腹泻和呕吐。

星形病毒的流行病学

星形病毒胃肠炎发生于世界各地的儿童。食源性和水源性暴发事件证明它经粪-口途径传播[338]。在大多数调查中分离病毒，最常见的血清型是1型。近几年星形病毒病的发病率大大增加，主要与诊断方法（如EIA和RT-PCR）的改进有关[339]。根据不同的计算方法，星形病毒可能引起3%~10%的小儿肠胃炎[275,340~348]。在温带，星形病毒感染率在冬季增加，这与RV和杯状病毒方式相似。

几个研究显示星形病毒比轮状病毒[325,343,344,347,349]更有可能造成幼儿（6个月以下）感染和疾病。这表明，与轮状病毒相比，母传免疫力可能对星形病毒不太有效。70%~90%的学龄儿童有星形病毒抗体[350~352]。在这些研究中血清型1抗体是最常见的。在同一出生队列的幼儿中，星形病毒感染的发病率与轮状病毒的相似，约0.2例/（人·年）[325]。

儿童日托中心[326]、学校[338]和医院[331]都暴发过星形病毒疾病。在这些情况下，RT-PCR研究已经表明，在出现症状之前或之后都可能排毒。

成人暴发星形病毒胃肠炎，可能会发生在疗养院[330,353,354]或新兵之中[355]。这些疫情远远比杯状病毒引起的疾病罕见，而且通常与较不常见的血清型如血清型3和血清型5相关。在日本的暴发事件似乎是与污染的食物有关[338]，另一个则是与一个浅水池有关[356]。

有报告称星形病毒是入侵免疫力低下宿主的重要病原体。对免疫缺陷[357,358]、HIV[359]和移植[344,360,361]患者的一些研究表明，很多有症状的感染发生在这些人群中，这种感染可能会显著延长。其他对HIV感染腹泻患者的调查中还没有发现大量的星形病毒感染[362]。

星形病毒的免疫

人们发现大多数有症状的星形病毒感染发生在幼儿，这表明获得性免疫具有保护作用。对埃及婴儿的纵向研究结果证明了感染后获得同型保护[325]。

成年志愿者研究也表明，血清中存在星形病毒特异性抗体，预示从疾病中得到了保护作用[329,330]。在某一病例中，使用免疫球蛋白与清除免疫缺陷成人[363]和骨髓移植接受者[364]的慢性、有症状的星形病毒感染相关，但类似的疗法未能在其他病例中获得成功[360]。

病毒与鼠单抗中和后会产生逃逸性突变，人们采用该方法确定并大致描绘出中和表位[365]。至少有一个这样的单克隆抗体在中和实验中与不同人血清型病毒有广泛的交叉反应，这意味着有可能存在一定程度的异型免疫。

细胞免疫也参与了预防星形病毒疾病。在成人的肠黏膜中已分离出星形病毒特异性的人类白细胞抗原（human leukocyte antigen，HLA）限制性 CD4 T 细胞[366]。T 细胞免疫缺陷[358]和化疗，会不均衡地降低 CD4 T 细胞的数量，引起星形病毒排毒延长[363]。CD8 和 CD16 T 细胞数量也与星形病毒排毒减少相关[360]。

星形病毒的控制和预防

在所有肠道传染病中，卫生标准在公共控制星形病毒感染方面发挥重要作用。在医院，腹泻患者应该被隔离，并密切观察以避免院内传播。用氯处理星形病毒后，它不再有感染性[327]，污染的表面用甲醇处理消毒也可灭活星形病毒。无症状的排毒使星形病毒感染和暴发的控制更加复杂。

最后，星形病毒疫苗将最有希望控制星形病毒感染。因为许多更严重的感染发生在非常小的婴儿，所以这种疫苗需要在早期就诱导免疫保护。也许进一步了解这种常见的感染最终会促进该疫苗的发展。

参 考 文 献

[1] Gordon I, Ingraham HS, Korns RF. Transmission of epidemic gastroenteritis to human volunteers by oral administration of fecal filtrates. J Exp Med 1947;86:409–422.

[2] Gordon I, Ingraham HS, Korns RF, Trussell RE. Gastroenteritis in man due to a filtrable agent. NY State J Med 1949;49:1918–1920.

[3] Kojima S, Fukumi H, Kusama H, et al. Studies on the causative agent of the infectious diarrhea: records of the experiments on human volunteers. Jpn Med J 1948;1:467–476.

[4] Reimann HA, Price AH, Hodges JH. The causes of epidemic diarrhea, nausea and vomiting (viral dysentery?) Proc Soc Exp Biol Med 1945;59:8–9.

[5] Yamamoto A, Zennyogi H, Yanagita K, Kato S. Research into the causative agent of epidemic gastroenteritis which prevailed in Japan in 1948. Jpn Med J 1948;1:379–384.

[6] Adams WR, Kraft LM. Epizootic diarrhea of infant mice: identification of the etiologic agent. Science 1963;141:359–360.

[7] Mebus C, Underdahl N, Rhodes M, Twiehaus M. Calf diarrhea (scours): reproduced with a virus from a field outbreak. Res Bull 1969;233:1–16.

[8] Malherbe H, Harwin R. The cytopathic effects of vervet monkey viruses. S Afr Med J 1963;37:407–411.

[9] Kapikian AZ, Wyatt RG, Dolin R, et al. Visualization by immune electron microscopy of a 27-nm particle associated with acute infectious nonbacterial gastroenteritis. J Virol 1972;10:1075–1081.

[10] Bishop RF, Davidson GP, Holmes IH, Ruck BJ. Virus particles in epithelial cells of duodenal mucosa

from children with acute non-bacterial gastroenteritis. Lancet 1973;2:1281–1283.

[11] Ward RL, Clark HF, Offit PA, Glass GI. Live vaccine strategies to prevent rotavirus disease. In: Levine MM, Kaper JB, Rappuoli R, Liu MA, Good MF, eds. New Generation Vaccines, 3rd ed.New York:Marcel Dekker, 2004:607–620.

[12] Tucker AW, Haddix AC, Bresee JS, et al. Cost-effectiveness analysis of a rotavirus immunization program for the United States. JAMA 1998;279:1371–1376.

[13] Kapikian AZ, Hoshino Y, Chanock RM.Rotaviruses. In: Knipe DM, Howley PM, Griffin DE, et al., eds. Fields Virology, 4th ed. Philadelphia: Lippincott Williams & Watkins, 2001:1787–1833.

[14] Murphy AM, Albrey MB, Hay PJ. Rotavirus infections in neonates. Lancet 1975;2:452–453.

[15] Bishop R, Barnes G, Cipriani E, et al. Clinical immunity after neonatal rotavirus infection: a prospective longitudinal study in young children. N Engl J Med 1983;309:72–76.

[16] Bhan MK, Lew JF, Sazawal S, et al. Protection conferred by neonatal rotavirus infection against subsequent rotavirus diarrhea. J Infect Dis 1993;168:282–287.

[17] Haffejee IE. Neonatal rotavirus infections. Rev Infect Dis 1991;13:957–962.

[18] Nakajima H, Nakagomi O, Kamisawa T, et al. Winter seasonality and rotavirus diarrhoea in adults. Lancet 2001;357:1950.

[19] Mikami T, Nakagomi T, Tsutsui R, et al. An outbreak of gastroenteritis during school trip caused by serotype G2 group A rotavirus. J Med Virol 2004;73:460–464.

[20] Research priorities for diarrhoeal diseases vaccines: memorandum from WHO meeting. Bull WHO 1991; 69:667–676.

[21] Shaw AL, Rothnagel R, Chen D, et al. Three-dimensional visualization of the rotavirus hemagglutinin structure. Cell 1993;74:693–701.

[22] Prasad BVV, Chiu W. Structure of rotavirus. Curr Top Microbiol Immunol 1994;185:9–29.

[23] Prasad BVV, Burns JW, Marietta E, et al. Localization of VP4 neutralization sites in rotavirus by threedimensional cryo-electron microscopy. Nature 1990; 343:476–479.

[24] Yeager M, Berriman JA, Baker TS, et al. Threedimensional structure of the rotavirus haemagglutinin VP4 by cryo-electron microscopy and difference map analysis. EMBO J 1994;13:1011–1018.

[25] Mattion NM, Mitchell DB, Both GW, Estes MK. Expression of rotavirus proteins encoded by alternative open reading frames of genome segment 11.Virology 1991; 181:295–304.

[26] Bridger JC. Detection by electron microscopy of caliciviruses, astroviruses and rotavirus-like particles in the faeces of piglets with diarrhoea. Vet Rec 1980;107:532.

[27] Saif LJ, Bohl EH, Theil KW, et al. Rotavirus-like, calicivirus-like, and 23–nm virus-like particles associated with diarrhea in young pigs. J Clin Microbiol 1980;12:105–111.

[28] Hung T, Wang C, Fang Z. et al.Waterborne outbreak of rotavirus diarrhea in adult in China caused by a novel rotavirus. Lancet 1984;26:1139–1142.

[29] Wang S, Cai S, Chen J, Li R, Jiang R. Etiologic studies of the 1983 and 1984 outbreaks of epidemic diarrhea in Guangxi. Intervirology 1985;24:140–146.

[30] Phan TG, Nishimura S, Okame M, et al.Virus diversity and an outbreak of group C rotavirus among infants and children with diarrhea in Maizuru City, Japan during 2002–2003. J Med Virol 2004;74:173–179.

[31] Ramig RF, Ward RL. Genomic segment reassortment in rotaviruses and other reoviridae. Adv Virus Res 1991;39:163–207.

[32] Yolken R, Arango-Jaramillo S, Eiden J, et al. Lack of genomic reassortant following infection of infant rats with group A and group B rotavirus. J Infect Dis 1988;158:1120–1123.

[33] Ward RL, Knowlton DR.Genotypic selection following coinfection of cultured cells with subgroup 1 and subgroup 2 human rotaviruses. J Gen Virol 1989;70:1691–1699.

[34] Nakagomi O, Nakagomi T. Interspecies transmission of rotaviruses studied from the perspective of genogroup. Microbiol Immunol 1993;37:337–348.

[35] Nakagomi O, Nakagomi T. Genetic diversity and similarity among mammalian rotaviruses in relation to interspecies transmission of rotavirus. Arch Virol 1991;120:43–55.

[36] Nakagomi O, Nakagomi T.Molecular evidence for naturally occurring single VP7 gene substitution reassortant between human rotaviruses belonging to two different genogroups. Arch Virol 1991;119:67–81.

[37] Ward RL, Nakagomi O, Knowlton DR, et al. Evidence for natural reassortants of human rotaviruses belonging to different genogroups. J Virol 1990;64:3219–3225.

[38] Hoshino Y, Wyatt RG, Greenberg HB, et al. Serotypic similarity and diversity of rotaviruses of mammalian and avian origin as studied by plaque-reduction neutralization. J Infect Dis 1984;149:694–702.

[39] Wyatt RG, Greenberg HB, James WD, et al. Definition of human rotavirus serotypes by plaque reduction assay. Infect Immun 1982;37:110–115.

[40] Ward R, Knowlton D, Schiff G, et al. Relative concentrations of serum neutralizing antibody to VP3 and VP7 proteins in adults infected with a human rotavirus. J Virol 1988;62:1543–1549.

[41] Ward RL, McNeal MM, Sander DS, et al. Immunodominance of the VP4 neutralization protein of rotavirus in protective natural infections of young children. J Virol 1993;67:464–468.

[42] Perez-Schael I, Blanco M,Vilar M, et al.Clinical studies of a quadrivalent rotavirus vaccine in Venezuelan infants. J Clin Microbiol 1990;28:553–558.

[43] Clark HF, Borian FE, Modesto K, et al. Serotype 1 reassortant of bovine rotavirus WC3 strain, strain W179–9, induces a polytypic antibody response in infants.Vaccine 1990;8:327–332.

[44] Gorziglia M, Larralde G, Kapikian AZ, et al. Antigenic relationships among human rotaviruses as determined by outer capsid protein VP4. Proc Natl Acad Sci USA 1990;87:7155–7159.

[45] Snodgrass DR, Hoshino Y, Fitzgerald TA, et al. Identification of four VP4 serological types (P serotypes) of bovine rotavirus using viral reassortants. J Gen Virol 1992;73:2319–2325.

[46] Estes MK, Cohen J.Rotavirus gene structure and function. Microbiol Rev 1989;53:410–449.

[47] Gentsch JR,Woods PA, Ramachandran M, et al.Review of G and P typing results from a global collection of rotavirus strains: implications for vaccine development. J Infect Dis 1996;174:S30–S36.

[48] Rao CD, Gowda K, Reddy BSY. Sequence analysis of VP4 and VP7 genes of nontypeable strains identifies a new pair of outer capsid proteins representing novel P and G genotypes in bovine rotaviruses. Virology 2000;276:104–113.

[49] Liprandi F, Gerder M, Bastidas Z, et al. A novel type of VP4 carried by a porcine rotavirus strain.Virology 2003;314:373–380.

[50] McNeal MM, Sestak K, Choi AH-C, et al. Development of a rotavirus shedding model in rhesus macaques using a homologous wild type rotavirus of a new P genotype. J Virol 2005;79:944–954.

[51] Barnes GL, Unicomb L, Bishop RF. Severity of rotavirus infection in relation to serotype, monotype and electropherotype. J Paediatr Child Health 1992;28: 54–57.

[52] Bern C, Unicomb L, Gentsch JR, et al. Rotavirus diarrhea in Bangladeshi children: correlation of disease severity with serotypes. J Clin Microbiol 1992;30: 3234–3238.

[53] Raul-Velazquez F, Calva JJ, Lourdes-Guerrero M, et al. Cohort study of rotavirus serotype patterns in

symptomatic and asymptomatic infections in Mexican children. Pediatr Infect Dis J 1993;12:54–61.

[54] Greenberg HB, Valdesuso J, Van Wyke K, et al. Production and preliminary characterization of monoclonal antibodies directed at two surface proteins of rhesus rotavirus. J Virol 1983;47:267–275.

[55] Taniguchi K, Urasawa T, Urasawa S, et al. Production of subgroup-specific monoclonal antibodies to an enzyme-linked immunosorbent assay for subgroup determination. J Med Virol 1984;14:115–125.

[56] Kalica AR, Greenberg HB, Espejo RT, et al. Distinctive ribonucleic acid patterns of human rotavirus subgroups 1 and 2. Infect Immunol 1981;33:958–961.

[57] Ludert JE, Mason BB, Angel J, et al. Identification of mutations in the rotavirus protein VP4 that alter sialic-acid-independent infection. J Gen Virol 1998; 79:725–729.

[58] Mendez E, Arias CF, López S. Binding to sialic acids is not an essential step for the entry of animal rotaviruses to epithelial cells in culture. J Virol 1993;67:5253–5259.

[59] Hewish MJ, Takada Y, Coulson BS. Integrins α2β1 and α4β1 can mediate SA11 rotavirus attachment and entry into cells. J Virol 2000;74:228–236.

[60] Graham KL, Halasz P, Tan Y, et al. Integrin-using rotaviruses bind alpha2beta1 integrin alpha2 I domain via VP4 DGE sequence and recognize alphaXbeta2 and alphavbeta3 by using VP7 during cell entry. J Virol 2003;77:9969–9978.

[61] Rolsma MD, Kuhlenschmidt TB, Gelberg HB, Kuhlenschmidt MS. Structure and function of a ganglioside receptor for porcine rotavirus. J Virol 1998;72: 9079–9091.

[62] Zárate S, Espinosa R, Romero P, Guerrero CA, Arias CF, López S. Integrin alpha2beta1 mediates the cell attachment of the rotavirus neuraminidase-resistant variant nar3.Virology 2000;278:50–54.

[63] Coulson BS, Londrigan SL, Lee DJ. Rotavirus contains integrin ligand sequences and a disintegrin-like domain that are implicated in virus entry into cells. Proc Natl Acad Sci USA 1997;94:5389–5394.

[64] Isa P, López S, Segovia L, Arias CF. Functional and structural analysis of the sialic acid-binding domain of rotaviruses. J Virol 1997;71:6749–6756.

[65] Zárate S, Cuadras MA, Espinosa R, et al. The interaction of rotaviruses with hsc70 during cell entry is mediated by VP5. J Virol 2003;77:7254–7260.

[66] Guerrero CA, Méndez E, Zárate S, Isa P, López S, Arias CF. Integrin alpha(v)beta(3) mediates rotavirus cell entry. Proc Natl Acad Sci USA 2000;97:14644–14649.

[67] Chen DY, Estes MK, Ramig RF. Specific interactions between rotavirus outer capsid proteins VP4 and VP7 determine expression of a cross-reactive, neutralizing VP4 specific epitope. J Virol 1992;66:432–439.

[68] Méndez E, Arias CF, López S. Interactions between the two surface proteins of rotavirus may alter the receptor-binding specificity of the virus. J Virol 1996;70: 1218–1222.

[69] Pralle A, Keller P, Florin E-L, Simons K, Horber JKH. Sphinolipid-cholesterol rafts diffuse as small entities in the plasma membrane of mammalian cells. J Cell Biol 2000;148:997–1007.

[70] Brown DA. Seeing is believing: visualization of rafts in model membranes. Proc Natl Acad Sci USA 2001;98:10517–10518.

[71] Isa P, Realpe M, Romero P, López S, Arias CF. Rotavirus RRV associates with lipid membrane microdomains during cell entry.Virology 2004;322:370–381.

[72] Quan CM, Doane FW.Ultrastructural evidence for the cellular uptake of rotavirus by endocytosis. Intervirology 1983;20:223–231.

[73] Ludert JE, Michelangeli F, Gil F, et al. Penetration and uncoating of rotaviruses in cultured cells. Intervirology 1987;27:95–101.

[74] Suzuki H, Kitaoka S, Konno T, et al. Two modes of human rotavirus entry into MA104 cells. Arch Virol

1985;85:25–34.

[75] Kaljot KT, Shaw RD, Rubin DH, Greenberg HB. Infectious rotavirus enters cells by direct cell membrane penetration, not by endocytosis. J Virol 1988;62:1136–1144.

[76] Fukuhara N, Yoshie O, Kitaoka S, et al. Evidence for endocytosis-independent infection of human rotavirus. Arch Virol 1987;97:93–99.

[77] Keljo DJ, Kuhn M, Smith A.Acidification of endosomes in not important for the entry of rotavirus into the cell. J. Pediatr Gastroenterol Nutr 1988;7:257–263.

[78] Martin S, Lorrot M, El Azher MA, Vasseur M. Ionic strength- and temperature-induced KCa shifts in the uncoating reaction of rotavirus strains RF and SA11: correlation with membrane permeabilization. J Virol 2002;76:552–559.

[79] Estes MK. Rotaviruses and their replication. In: Knipe DM,Howley PM,Griffin DE, et al., eds. Fields Virology, 4th ed. Philadelphia: Lippincott Williams & Wilkins, 2001:1747–1785.

[80] Denisova E, Dowling W, LaMonica R, et al. Rotavirus Capsid Protein VP5* permeabilizes membranes. J Virol 1999;73:3147–3153.

[81] Cuadras MA, Arias CF, Lopez S. Rotaviruses induce an early membrane permeabilization of MA104 cells and do not require a low intracellular Ca2+ concentration to initiate their replication cycle. J Virol 1997;71: 9065–9074.

[82] Liprandi F, Moros Z, Gerder M, et al. Productive penetration of rotavirus in cultured cells induces coentry of the translation inhibitor alpha-sarcin. Virology 1997;237:430–438.

[83] Lawton JA, Estes MK, Prasad BV. Three-dimensional visualization of mRNA release from actively transcribing rotavirus particles. Nat Struct Biol 1997;4: 118–121.

[84] Silvestri LS, Taraporewala ZF, Patton JT. Rotavirus replication: plus-sense templates for double-stranded RNA synthesis are made in viroplasms. J Virol 2004; 78:7763–7774.

[85] Vende P, Piron M, Castagne N, Poncet D. Efficient Translation of rotavirus mRNA requires simultaneous interaction of NSP3 with the eukaryotic translation initiation factor eIF4G and the mRNA 3′ end. J Virol 2000;74:7064–7071.

[86] Piron M, Vende P, Cohen, Poncet D. Rotavirus RNAbinding protein NSP3 interacts with eIF4GI and evicts the poly (A) binding protein from eIF4F. EMBO J 1998;17:5811–5821.

[87] Padilla-Noriega L. Paniagua O, Guzman-Leon S. Rotavirus protein NSP3 shuts off host protein synthesis. Virology 2002;298:1–7.

[88] Fabbretti E, Afrikanova I, Vascotto F, Burrone O. Two non-structural rotavirus proteins, NSP2 and NSP5, form viroplasm-like structures in vivo. J Gen Virol 1999;80:333–339.

[89] Berois M, Sapin C, Erk I, Poncet D, Cohen J. Rotavirus nonstructural protein NSP5 interacts with major core protein VP2. J Virol 2003;77:1757–1763.

[90] Mohan KVK, Muller J, Atreya CD. The N- and C-terminal regions of rotavirus NSP5 are the critical determinants for the formation of viroplasm-like structures independent of NSP2. J Virol 2003;77: 12184–12192.

[91] Taraporewala ZF, Patton JT. Nonstructural proteins involved in genome packaging and replication of rotaviruses and other members of the reoviridae. Virus Res 2004;101:57–66.

[92] Patton JT, Kearney K, Taraporewala Z. Rotavirus genome replication: role of the RNA—binding protein. In: Desselberger U, Gray J, eds. Viral Gastroenteritis, vol. 9. The Netherlands: Elsevier Science, 2003:165–183.

[93] Taniguchi K, Kojima K, Urasawa S. Nondefective rotavirus mutants with an NSP1 gene which has a

deletion of 500 nucleotides, including a cysteine-rich zinc finger motif-encoding region (nucleotides 156 to 248) or which has a nonsense codon at nucleotides 153 to 155. J Virol 1996;70:4125–4130.

[94] Graff JW, Mitzel DN, Weisend CM, Flenniken ML, Hardy ME. Interferon regulatory factor 3 is a cellular partner of rotavirus NSP1. J Virol 2002;76:9545–9550.

[95] Gonzalez RA, Espinosa R, Romero P, López S,Arias CF. Relative localization of viroplasmic and endoplasmic reticulum-resident rotavirus proteins in infected cells. Arch Virol 2000;145:1963–1973.

[96] Petrie BL, Greenberg HB, Graham DY, Estes MK. Ultrastructural localization of rotavirus antigens using colloidal gold.Virus Res 1984;1:133–152.

[97] Delmas O, Durand-Schneider AM, Cohen J, Colard O, Trugnan G. Spike protein VP4 assembly with maturing rotavirus requires a postendoplasmic reticulum event in polarized Caco-2 cells. J Virol 2004;78: 10987–10994.

[98] Perez JF, Chemello ME, Liprandi F, Ruiz MC, Michelangeli F. Oncosis in MA104 cells induced by rotavirus infection through an increase in intracellular Ca^{2+} concentration.Virology 1998;252:17–27.

[99] Superti F. Ammendolia MG, Tinari A, et al. Induction of apoptosis in HT-29 cells infected with SA-11 rotavirus. J Med Virol 1996;50:325–334.

[100] Jourdan N, Maurice M, Delautier D, Quero AM, Servin AL, Trugnan G. Rotavirus is released from the apical surface of cultured human intestinal cells through nonconventional vesicular transport that bypasses the golgi apparatus. J Virol 1997;71:8268–8278.

[101] Cuadras MA. Greenberg HB. Rotavirus infectious particles use lipid rafts during replication for transport to the cell surface in vitro and in vivo. Virology 2003;313:308–321.

[102] Musalem C, Espejo RT. Release of progeny virus from cells infected with simian rotavirus SA11. J Gen Virol 1985;66:2715–2724.

[103] Rodriguez WJ, Kim HW, Arrobio JO, et al. Clinical features of acute gastroenteritis associated with human reovirus-like agent in infants and young children. J Pediatr 1977;91:188–193.

[104] Bernstein DI, Ward RL. Rotaviruses. In: Feigin RD, Cherry JD, Demmler GJ, Kaplan SL, eds. Textbook of Pediatric Infectious Diseases, 5th ed. Philadelphia: Saunders, 2004:2110–2133.

[105] Honeyman MC, Coulson BS, Stone NL, et al. Association between rotavirus infection and pancreatic islet autoimmunity in children at risk of developing type 1 diabetes. Diabetes 2000;49:1319–1324.

[106] Blomqvist M, Juhela S, Erkkila S, et al.Rotavirus infections and development of diabetes-associated autoantibodies during the first 2 years of life. Clin Exp Immunol 2002;128:511–515.

[107] Murphy TV, Gargiullo PM, Massoudi MS, et al. Intussusception among infants given an oral rotavirus vaccine. N Eng J Med 2001;344:564–572.

[108] Parashar UD, Holman RC, Cummings KC, et al. Trends in intussusception-associated hospitalizations and deaths among U.S. infants. Pediatrics 2000;106: 1413–1421.

[109] Rennels MB, Parashar UD, Holman RC, et al. Lack of an apparent association between intussusception and wild or vaccine rotavirus infection. Pediatr Infect Dis J 1998;17:924–925.

[110] Mebus CA, Stair EL, Underdahl NR, et al. Pathology of neonatal calf diarrhea induced by a reo-like virus. Vet Pathol 1974;8:490–505.

[111] Pearson GR, McNulty MS. Ultrastructural changes in small intestinal epithelium of neonatal pigs infected with pig rotavirus. Arch Virol 1979;59:127–136.

[112] Torres-Medina A. Effect of combined rotavirus and Escherichia coli in neonatal gnotobiotic calves. Am J Vet Res 1984;45:643–651.

[113] Boshuizen JA, Reimerink HJ, Korteland-van Male AM, et al. Changes in small intestinal homeostasis

morphology and gene expression during rotavirus infection of infant mice. J Virol 2003;77:13005–13016.

[114] Suzuki H, Konno T. Reovirus-like particles in jejunal mucosa of a Japanese infant with acute infectious nonbacterial gastroenteritis. Tohoku J Exp Med 1975;115: 199–221.

[115] Holmes IH, Ruck BJ, Bishop RF, et al. Infantile enteritis viruses: morphogenesis and morphology. J Virol 1975;16:937–943.

[116] Davidson GP, Gall DG, Petric M, et al. Human rotavirus enteritis induced in conventional piglets: intestinal structure and transport. J Clin Invest 1977;60:1402–1409.

[117] Graham DY, Sackman JW, Estes MK. Pathogenesis of rotavirus-induced diarrhea: preliminary studies in miniature swine piglet. Dig Dis Sci 1984;29:1028–1035.

[118] Collins J, Starkey WG, Wallis TS, et al. Intestinal enzyme profiles in normal and rotavirus-infected mice. J Pediatr Gastroenterol Nutr 1988;7:264–272.

[119] Ball JM, Peng T, Zeng CQY, Morris AP, Estes MK. Agedependent diarrhea induced by a rotaviral nonstructural glycoprotein. Science 1996;272:101–104.

[120] Morris AP, Scott JK, Ball JM, et al. NSP4 elicits agedependent diarrhea and Ca^{2+}-mediated I^- influx into intestinal crypts of CF mice. Am J Physiol 1999;277:G431–G444.

[121] Tian P, Estes MK, Hu Y, et al. The rotavirus nonstructural glycoprotein NSP4 mobilizes Ca^{2+} from the endoplasmic reticulum. J Virol 1995;69:5763–5772.

[122] Tian P, Hu Y, Schilling WP, et al. The nonstructural glycoprotein of rotavirus affects intracellular calcium levels. J Virol 1994;68:251–257.

[123] Dong Y, Zeng CQY, Ball JM, Estes MK, Morris AP. The rotavirus enterotoxin NSP4 mobilizes intracellular calcium in human intestinal cells by stimulating phospholipase C-mediated inositol 1,4,5–triphosphate production. Proc Natl Acad Sci USA 1997;94:3960–3965.

[124] Browne EP, Bellamy AR, Taylor JA. Membranedestabilizing activity of rotavirus NSP4 is mediated by a membrane-proximal amphipathic domain. J Gen Virol 2000;81:1955–1959.

[125] Tian P, Ball JM, Zeng CQY, Estes MK. The rotavirus nonstructural glycoprotein NSP4 possesses membrane destabilization activity. J Virol 1996;70:6973–6981.

[126] Brunet J-P, Cotte-Lafitte J, Linxe C, et al. Rotavirus infection induces an increase in intracellular calcium concentration in human intestinal epithelial cells: role in microvillar actin alteration. J Virol 2000;74: 2323–2332.

[127] Brunet J-P, Jourdan N, Cotte-Lafitte J, et al. Rotavirus infection induces cytoskeleton disorganization in human intestinal epithelial cells: implication of an increase in intracellular calcium concentration. J Virol 2000;74:10801–10806.

[128] Perez JF, Ruiz M-C, Chemello ME, Michelangeli F. Characterization of a membrane calcium pathway induced by rotavirus infection in cultured cells. J Virol 1999;73:2481–2490.

[129] Lundgren O, Peregrin AT, Persson K, et al. Role of the enteric nervous system in the fluid and electrolyte secretion of rotavirus diarrhea. Science 2000;287:491–495.

[130] Horie Y, Nakagomi O, Koshimura Y, et al. Diarrhea induction by rotavirus NSP4 in the homologous mouse model system. Virology 1999;262:398–407.

[131] Zhang M, Zeng CQY, Dong Y, et al. Mutations in rotavirus nonstructural glycoprotein NSP4 are associated with altered virus virulence. J Virol 1998;72:3666–3672.

[132] Angel J, Tang B, Feng N, Greenberg HB, Bass D. Studies of the role for NSP4 in the pathogenesis of homologous murine rotavirus diarrhea. J Infect Dis 1998;177:455–458.

[133] Lee C-N, Wang Y-L, Kao C-L, et al. NSP4 gene analysis of rotaviruses recovered from infected children

with and without diarrhea. J Clin Microbiol 2000;38:4471–4477.

[134] Ward RL, Mason BB, Bernstein DI, et al. Attenuation of a human rotavirus vaccine candidate did not correlate with mutations in the NSP4 protein gene. J Virol 1997;71:6267–6270.

[135] Offit PA, Blavat G, Greenberg HB, et al. Molecular basis of rotavirus virulence role of gene segment 4. J Virol 1986;57:46–49.

[136] Broome RL, Vo PT, Ward RL, et al. Murine rotavirus genes encoding outer capsid proteins VP4 and VP7 are not major determinants of host range restriction and virulence. J Virol 1993;67:2448–2455.

[137] Bridger JC, Tauscher GI, and Desselberger U. Viral determinants of rotavirus pathogenicity in pigs: evidence that the fourth gene of a porcine rotavirus confers diarrhea in the homologous host. J Virol 1998;72:6929–6931.

[138] Hoshino Y, Saif LJ, Kang S-Y, et al. Identification of group A rotavirus genes associated with virulence of a porcine rotavirus and host range restriction of a human rotavirus in the gnotobiotic piglet model. Virology 1995;209:274–280.

[139] McNeal MM, Ward RL. Long-term production of rotavirus antibody and protection against reinfection following a single infection of neonatal mice with murine rotavirus. Virology 1995;211:474–480.

[140] Bridger JC. A definition of bovine rotavirus virulence. J Gen Virol 1994;75:2807–2812.

[141] Kirstein CG, Clare DA, Lecce JG. Development of resistance of enterocytes to rotavirus in neonatal agammaglobulinemic piglets. J Virol 1985;55:567–573.

[142] Riepenhoff-Talty M, Lee PC, Carmody PJ, et al. Agedependent rotavirus-enterocyte interactions. Proc Soc Exp Biol Med 1982;170:146–154.

[143] Varshney KC, Bridger JC, Parson KR, et al. The lesions of rotavirus infection in 1– and 10–day-old gnotobiotic calves. Vet Pathol 1995;32:619–627.

[144] Lebenthal E, Lee PC. Development of functional response in human exocrine pancreas. Pediatrics 1980; 66:556–560.

[145] Zheng BJ, Lo SKF, Tam JSL, et al. Prospective study of community-acquired rotavirus infection. J Clin Microbiol 1989;27:2083–2090.

[146] Ward RL, Bernstein DI, Shukla R, et al. Effects of antibody to rotavirus on protection of adults challenged with a human rotavirus. J Infect Dis 1989;159:79–88.

[147] Chiba S, Yokoyama T, Nakata S, et al. Protective effect of naturally acquired homotypic and heterotypic rotavirus antibodies. Lancet 1986;2:417–421.

[148] Hjelt K, Graubelle PC, Paerregaard A, et al. Protective effect of pre-existing rotavirus-specific immunoglobulin A against naturally acquired rotavirus infection in children. J Med Virol 1987;21:39–47.

[149] Bernstein DI, Smith VE, Sander DS, Pax KA, Schiff GM, Ward RL. Evaluation of WC3 rotavirus vaccine and correlates of protection in healthy infants. J Infect Dis 1990;162:1055–1062.

[150] Valazques FR, Matson DO, Guerrero ML, et al. Serum antibody as a marker of protection against natural rotavirus infection and disease. J Infect Dis 2000; 182:1602–1609.

[151] Matson DO, O'Ryan ML, Herrera I, Pickering LK, Estes MK. Fecal antibody responses to symptomatic and asymptomatic rotavirus. J Infect Dis 1993;167:577–583.

[152] Coulson BS, Grimwood K, Hudson IL, Barnes GL, Bishop RF. Role of coproantibody in clinical protection of children during reinfection with rotavirus. J Clin Microbiol 1992;30:1678–1684.

[153] Graham A, Kudesia G, Allen AM, et al. Reassortment of human rotavirus possessing genome rearrangements with bovine rotavirus: evidence of host cell selection. J Gen Virol 1987;68:115–122.

[154] Gombold JL, Ramig RF. Analysis of reassortment of genome segments in mice mixedly infected with

rotaviruses SA11 and RRV. J Virol 1986;57:110–116.

[155] Bridger JC, Dhaliwal W, Adamson MJV, Howard CR. Determinants of rotavirus host range restriction—a heterologous bovine NSP1 gene does not affect replication kinetics in the pig. Virology 1998;245:47–52.

[156] Haffejee IE. The epidemiology of rotavirus infections: a global perspective. J Pediatr Gastroent Nutr 1995;20: 275–286.

[157] Ward RL, Knowlton DR, Pierce MJ. Efficiency of human rotavirus propagation in cell culture. J Clin Microbiol 1984;19:748–753.

[158] Keswick BH, Pickering LK, Dupont HL, et al. Survival and detection of rotaviruses on environmental surfaces in day care centers. Appl Environ Microbiol 1983;46:813–816.

[159] Estes MK, Graham DY, Smith EM, et al. Rotavirus stability and inactivation. J Gen Virol 1979;43:403–409.

[160] Butz AM, Fosarelli P, Dick J, et al. Prevalence of rotavirus on high-risk fomites in daycare facilities. Pediatrics 1993;92:202–205.

[161] Shaw R, Merchant A, Groene W, Cheng EH. Persistence of intestinal antibody response to heterologous rotavirus infection in a murine model beyond 1 year. J Clin Microbiol 1993;31:188–191.

[162] Feng N, Burns JW, Bracy L, Greenberg HB. Comparison of mucosal and systemic humoral immune responses and subsequent protection in mice orally inoculated with a homologous or a heterologous rotavirus. J Virol 1994;68:7766–7773.

[163] McNeal MM, Broome RL, Ward RL. Active immunity against rotavirus infection in mice is correlated with viral replication and titers of serum rotavirus IgA following vaccination. Virology 1994;204:642–650.

[164] Chiba S, Yokoyama T, Nakata S, et al. Protective effect of naturally acquired homotypic and heterotypic rotavirus antibodies. Lancet 1986;2:417–421.

[165] Hoshino Y, Saif LJ, Sereno MM, Chanock RM, Kapikian AZ. Infection immunity of piglets to either VP3 or VP7 outer capsid protein confers resistance to challenge with a virulent rotavirus bearing the corresponding antigen. J Virol 1988;62:744–748.

[166] Ward RL, McNeal MM, Sheridan JF. Evidence that active protection following oral immunization of mice with live rotavirus is not dependent on neutralizing antibody.Virology 1992;188:57–66.

[167] Flores J, Perez-Schael I, Gonzales M, et al. Protection against severe rotavirus diarrhoea by rhesus rotavirus vaccine in Venezuelan infants. Lancet 1987;1:882–884.

[168] Santosham M, Letson GW,Wolff M, et al. A field study of the safety and efficacy of two candidate rotavirus vaccines in a Native American population. J Infect Dis 1991;163:483–487.

[169] Ward RL, Knowlton DR, Zito ET, Davidson BL, Rappaport R, Mack ME. Serological correlates of immunity in a tetravalent reassortant rotavirus vaccine trial. J Infect Dis 1997;176:570–577.

[170] Burns JW, Siadat-Pajouh M, Krishnaney AA, Greenberg HB. Protective effect of rotavirus VP6–specific IgA monoclonal antibodies that lack neutralizing activity. Science 1996;272:104–107.

[171] Feng N, Lawton JA, Gilbert J, et al. Inhibition of rotavirus biogenesis by a non-neutralizing, rotavirus VP6–specific IgA mAb. J Clin Invest 2002;109:1203–1213.

[172] O'Neal CM, Crawford SE, Estes ME, Conner ME. Rotavirus VLPs administered mucosally induce protective immunity. J Virol 1997;71:8707–8717.

[173] Choi AHC, Basu M, McNeal MM, Clements JD, Ward RL. Antibody-independent protection against rotavirus infection of mice stimulated by intranasal immunization with chimeric VP4 or VP6 protein. J Virol 1999;73:7574–7581.

[174] Offit P, Dudzik K. Rotavirus-specific cytotoxic T lymphocytes passively protect against gastroenteritis in suckling mice. J Virol 1990;64:6325–6328.

[175] Dharakul T, Rott L, Greenberg H. Recovery from chronic rotavirus infection in mice with severe combined immunodeficiency: virus clearance mediated by adoptive transfer of immune CD8+ T lymphocytes. J Virol 1990;64:4375–4382.

[176] Ward RL, McNeal MM, Sheridan JF. Development of an adult mouse model for studies on protection against rotavirus. J Virol 1990;64:5070–5075.

[177] Feng N, Vo PT, Chung D, Hoshino Y, Greenberg HB. Heterotypic protection following oral immunization with live heterologous rotaviruses in the mouse model. J Infect Dis 1997;175:330–341.

[178] Moser CA, Cookinham S, Coffin SE, Clark HF, Offit PA. Relative importance of rotavirus-specific effector and memory B cells in protection against challenge. J Virol 1998;72:1108–1114.

[179] Franco MA, Greenberg HB. Role of B cells and cytotoxic T lymphocytes in clearance of and immunity to rotavirus infection in mice. J Virol 1995;69:7800–7806.

[180] McNeal MM, Barone KS, Rae MN, Ward RL. Effector functions of antibody and CD8+ cells in resolution of rotavirus infection and protection against reinfection in mice. Virology 1995;214:387–397.

[181] Coffin SE, Clark SL, Bos NA, Brubaker JO, Offit PA. Migration of antigen-presenting B cells from peripheral to mucosal lymphoid tissues may induce intestinal antigen-specific IgA following parental immunization. J Immunol 1999;163:3064–3070.

[182] O'Neal CM, Harriman GR, Conner ME. Protection of the villus epithelial cells in the small intestine infection does not require immunoglobulin A. J Virol 2000;74:4102–4109.

[183] Kuklin NA, Rott L, Feng N, et al. Protective intestinal anti-rotavirus B cell immunity is dependent on $\alpha 4\beta 7$ integrin expression but does not require IgA antibody production. J Immunol 2001;166:1894–1902.

[184] Choi AHC, Basu M, McNeal MM, et al. Functional mapping of protective domains and epitopes in the rotavirus VP6 protein. J Virol 2000;74:11574–11580.

[185] McNeal, MM, VanCott JL, Choi AHC, et al. CD4 T cells are the only lymphocytes needed to protect mice against rotavirus shedding after intranasal immunization with a chimeric VP6 protein and the adjuvant LT(R192G). J Virol 2002;76:560–568.

[186] Bernstein DI, Sack DA, Rothstein E, et al. Efficacy of live, attenuated, human rotavirus vaccine 89–12 in infants: a randomized placebo-controlled trial. Lancet 1999;354:287–290.

[187] Ciarlet M, Crawford SE, Barone C, Bertolotti-Ciarlet A, Estes MK, Conner ME. Subunit rotavirus vaccine administered parenterally to rabbits induces active protective immunity. J Virol 1998;72:9233–9246.

[188] Coste A, Sirard JC, Johansen K, Cohen J, Kraehenbuhl JP. Nasal immunization of mice with virus-like particles protects offspring against rotavirus diarrhea. J Virol 2000;74:8966–8971.

[189] Yuan L, Iosef C, Azevedo MSP, et al. Protective immunity and antibody-secreting cell responses elicited by combined oral attenuated Wa human rotavirus and intranasal Wa 2/6–VLPs with mutant Escherichia coli heat-labile toxin in gnotobiotic pigs. J Virol 2001;75:9229–9238.

[190] Ward RL, Clemens JD, Sack DA, et al. Culture-adaptation of group A rotaviruses causing diarrheal illnesses in Bangladesh during 1985–1986. J Clin Microbiol 1991;29:1915–1923.

[191] Green KY, Ando T, Balayan MS, et al. Taxonomy of the caliciviruses. J Infect Dis 2000;181:S322–330.

[192] Liu BL, Clarke IN, Caul EO, Lambden PR. Human enteric caliciviruses have a unique genome structure and are distinct from the Norwalk-like viruses. Arch Virol 1995;140:1345–1356.

[193] Adler J, Zickl R. Winter vomiting disease. J Infect Dis 1969;119:668–673.

[194] Dolin R. Norwalk agent-like particles associated with gastroenteritis in human beings. J Am Vet Med

Assoc 1978;173:615–619.

[195] Dolin R, Reichman RC, Roessner KD, et al. Detection by immune electron microscopy of the Snow Mountain agent of acute viral gastroenteritis. J Infect Dis 1982;146:184–189.

[196] Thornhill TS, Wyatt RG, Kalica AR, Dolin R, Chanock RM, Kapikian AZ. Detection by immune electron microscopy of 26– to 27–nm viruslike particles associated with two family outbreaks of gastroenteritis. J Infect Dis 1977;135:20–27.

[197] Wyatt RG, Dolin R, Blacklow NR, et al. Comparison of three agents of acute infectious nonbacterial gastroenteritis by cross-challenge in volunteers. J Infect Dis 1974;129:709–714.

[198] Chiba S, Sakuma Y, Kogasaka R, et al. An outbreak of gastroenteritis associated with calicivirus in an infant home. J Med Virol 1979;4:249–254.

[199] Jiang X, Graham DY, Wang KN, Estes MK. Norwalk virus genome cloning and characterization. Science 1990;250:1580–1583.

[200] Jiang X, Wang M, Wang K, Estes MK. Sequence and genomic organization of Norwalk virus. Virology 1993;195:51–61.

[201] De Leon R, Matsui SM, Baric RS, et al. Detection of Norwalk virus in stool specimens by reverse transcriptasepolymerase chain reaction and nonradioactive oligoprobes. J Clin Microbiol 1992;30:3151–3157.

[202] Jiang X, Wang J, Graham DY, Estes MK. Detection of Norwalk virus in stool by polymerase chain reaction. J Clin Microbiol 1992;30:2529–2534.

[203] Jiang X, Wang M, Graham DY, Estes MK. Expression, self-assembly, and antigenicity of the Norwalk virus capsid protein. J Virol 1992;66:6527–6532.

[204] Baric RS, Yount B, Lindesmith L, et al. Expression and self-assembly of Norwalk virus capsid protein from Venezuelan equine encephalitis virus replicons. J Virol 2002;76:3023–3030.

[205] Mason HS, Ball JM, Shi JJ, Jiang X, Estes MK, Arntzen CJ. Expression of Norwalk virus capsid protein in transgenic tobacco and potato and its oral immunogenicity in mice. Proc Natl Acad Sci USA 1996;93:5335–5340.

[206] Graham DY, Jiang X, Tanaka T, Opekun AR, Madore HP, Estes MK. Norwalk virus infection of volunteers: new insights based on improved assays. J Infect Dis 1994;170:34–43.

[207] Monroe SS, Stine SE, Jiang X, Estes MK, Glass RI. Detection of antibody to recombinant Norwalk virus antigen in specimens from outbreaks of gastroenteritis. J Clin Microbiol 1993;31:2866–2872.

[208] Huang P, Farkas T, Marionneau S, et al. Noroviruses bind to human ABO, Lewis, and secretor histo-blood group antigens: identification of 4 distinct strainspecific patterns. J Infect Dis 2003;188:19–31.

[209] Marionneau S, Ruvoen N, Le Moullac-Vaidye B, et al. Norwalk virus binds to histo-blood group antigens present on gastroduodenal epithelial cells of secretor individuals. Gastroenterology 2002;122:1967–1977.

[210] Gray JJ, Cunliffe C, Ball J, Graham DY, Desselberger U, Estes MK. Detection of immunoglobulin M (IgM), IgA, and IgG Norwalk virus-specific antibodies by indirect enzyme-linked immunosorbent assay with baculovirus-expressed Norwalk virus capsid antigen in adult volunteers challenged with Norwalk virus. J Clin Microbiol 1994;32:3059–3063.

[211] Green KY, Lew JF, Jiang X, Kapikian AZ, Estes MK. Comparison of the reactivities of baculovirusexpressed recombinant Norwalk virus capsid antigen with those of the native Norwalk virus antigen in serologic assays and some epidemiologic observations. J Clin Microbiol 1993;31:2185–2191.

[212] Jiang X, Cubitt D, Hu J, et al. Development of an ELISA to detect MX virus, a human calicivirus in the Snow Mountain agent genogroup. J Gen Virol 1995;76:2739–2747.

[213] Jiang X, Wang J, Estes MK. Characterization of SRSVs using RT-PCR and a new antigen ELISA. Arch Virol 1995;140:363–374.

[214] Parker S, Cubitt D, Jiang JX, Estes M. Efficacy of a recombinant Norwalk virus protein enzyme immunoassay for the diagnosis of infections with Norwalk virus and other human "candidate" caliciviruses. J Med Virol 1993;41:179–184.

[215] Parker SP, Cubitt WD. Measurement of IgA responses following Norwalk virus infection and other human caliciviruses using a recombinant Norwalk virus protein EIA. Epidemiol Infect 1994;113:143–151.

[216] Parker SP, Cubitt WD, Jiang X. Enzyme immunoassay using baculovirus-expressed human calicivirus (Mexico) for the measurement of IgG responses and determining its seroprevalence in London, UK. J Med Virol 1995;46:194–200.

[217] Ball JM, Estes MK, Hardy ME, et al. Recombinant Norwalk virus-like particles as an oral vaccine. Arch Virol 1996;12:243–249.

[218] Ball JM, Graham AR, Opekun MA, et al. Recombinant Norwalk virus-like particles given orally to volunteers: phase I study. Gastroenterology 1999;117:40–48.

[219] Ball JM, Hardy ME, Atmar RL, Conner ME, Estes MK. Oral immunization with recombinant Norwalk viruslike particles induces a systemic and mucosal immune response in mice. J Virol 1998;72:1345–1353.

[220] Prasad BV, Hardy ME, Dokland T, Bella J, Rossmann MG, Estes MK. X-ray crystallographic structure of the Norwalk virus capsid. Science 1999;286:287–290.

[221] Prasad BV, Rothnagel R, Jiang X, Estes MK. Threedimensional structure of baculovirus-expressed Norwalk virus capsids. J Virol 1994;68:5117–5125.

[222] Prasad BV, Hardy ME, Estes MK. Structural studies of recombinant Norwalk capsids. J Infect Dis 2000;181: S317–321.

[223] Tan M, Hegde RS, Jiang X. The P domain of norovirus capsid protein forms dimer and binds to histo-blood group antigen receptors. J Virol 2004;78:6233–6242.

[224] Tan M, Huang P, Meller J, Zhong W, Farkas T, Jiang X. Mutations within the P2 domain of norovirus capsid affect binding to human histo-blood group antigens: evidence for a binding pocket. J Virol 2003;77:12562–12571.

[225] Greenberg HB, Valdesuso JR, Kalica AR, et al. Proteins of Norwalk virus. J Virol 1981;37:994–999.

[226] Matson DO, Zhong WM, Nakata S, et al. Molecular characterization of a human calicivirus with sequence relationships closer to animal caliciviruses than other known human caliciviruses. J Med Virol 1995;45:215–222.

[227] Dastjerdi AM, Green J, Gallimore CI, Brown DW, Bridger JC. The bovine Newbury agent-2 is genetically more closely related to human SRSVs than to animal caliciviruses. Virology 1999;254:1–5.

[228] Guo M, Chang KO, Hardy ME, Zhang Q, Parwani AV, Saif LJ. Molecular characterization of a porcine enteric calicivirus genetically related to Sapporo-like human caliciviruses. J Virol 1999;73:9625–9631.

[229] Sugieda M, Nagaoka H, Kakishima Y, Ohshita T, Nakamura S, Nakajima S. Detection of Norwalk-like virus genes in the caecum contents of pigs. Arch Virol 1998;143:1215–1221.

[230] van der Poel WH, Vinje J, van der Heide R, Herrera MI, Vivo A, Koopmans MP. Norwalk-like calicivirus genes in farm animals. Emerg Infect Dis 2000;6:36–41.

[231] Katayama K, Shirato-Horikoshi H, Kojima S, et al. Phylogenetic analysis of the complete genome of 18 Norwalk-like viruses. Virology 2002;299:225–239.

[232] Ando T, Noel JS, Fankhauser RL. Genetic classification of "Norwalk-like viruses." J Infect Dis 2000;181:S336–348.

[233] Schuffenecker I, Ando T, Thouvenot D, Lina B, Aymard M. Genetic classification of "Sapporo-like viruses." Arch Virol 2001;146:2115–2132.

[234] Karst SM, Wobus CE, Lay M, Davidson J, Virgin HWT. STAT1–dependent innate immunity to a Norwalk-like virus. Science 2003;299:1575–1578.

[235] Jiang X, Matson DO, Cubitt WD, Estes MK. Genetic and antigenic diversity of human caliciviruses (HuCVs) using RT-PCR and new EIAs. Arch Virol 1996;12:251– 262.

[236] Jiang X. Development of serological and molecular tests for the diagnosis of calicivirus infections. In: Desselberger U, Gray J, eds. Viral Gastroenteritis, 1st ed. Amsterdam: Elsevier Science BV, 2003:505–522.

[237] Jiang X, Wilton N, Zhong WM, et al. Diagnosis of human caliciviruses by use of enzyme immunoassays. J Infect Dis 2000;181:S349–S359.

[238] White LJ, Ball JM, Hardy ME, Tanaka TN, Kitamoto N, Estes MK. Attachment and entry of recombinant Norwalk virus capsids to cultured human and animal cell lines. J Virol 1996;70:6589–6597.

[239] Duizer E, Schwab KJ, Neill FH, Atmar RL, Koopmans MP, Estes MK. Laboratory efforts to cultivate noroviruses. J Gen Virol 2004;85:79–87.

[240] Flynn WT, Saif LJ. Serial propagation of porcine enteric calicivirus-like virus in primary porcine kidney cell cultures. J Clin Microbiol 1988;26:206–212.

[241] Guo M, Hayes J, Cho KO, Parwani AV, Lucas LM, Saif L. Comparative pathogenesis of tissue culture-adapted and wild-type Cowden porcine enteric calicivirus (PEC) in gnotobiotic pigs and induction of diarrhea by intravenous inoculation of wild-type PEC. J Virol 2001;75:9239–9251.

[242] Guo M, Saif LJ. Pathogenesis of enteric calicivirus infections. In: Desselberger U, Gray J, eds. Viral Gastroenteritis, 1st ed. Amsterdam: Elsevier Science BV, 2003:489–503.

[243] Chang KO, Sosnovtsev SV, Belliot G, et al. Bile acids are essential for porcine enteric calicivirus replication in association with down-regulation of signal transducer and activator of transcription 1. Proc Natl Acad Sci USA 2004;101:8733–8738.

[244] Wobus CE, Karst SM, Thackray LB, et al. Replication of norovirus in cell culture reveals a tropism for dendritic cells and macrophages. PLoS Biol 2004;2:e432.

[245] Dolin R, Levy AG, Wyatt RG, Thornhill TS, Gardner JD. Viral gastroenteritis induced by the Hawaii agent. Jejunal histopathology and serologic response. Am J Med 1975;59:761–768.

[246] Parrino TA, Schreiber DS, Trier JS, Kapikian AZ, Blacklow NR. Clinical immunity in acute gastroenteritis caused by Norwalk agent. N Engl J Med 1977; 297:86–89.

[247] Thornhill TS, Kalica AR, Wyatt RG, Kapikian AZ, Chanock RM. Pattern of shedding of the Norwalk particle in stools during experimentally induced gastroenteritis in volunteers as determined by immune electron microscopy. J Infect Dis 1975;132:28–34.

[248] Rockx B, De Wit M, Vennema H, et al. Natural history of human calicivirus infection: a prospective cohort study. Clin Infect Dis 2002;35:246–253.

[249] Pang XL, Joensuu, J, Vesikari T. Human calicivirus associated sporadic gastroenteritis in Finnish children less than two years of age followed prospectively during a rotavirus vaccine trial. Pediatr Infect Dis J 1999;18:420–426.

[250] Pang XL, Zeng SQ, Honma S, Nakata S, Vesikari T. Effect of rotavirus vaccine on Sapporo virus gastroenteritis in Finnish infants. Pediatr Infect Dis J 2001;20:295–300.

[251] Flynn WT, Saif LJ, Moorhead PD. Pathogenesis of porcine enteric calicivirus-like virus in four-day-old gnotobiotic pigs. Am J Vet Res 1988;49:819–825.

[252] Hardy ME, White LJ, Ball JM, Estes MK. Specific proteolytic cleavage of recombinant Norwalk virus capsid protein. J Virol 1995;69:1693–1698.

[253] Ruvoen-Clouet N, Ganiere JP, Andre-Fontaine G, Blanchard D, Le Pendu J. Binding of rabbit hemorrhagic disease virus to antigens of the ABH histoblood group family. J Virol 2000;74:11950–11954.

[254] Hutson AM, Atmar RL, Marcus DM, Estes MK. Norwalk virus-like particle hemagglutination by binding to histo-blood group antigens. J Virol 2003;77:405–415.

[255] Hutson AM, Atmar RL, Graham DY, Estes MK. Norwalk virus infection and disease is associated with ABO histo-blood group type. J Infect Dis 2002;185:1335–1337.

[256] Hennessy E, Green AD, Connor MP, Darby R, MacDonald P. Norwalk virus infection and disease is associated with ABO histo-blood group type. J Infect Dis 2003;188:176–177.

[257] Lindesmith L, Moe C, Marionneau S, et al. Human susceptibility and resistance to Norwalk virus infection. Nature Med 2003;9:548–553.

[258] Blacklow NR, Cukor G, Bedigian MK, et al. Immune response and prevalence of antibody to Norwalk enteritis virus as determined by radioimmunoassay. J Clin Microbiol 1979;10:903–909.

[259] Nakata S, Chiba S, Terashima H, Yokoyama T, Nakao T. Humoral immunity in infants with gastroenteritis caused by human calicivirus. J Infect Dis 1985;152:274–279.

[260] Evans MR, Meldrum R, Lane W, et al. An outbreak of viral gastroenteritis following environmental contamination at a concert hall. Epidemiol Infect 2002;129: 355–360.

[261] Marks PJ, Vipond IB, Carlisle D, Deakin D, Fey RE, Caul EO. Evidence for airborne transmission of Norwalklike virus (NLV) in a hotel restaurant. Epidemiol Infect 2000;124:481–487.

[262] Marks PJ, Vipond IB, Regan FM, Wedgewood K, Fey RE, Caul EO. A school outbreak of Norwalk-like virus: evidence for airborne transmission. Epidemiol Infect 2003;131:727–736.

[263] Cubitt WD, Green KY, Payment P. Prevalence of antibodies to the Hawaii strain of human calicivirus as measured by a recombinant protein based immunoassay. J Med Virol 1998;54:135–139.

[264] Gray JJ, Jiang X, Morgan-Capner P, Desselberger U, Estes MK. Prevalence of antibodies to Norwalk virus in England: detection by enzyme-linked immunosorbent assay using baculovirus-expressed Norwalk virus capsid antigen. J Clin Microbiol 1993;31:1022–1025.

[265] Jiang X, Matson DO, Velazquez FR, et al. Study of Norwalk-related viruses in Mexican children. J Med Virol 1995;47:309–316.

[266] Jing Y, Qian Y, Huo Y, Wang LP, Jiang X. Seroprevalence against Norwalk-like human caliciviruses in Beijing, China. J Med Virol 2000;60:97–101.

[267] Numata K, Nakata S, Jiang X, Estes MK, Chiba S. Epidemiological study of Norwalk virus infections in Japan and Southeast Asia by enzyme-linked immunosorbent assays with Norwalk virus capsid protein produced by the baculovirus expression system. J Clin Microbiol 1994;32:121–126.

[268] Parker SP, Cubitt WD, Jiang XJ, Estes MK. Seroprevalence studies using a recombinant Norwalk virus protein enzyme immunoassay. J Med Virol 1994;42:146–150.

[269] Farkas T, Jiang X, Guerrero ML, et al. Prevalence and genetic diversity of human caliciviruses (HuCVs) in Mexican children. J Med Virol 2000;62:217–223.

[270] Foley B, O'Mahony J, Morgan SM, Hill C, Morgan JG. Detection of sporadic cases of Norwalk-like virus (NLV) and astrovirus infection in a single Irish hospital from 1996 to 1998. J Clin Virol 2000;17:109–117.

[271] Kirkwood CD, Bishop RF. Molecular detection of human calicivirus in young children hospitalized with acute gastroenteritis in Melbourne, Australia, during 1999. J Clin Microbiol 2001;39:2722–2424.

[272] Marie-Cardine A, Gourlain K, Mouterde O, et al. Epidemiology of acute viral gastroenteritis in children

hospitalized in Rouen, France. Clin Infect Dis 2002; 34:1170–1178.

[273] Subekti DS, Tjaniadi P, Lesmana M, et al. Characterization of Norwalk-like virus associated with gastroenteritis in Indonesia. J Med Virol 2002;67:253–258.

[274] Roman E, Negredo A, Dalton RM, Wilhelmi I, Sanchez-Fauquier A. Molecular detection of human calicivirus among Spanish children with acute gastroenteritis. J Clin Microbiol 2002;40:3857–3859.

[275] Bon F, Fascia P, Dauvergne M, et al. Prevalence of group A rotavirus, human calicivirus, astrovirus, and adenovirus type 40 and 41 infections among children with acute gastroenteritis in Dijon, France. J Clin Microbiol 1999;37:3055–3058.

[276] Iritani N, Seto Y, Kubo H, et al. Prevalence of Norwalklike virus infections in cases of viral gastroenteritis among children in Osaka City, Japan. J Clin Microbiol 2003;41:1756–1759.

[277] Martinez N, Espul C, Cuello H, et al. Sequence diversity of human caliciviruses recovered from children with diarrhea in Mendoza, Argentina, 1995–1998. J Med Virol 2002;67:289–298.

[278] O'Ryan ML, Mamani N, Gaggero A, et al. Human caliciviruses are a significant pathogen of acute sporadic diarrhea in children of Santiago, Chile. J Infect Dis 2000;182:1519–1522.

[279] Bereciartu A, Bok K, Gómez J. Identification of viral agents causing gastroenteritis among children in Buenos Aires, Argentina. J Clin Virol 2002;25:197–203.

[280] Bonrud P, Volmer A, Dosch T, et al. Leads from the MMWR. Viral gastroenteritis—South Dakota and New Mexico. JAMA 1988;259:1459–1460.

[281] Qiao H, Nilsson M, Abreu ER, et al. Viral diarrhea in children in Beijing, China. J Med Virol 1999;57:390–396.

[282] Subekti D, Lesmana M, Tjaniadi P, et al. Incidence of Norwalk-like viruses, rotavirus and adenovirus infection in patients with acute gastroenteritis in Jakarta, Indonesia. FEMS Immunol Med Microbiol 2002;33:27–33.

[283] Wolfaardt M, Taylor MB, Booysen HF, Engelbrecht L, Grabow WO, Jiang X. Incidence of human calicivirus and rotavirus infection in patients with gastroenteritis in South Africa. J Med Virol 1997;51:290–296.

[284] Buesa J, Collado B, Lopez-Andujar P, et al. Molecular epidemiology of caliciviruses causing outbreaks and sporadic cases of acute gastroenteritis in Spain. J Clin Microbiol 2002;40:2854–2859.

[285] de Wit MA, Koopmans MP, Kortbeek LM, et al. Sensor, a population-based cohort study on gastroenteritis in the Netherlands: incidence and etiology. Am J Epidemiol 2001;154:666–674.

[286] McIver CJ, Hansman G, White P, Doultree JC, Catton M, Rawlinson WD. Diagnosis of enteric pathogens in children with gastroenteritis. Pathology 2001;33:353–358.

[287] Oh DY, Gaedicke G, Schreier E. Viral agents of acute gastroenteritis in German children: prevalence and molecular diversity. J Med Virol 2003;71:82–93.

[288] Sakai Y, Nakata S, Honma S, Tatsumi M, Numata-Kinoshita K, Chiba S. Clinical severity of Norwalk virus and Sapporo virus gastroenteritis in children in Hokkaido, Japan. Pediatr Infect Dis J 2001;20:849–853.

[289] Schnagl RD, Barton N, Patrikis M, Tizzard J, Erlich J, Morey F. Prevalence and genomic variation of Norwalk-like viruses in Central Australia in 1995–1997. Acta Virol 2000;44:265–271.

[290] Simpson R, Aliyu S, Iturriza-Gomara M, Desselberger U, Gray J. Infantile viral gastroenteritis: On the way to closing the diagnostic gap. J Med Virol 2003;70: 258–262.

[291] Traore O, Belliot G, Mollat C, et al. RT-PCR identification and typing of astroviruses and Norwalk-like viruses in hospitalized patients with gastroenteritis: evidence of nosocomial infections. J Clin Virol

2000;17:151–158.

[292] Fankhauser RL, Monroe SS, Noel JS, et al. Epidemiologic and molecular trends of "Norwalk-like viruses" associated with outbreaks of gastroenteritis in the United States. J Infect Dis 2002;186:1–7.

[293] Thornton SV, Davies DV, Chapman F, et al. Detection of Norwalk-like virus infection aboard two U.S. Navy ships. Mil Med 2002;167:826–830.

[294] Vinje J, Vennema L, Maunula L, et al. International collaborative study to compare reverse transcriptase PCR assays for detection and genotyping of noroviruses. J Clin Microbiol 2003;41:1423–1433.

[295] Okada M, Shinozake K, Ogawa T, Kaiho I. Molecular epidemiology and phylogenetic analysis of Sapporolike viruses. Arch Virol 2002;147:1445–1551.

[296] Chakrabarti S, Collingham KE, Stevens RH, et al. Isolation of viruses from stools in stem cell transplant recipients: a prospective surveillance study. Bone Marrow Transplant 2000;25:277–282.

[297] Kaufman SS, Chatterjee NK, Fuschino ME, et al. Calicivirus enteritis in an intestinal transplant recipient. Am J Transplant 2003;3:764–768.

[298] Cegielski JP, Msengi AE, Miller SE. Enteric viruses associated with HIV infection in Tanzanian children with chronic diarrhea. Pediatr AIDS HIV Infect 1994;5:296–299.

[299] Wardley RC, Povey RC. The clinical disease and patterns of excretion associated with three different strains of feline caliciviruses. Res Vet Sci 1977;23:7–14.

[300] Farkas T, Thornton SA, Wilton N, Zhong W, Altaye M, Jiang X. Homologous versus heterologous immune responses to Norwalk-Like viruses among crew members after acute gastroenteritis outbreaks on 2 US Navy vessels. J Infect Dis 2003;187:187–193.

[301] Estes MK, Ball JM, Guerrero RA, et al. Norwalk virus vaccines: challenges and progress. J Infect Dis 2000; 181:S367–373.

[302] Richter L, Mason HS, Arntzen CJ. Transgenic plants created for oral immunization against diarrheal diseases. J Travel Med 1996;3:52–56.

[303] Harrington PR, Yount B, Johnston RE, Davis N, Moe C, Baric RS. Systemic, mucosal, and heterotypic immune induction in mice inoculated with Venezuelan equine encephalitis replicons expressing Norwalk virus-like particles. J Virol 2002;76:730–742.

[304] Tacket CO, Mason HS, Losonsky G, Estes MK, Levine MM, Arntzen CJ. Human immune responses to a novel Norwalk virus vaccine delivered in transgenic potatoes. J Infect Dis 2000;182:302–305.

[305] Guerrero R, Ball J, Estes M. Immunogenicity in mice of recombinant Norwalk virus-like particles administered by mucosal routes. J Pediatr Gastroenterol Nutr 1998;26:547.

[306] Estes MK, Ball JM, Crawford SE, et al. Virus-like particle vaccines for mucosal immunization. Adv Exp Med Biol 1997;412:387–395.

[307] Periwal SB, Kourie KR, Ramachandaran N, et al. A modified cholera holotoxin CT-E29H enhances systemic and mucosal immune responses to recombinant Norwalk virus-virus like particle vaccine. Vaccine 2003;21:376–385.

[308] Prasad BV, Hardy ME, Jiang X, Estes MK. Structure of Norwalk virus. Arch Virol 1996;12:237–242.

[309] Monroe SS, Jiang B, Stine SE, et al. Subgenomic RNA sequence of human astrovirus supports classification of Astroviridae as a new family of RNA viruses. J Virol 1993;67:3611–3614.

[310] Madeley CR, Cosgrove BP. Viruses in infantile gastroenteritis. Lancet 1975;2:124.

[311] Lee TW, Kurtz JB. Serial propagation of astrovirus in tissue culture with the aid of trypsin. J Gen Virol 1981; 57:421–424.

[312] Risco C, Carrascosa JL, Pedregosa AM, et al. Ultrastructure of human astrovirus serotype 2. J Gen Virol

1995;76:2075–2080.

[313] Matsui M, Greenberg HB.Astroviruses. In: Knipe DM, Howley PM, eds. Fields Virology. Philadelphia: Lippincott Williams & Wilkins, 2001:875–916.

[314] Qureshi MA, Saif YM, Heggen-Peay CL, et al. Induction of functional defects in macrophages by a poultry enteritis and mortality syndrome-associated turkey astrovirus. Avian Dis 2001;45:853–861.

[315] Imada T, Yamaguchi S, Mase M, et al. Avian nephritis virus (ANV) as a new member of the family Astroviridae and construction of infectious ANV cDNA. J Virol 2000;74:8487–8493.

[316] Gough RE, Collins MS, Borland E, et al.Astrovirus-like particles associated with hepatitis in ducklings. Vet Rec 1984;114:279.

[317] Jiang B, Monroe SS, Koonin EV, et al. RNA sequence of astrovirus: distinctive genomic organization and a putative retrovirus-like ribosomal frameshifting signal that directs the viral replicase synthesis. Proc Nat Acad Sci USA 1993;90:10539–10543.

[318] Kiang D, Matsui SM. Proteolytic processing of a human astrovirus nonstructural protein. J Gen Virol 2002;83:25–34.

[319] Lewis TL, Matsui SM. An astrovirus frameshift signal induces ribosomal frameshifting in vitro. Arch Virol 1995;140:1127–1135.

[320] Donelli G, Superti F, Tinari A, et al. Mechanism of astrovirus entry into Graham 293 cells. J Med Virol 1992;38:271–277.

[321] Aroonprasert D, Fagerland JA, Kelso NE, et al. Cultivation and partial characterization of bovine astrovirus. Vet Microbiol 1989;19:113–125.

[322] Bass DM, Qiu S. Proteolytic processing of the astrovirus capsid. J Virol 2000;74:1810–1814.

[323] Mendez E, Fernandez-Luna T, Lopez S, et al. Proteolytic processing of a serotype 8 human astrovirus ORF2 polyprotein. J Virol 2002;76:7996–8002.

[324] Mendez E, Salas-Ocampo E, Arias CF.Caspases mediate processing of the capsid precursor and cell release of human astroviruses. J Virol 2004;78:8601–8608.

[325] Naficy AB, Rao MR, Holmes JL, et al.Astrovirus diarrhea in Egyptian children. J Infect Dis 2000;182:685–690.

[326] Mitchell DK, Van R, Morrow AL, et al. Outbreaks of astrovirus gastroenteritis in day care centers. J Pedriatr 1993;123:725–732.

[327] Traore O, Belliot G, Mollat C, et al. RT-PCR identification and typing of astroviruses and Norwalk-like viruses in hospitalized patients with gastroenteritis: evidence of nosocomial infections. J Clin Virol 2000;17:151–158.

[328] Phillips AD, Rice S,Walker-Smith JA.Astrovirus within the human small intestinal mucosa. Gut 1982;23: A923–A924.

[329] Kurtz JB, Lee TW, Craig JW, et al. Astrovirus infection in volunteers. J Med Virol 1979;3:221–230.

[330] Midthun K, Greenberg HB, Kurtz JB, et al. Characterization and seroepidemiology of a type 5 astrovirus associated with an outbreak of gastroenteritis in Marin County, California. J Clin Microbiol 1993;31:955–962.

[331] Sebire, NJ, Malone M, Shah N, et al. Pathology of astrovirus associated diarrhoea in a paediatric bone marrow transplant recipient. J Clin Pathol 2004;57:1001–1003.

[332] Gray EW, Angus KW, Snodgrass DR. Ultrastructure of the small intestine in astrovirus-infected lambs. J Gen Virol 1980;49:71–82.

[333] Hall GA. Comparative pathology of infection by novel diarrhoea viruses. Ciba Fdn Sym 1987;128:192–

[334] Snodgrass DR, Angus KW, Gray EW, et al. Pathogenesis of diarrhoea caused by astrovirus infections in lambs. Arch Virol 1979;60:217–226.

[335] Woode GN, Pohlenz JF, Gourley NE, et al. Astrovirus and Breda virus infections of dome cell epithelium of bovine ileum. J Clin Microbiol 1984;19:623–630.

[336] Baxendale W, Mebatsion T. The isolation and characterisation of astroviruses from chickens. Avian Path 2004;33:364–370.

[337] Koci MD, Moser LA, Kelley LA, et al. Astrovirus induces diarrhea in the absence of inflammation and cell death. J Virol 2003;77:11798–11808.

[338] Oishi I, Yamazaki K, Kimoto T, et al. A large outbreak of acute gastroenteritis associated with astrovirus among students and teachers in Osaka, Japan. J Infect Dis 1994;170:439–443.

[339] Glass RI, Noel J, Mitchell D, et al. The changing epidemiology of astrovirus-associated gastroenteritis: a review. Arch Virol 1996;12:287–300.

[340] Herrmann JE, Taylor DN, Echeverria P, et al. Astroviruses as a cause of gastroenteritis in children. N Engl J Med 1991;324:1757–1760.

[341] Cruz JR, Bartlett AV, Herrmann JE, et al. Astrovirusassociated diarrhea among Guatemalan ambulatory rural children. J Clin Microbiol 1992;30:1140–1144.

[342] Unicomb LE, Banu NN, Azim T, et al. Astrovirus infection in association with acute, persistent and nosocomial diarrhea in Bangladesh. Pedriatr Infect Dis J 1998;17:611–614.

[343] Shastri S, Doane AM, Gonzales J, et al. Prevalence of astroviruses in a children's hospital. J Clin Microbiol 1998;36:2571–2574.

[344] Rodriguez-Baez N, O'Brien R, Qiu SQ, et al. Astrovirus, adenovirus, and rotavirus in hospitalized children: prevalence and association with gastroenteritis. J Pediatr Gastroenterol Nutr 2002;35:64–68.

[345] Schnagl RD, Belfrage K, Farrington R, et al. Incidence of human astrovirus in central Australia (1995 to 1998) and comparison of deduced serotypes detected from 1981 to 1998. J Clin Microbiol 2002;40:4114–4120.

[346] Dalton RM, Roman ER, Negredo AA, et al. Astrovirus acute gastroenteritis among children in Madrid, Spain. Pedriatr Infect Dis J 2002;21:1038–1041.

[347] Liu CY, Shen KL, Wang SX, et al. Astrovirus infection in young children with diarrhea hospitalized at Beijing Children's Hospital. Chin Med J 2004;117:353–356.

[348] Phan TG, Okame M, Nguyen TA, et al. Human astrovirus, norovirus (GI, GII), and sapovirus infections in Pakistani children with diarrhea. J Med Virol 2004;73:256–261.

[349] Espul C, Martinez N, Noel JS, et al. Prevalence and characterization of astroviruses in Argentinean children with acute gastroenteritis. J Med Virol 2004;72:75–82.

[350] Mitchell DK, Matson DO, Cubitt WD, et al. Prevalence of antibodies to astrovirus types 1 and 3 in children and adolescents in Norfolk, Virginia. Pediatr Infect Dis J 1999;18:249–254.

[351] Koopmans, MP, Bijen MH, Monroe SS, et al. Agestratified seroprevalence of neutralizing antibodies to astrovirus types 1 to 7 in humans in the Netherlands. Clin Diag Lab Immunol 1998;5:33–37.

[352] Kriston S, Willcocks MM, Carter MJ, et al. Seroprevalence of astrovirus types 1 and 6 in London, determined using recombinant virus antigen. Epidemiol Infect 1996;117:159–164.

[353] Lewis DC, Lightfoot NF, Cubitt WD, et al. Outbreaks of astrovirus type 1 and rotavirus gastroenteritis in a geriatric in-patient population. J Hosp Infect 1989;14:9–14.

[354] Gray JJ, Wreghitt TG, Cubitt WD, et al. An outbreak of gastroenteritis in a home for the elderly associated

with astrovirus type 1 and human calicivius. J Med Virol 1987;23:377–381.

[355] Belliot G, Laveran H, Monroe SS. Outbreak of gastroenteritis in military recruits associated with serotype 3 astrovirus infection. J Med Virol 1997;51:101–106.

[356] Maunula L, Kalso S, Von Bonsdorff CH, et al. Wading pool water contaminated with both noroviruses and astroviruses as the source of a gastroenteritis outbreak. Epidemiol Infect 2004;132:737–743.

[357] Noel J and Cubitt D. Identification of astrovirus serotypes from children treated at the Hospitals for Sick Children, London 1981–93. Epidemiol Infect 1994;113:153–159.

[358] Wood DJ, David TJ, Chrystie IL, et al. Chronic enteric virus infection in two T-cell immunodeficient children. J Med Virol 1988;24:435–444.

[359] Grohmann GS, Glass RI, Pereira HG, et al. Enteric viruses and diarrhea in HIV-infected patients. Enteric opportunistic infections working group. N Engl J Med 1993;329:14–20.

[360] Cubitt WD, Mitchell DK, Carter MJ, et al. Application of electron microscopy, enzyme immunoassay, and RT-PCR to monitor an outbreak of astrovirus type 1 in a paediatric bone marrow transplant unit. J Med Virol 1999;57:313–321.

[361] Cox GJ, Matsui SM, Lo RS, et al. Etiology and outcome of diarrhea after marrow transplantation: a prospective study. Gastroenterology 1994;107:1398–1407.

[362] Liste MB, Natera I, Suarez JA, et al. Enteric virus infections and diarrhea in healthy and human immunodeficiency virus-infected children. J Clin Microbiol 2000;38:2873–2877.

[363] Coppo P, Scieux C, Ferchal F, et al. Astrovirus enteritis in a chronic lymphocytic leukemia patient treated with fludarabine monophosphate. Annals Hematol 2000;79:43–45.

[364] Yuen KY, Woo PC, Liang RH, et al. Clinical significance of alimentary tract microbes in bone marrow transplant recipients. Diag Microbiol Infect Dis 1998;30: 75–81.

[365] Bass DM, Upadhyayula U. Characterization of human serotype 1 astrovirus-neutralizing epitopes. J Virol 1997;71:8666–8671.

[366] Molberg O, Nilsen EM, Sollid LM, et al. $CD4^+$ T cells with specific reactivity against astrovirus isolated from normal human small intestine (see comment). Gastroenterology 1998;114:115–122.

第5章
病毒性疾病的口腔表现
Denis P. Lynch

口腔是由软、硬两种组织构成的独特的生态系统。口腔、口咽部及邻近的唾液腺软组织对不同病毒感染特别敏感,其中部分病毒感染具有位点特异性。从简单的复层鳞状上皮如唇黏膜到高度特化组织如背侧舌组成口腔黏膜。腺组织分为浆液型、黏液型和混合型。此外,口腔能够表现出许多因HIV而诱发的免疫抑制所产生的继发性细菌、真菌和病毒性感染及肿瘤。因此,口腔的表现对反映病毒介导的免疫抑制进程而言起到"生物晴雨表"的作用。

在口腔病毒性疾病中,不同病原体的传染性差异显著。口腔传染的后遗症的严重程度也各有不同,从无关紧要到具有潜在致死性。这不仅是牙科保健工作者需要关注的,也是任何负责口腔检查或口腔组织处理的健康工作者需要关注的。特别需要说明的是,与大多数医师相比,皮肤科医师更有可能参与到口腔和邻近组织的检查及口腔软组织病变的后续诊断和治疗。

本章包括四部分内容。第一部分介绍重要的口腔疾病、损伤和病毒病原学概况,重点是流行病学,特殊病毒感染的病理生理学将在其他章节阐述。第二部分介绍病毒感染引起的口腔病变的临床表现,重点阐述特殊病毒口腔病变的鉴别诊断。第三部分介绍病毒引起的口腔病变的诊断方法。第四部分介绍现行治疗处置策略的概要及其与长期预后的关系。

本章最后总结了HIV感染的口腔表现,包括因HIV感染导致的免疫抑制个体重要的非病毒性感染和口腔肿瘤。

疱疹病毒

疱疹病毒是引起口腔疾病的最庞大的病毒家族(表5.1)[1]。已知有8个型别的疱疹病毒对人类致病,它们均与口腔疾病具有不同程度的显著相关性。单纯疱疹病毒1型(herpes simplex virus-1,HSV-1)是最常见的口腔和经口感染的病毒;HSV-2通常感染生殖器,但是也有关于口腔病变的报道。

表 5.1　病毒性疾病的口腔表现

病毒家族	病毒	疾病
疱疹病毒	HSV-1（疱疹1）	原发性疱疹性龈口炎
		复发性口内疱疹
		唇疱疹（热病性疱疹或感冒疮）
	HSV-2（疱疹2）	与 HSV-1 无明显区别
	VZV（疱疹3）	水痘（禽痘）
		带状疱疹（蛇盘疮）
	EBV（疱疹4）	单核细胞增多症
		伯基特淋巴瘤
		鼻咽癌
		口腔毛状白斑
	CMV（疱疹5）	涎腺增大
		口腔阿弗他溃疡
	KSHV（疱疹8）	卡波西肉瘤
乳头瘤病毒	乳头瘤病毒	口腔疣
		尖锐湿疣
		局灶性上皮细胞增多症（Heck 氏病）
副黏液病毒	麻疹病毒	麻疹
腮腺炎	腮腺炎病毒	腮腺炎
小 RNA 病毒	柯萨奇病毒	手足口病
		疱疹性咽峡炎

原发性水痘 - 带状疱疹病毒（varicella-zoster virus，VZV）（或疱疹3）感染或水痘的口腔表现被皮肤表现所掩盖，然而复发性 VZV 感染可同时出现面部和口腔内部的临床症状及体征。EB 病毒（Epstein-Barr virus，EBV 或疱疹4）感染与传染性单核细胞增多症、伯基特淋巴瘤、鼻咽癌和毛状白斑的发生有关。巨细胞病毒（cytomegalovirus，CMV 或疱疹5）感染可导致涎腺增大，最近发现在 HIV 感染的免疫抑制个体中也会发生 CMV 相关性溃疡。人疱疹病毒 6 型（HHV-6，疱疹6）是幼儿急疹（猝发疹）的病原体，与特异性口腔病变的关系仍不明确。HHV-7 型（疱疹7）还未发现引发口腔黏膜表现。有证据表明，HHV-8 型（疱疹8）在 AIDS 患者中是卡波西肉瘤（Kaposi's sarcoma，KS）的病原体。

HSV-1

HSV-1 是最常见的感染人类的疱疹病毒[2~5]。由于在感染初期，口腔病变大多数发生在齿龈，所以通常被称为原发性疱疹性龈口炎，但是感染也可能会累及唇红部和口腔内黏膜的任何位置。虽然 HSV-1 感染导致皮肤棘层松解伴随小囊泡形成，但是完整的口腔内小囊泡罕见，可能由于说话、进食和吞咽等动作的摩擦导致小囊泡发生破裂。

病毒的激活与很多诱导因素有关，如与唇疱疹发生最为密切的因素是紫外线暴露（表5.2）[6]。所有这些因素都会对感染患者产生某种应激，而每个个体对于这些应激的反应又是千差万别的。

活化后的 HSV-1 可以沿着神经轴突运送到身体远端的上皮细胞完成远距离传播，并在此复制，导致皮肤棘层松解和典型的小囊泡丛生，其原因不是完全清楚。继发感染范围比较局限，并少有全身表现。有趣的是，复发性病变经常在相同的解剖学位置发生。激活因素列于表5.2 中。

表 5.2　常见的导致潜伏 HSV-1 激活因素

紫外线（阳光）
情绪紧张
内分泌波动（月经和怀孕）
发烧
物理外伤
免疫抑制
上呼吸道感染
过敏
胃肠道紊乱

口腔表现

即使在其他方面健康的儿童中，原发性疱疹性龈口炎仍然具有相当典型的临床表现[7]。通常婴幼儿会表现为中度发热，并伴有头痛、精神萎靡、吞咽困难、间歇性关节痛和颈部淋巴结肿大[8]。小囊泡可能会发生在唇红部和口周皮肤等部位（图 5.1），但是口腔内病变（尤其是齿龈）常常占主导地位（图 5.2~图 5.4）[9]。与口腔复发性疱疹性病变不同，原发性感染同时累及角质化和非角质化的口腔黏膜，而咽部常常幸免。病变通常在第 10~14 天消退，此时病毒移行到周围神经节并且休眠[10]。

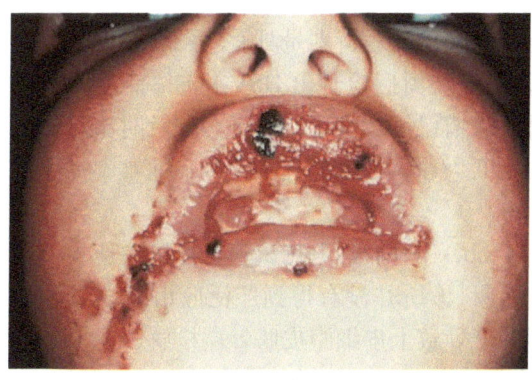

图 5.1　原发性 HSV-1 感染。唇红部流血、结痂和囊泡破裂的症状让人回忆起发生于成人的多形性红斑。

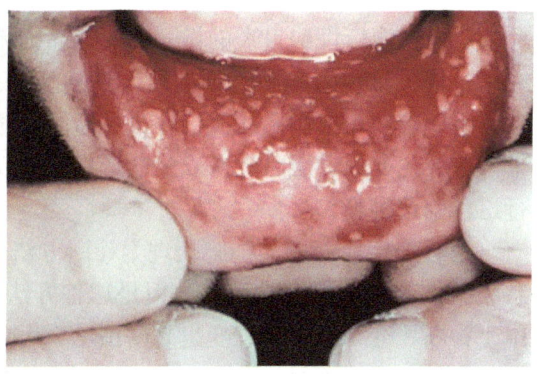

图 5.2　原发性 HSV-1 感染。在角质化牙龈（如硬腭和齿龈）没有共发病变，下唇黏膜上的破裂小囊泡在临床表现上与非病毒性的疱疹样口疮没有明显区别（Source: Courtesy of J. Robert Newland, D.D.S., M.S., University of Texas, Houston Health Science Center, Dental Branch）。

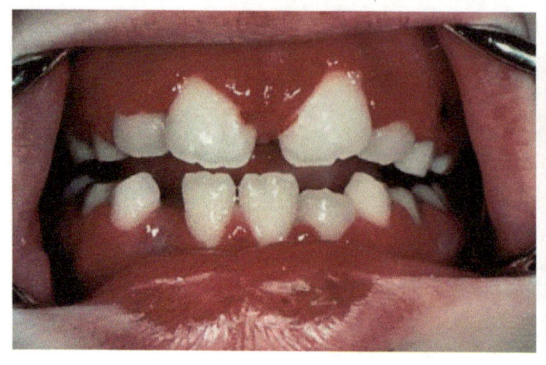 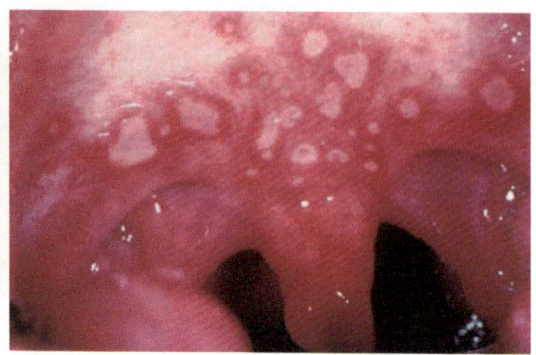

图 5.3　原发性 HSV-1 感染。齿龈小囊泡和继发性溃疡是原发性疱疹性龈口炎的临床标志（Source: Courtesy of J. Robert Newland, D.D.S., M.S., University of Texas, Houston Health Science Center, Dental Branch）。

图 5.4　原发性 HSV-1 感染。原发性疱疹性龈口炎也可发生于成人，累及软腭，导致吞咽困难。

复发性病变，尤其是在唇红部，与显著的个性化的前驱症状相关，经常被描述为麻刺感、紧缩感、烧灼感或者瘙痒。在前驱症状出现的 24h 内，多发的小囊泡出现并迅速合并、破裂而形成典型的热病性疱疹或感冒疮（图 5.5）。在免疫抑制个体中，病毒被激活的频率也会增加。

复发性口腔病变局限于角质化黏膜，即附着龈（图 5.6 和图 5.7）和硬腭（图 5.8 和图 5.9）。这一点与复发性阿弗他溃疡不同，后者仅发生在非角质化黏膜[11, 12]。复发性口腔内病变很少有前驱症状的报道，并且完整小囊泡也明显少见。口腔内病变的临床过程与唇红部和口周损伤平行发生，14 天内可完全消退。

诊断

原发性疱疹性龈口炎的诊断主要依靠临床症状和体征，特别是具有病毒暴露史的有力证据，如父母或者同胞近期的复发性病变史。发病 2 周后检测出 HSV-1 抗体滴度 4 倍升高也可以确诊，但利用此方法作出论断结论时，病情已经缓解了。由于必须及时治疗，对于一些其他方面健康且无并发症的病例，如仅推断为原发性疱疹性龈口炎，通常不需要进行这种确诊实验。

尽管疱疹性病变的细胞病理学诊断方法（Tzanck test，察内克试验）可以快速检测被感染上皮细胞的病理性改变，但是这种方法在牙科诊所并没有得到广泛应用[13]。即使不用于诊断，这种病理性改变也高度预示着病毒感染导致上皮细胞皮肤棘层松解。

虽然病毒培养是诊断 HSV-1 口腔感染的"金标准"，但是由于费用高和诊断延迟的原因，并没有得到广泛应用。然而，在特殊情况下可使用此方法，如免疫抑制患者出现持续的囊泡性溃疡病变[14]。当样本中 HSV-1 感染水平较低时，可以使用聚合酶链反应（polymerase chain reaction，PCR）技术放大病毒拷贝数来进行检测[15]。

鉴别诊断

原发性疱疹性龈口炎在临床上有时候会与小脓疱疹混淆，特别是当病变主要发生在口周，而不是口内时。成人原发性疱疹性龈口炎有时被误诊为多形性红斑[16]。遇到这种情况应特别慎重，因为这样的患者通常会使用皮质激素进行治疗，而这种治疗可能会加重潜

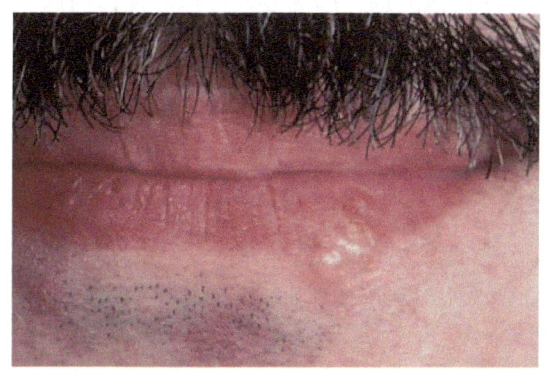

图 5.5 复发性 HSV-1 感染。典型的复发性疱疹病变发生于下唇的唇红部和周围皮肤，首先是瘙痒、烧灼感、刺痛感或紧缩感等前驱症状，然后是疱疹样小囊泡暴发、合并和破裂。

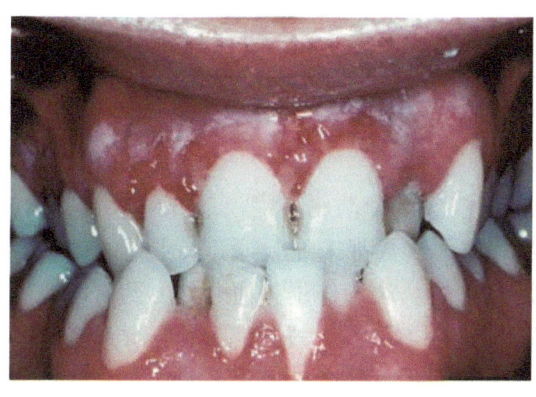

图 5.6 复发性 HSV-1 感染。复发性口腔内 HSV-1 感染的特征是偶发的小囊泡和齿龈溃疡。这些病变与寻常型天疱疮的齿龈病变相似（Source: Courtesy of J. Robert Newland, D.D.S., M.S., University of Texas, Houston Health Science Center, Dental Branch）。

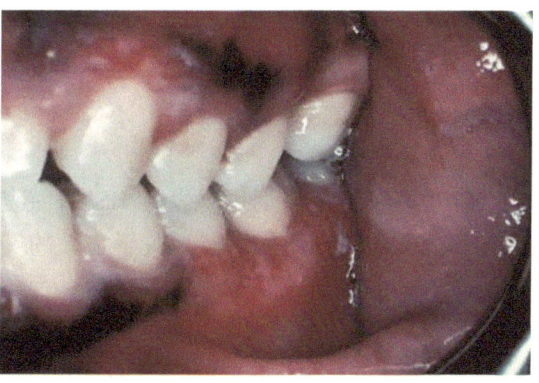

图 5.7 口腔内 HSV-1 复发性感染。牙科手术过程中的意外创伤可能会加速口腔内 HSV-1 的复发性感染，在实施前后全身注射阿昔洛韦可用来预防此类复发性感染。

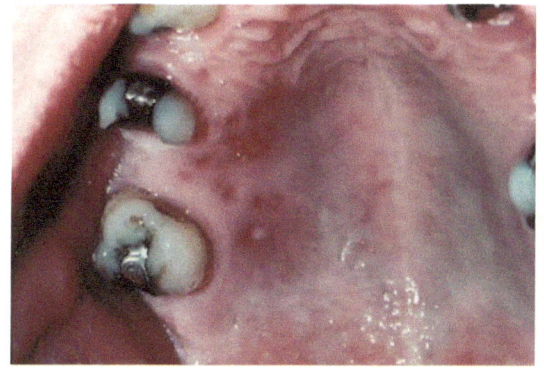

图 5.8 复发性 HSV-1 感染。复发性口腔内 HSV-1 感染可能累及上腭，并且无唇疱疹史。

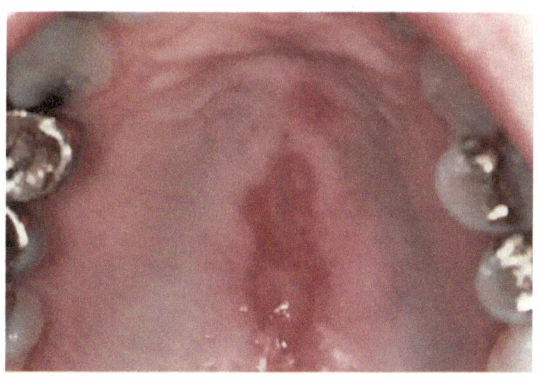

图 5.9 复发性 HSV-1 感染。破损的囊泡迅速合并成被假膜覆盖的不规则的浅表糜烂。

在的原发性病毒感染。

唇疱疹的临床诊断并不难,因为患者病史经常可以用来确诊[17]。通过病变的解剖位置不同可以明显地区别疱疹性口内病变和复发性阿弗他溃疡,因为复发性疱疹性口内病变只发生在角质化黏膜(附着龈和硬腭),而复发性阿弗他溃疡只发生在非角质化黏膜(唇、口颊黏膜、牙槽龈、舌、口底、软腭和口咽部)[18, 19]。表5.3提供了更多的鉴别诊断信息。

表5.3 复发性HSV-1和HSV-2损害的鉴别诊断

阿弗他溃疡:	仅发生在非角质化黏膜(唇、颊、舌、齿龈黏膜、软腭和口咽部),且前期无囊泡。
小脓疱疹:	通常主要累及口周和邻近的面部皮肤。
多形性红斑:	累及唇红部的血性突起的小囊泡和大囊泡;常发生于可见皮肤的特征性的牛眼状病变、同心圆状靶形和虹膜样病变。
唇疱疹:	刺痛、烧灼或悸动等前驱症状;聚集性小水泡。
水痘-带状疱疹:	口内水痘-带状疱疹病变不常见于原发性感染(水痘);复发性病变(带状疱疹)表现为疼痛、沿皮节分布的单侧疱疹。

治疗和预后

针对原发性,特别是复发性HSV-1感染有很多的治疗药物[20~28](表5.4)。虽然有许多非处方药可以使用,但是关于它们的实际疗效大多数都未经验证,其主要的效果似乎是某一个症状的减轻和安慰剂效应,而不是真正的杀病毒作用。而非处方药(OTC)Abreva™(10%二十二烷醇)与治疗唇疱疹的处方药霜和药膏的治疗指数相同(表5.5)[29]。

表5.4 口腔HSV-1型感染的治疗性药物

药物	剂型	使用方式
无环鸟苷(Zovirax™)	胶囊	全身
无环鸟苷(Zovirax™)	软膏	局部
无环鸟苷(Zovirax™)	霜剂	局部
喷昔洛韦(Denavir™)	霜剂	局部
更昔洛韦(Cytovene™)	胶囊	全身
	粉剂	静脉
万乃洛韦(Valtrex™)	糖衣片	全身
泛昔洛韦(Famvir™)	片剂	全身
膦甲酸钠(Foscavir™)	溶液	静脉
疱疹净(Stoxil™)	眼科软膏	局部
阿糖腺苷(Vira-A™)	眼科软膏	局部
曲氟尿苷(Viroptic™)	眼科溶液	局部

虽然美国食品药品管理局（Food and Drug Administration，FDA）没有批准用于无并发症的原发性和复发性口腔 HSV-1 感染的全身性抗病毒治疗药物（如阿昔洛韦），但是经验和初步报告表明，早期使用阿昔洛韦进行全身治疗干预，在很大程度上可以减轻原发性疱疹性龈口炎的临床症状和体征[30]。

虽然全身性使用阿昔洛韦也可用于复发性唇疱疹治疗，但是如果这种治疗不是在前驱症状刚开始时则是无效的[31]。据报道，全身应用阿昔洛韦可以有效预防并阻止 HSV-1 复发性感染，但是也会加速其他症状的出现，如多形性红斑[32]。因此，处理阿昔洛韦耐药性 HSV 感染的方案也已经形成[33]。表 5.6 列出了 HSV-1 的对症治疗方法。

表 5.5 在口腔 HSV-1 复发感染治疗中应用的非处方制剂

抗病毒药
Abreva™（10% 二十二烷醇）
阻断和镇静剂
Orabase™
Orabase™（添加苯佐卡因）
Anbesol™ 凝胶
Anbesol™ 液体
Zilactin™ 和 Zilactin-B™ 凝胶
Zilactin-L™ 液体
Campho-Phenique™ 凝胶
干燥剂
乙醇
乙醚
氯仿
紫外线阻断剂
Chap-Stick™ Sunblock 15 balm
Herpecin-L™ balm
Pre-Sun-15™ lotion
Pre-Sun-15™ 唇胶

表 5.6 常见 HSV-1 的治疗方法

原发性疱疹性龈口炎	
普通口腔不适	局部麻醉，对乙酰氨基酚黏膜涂层剂（Kaopectate™ 和 Magnesia™ 乳液）
脱水	补水
	冰棍、冰块用于缓解痛苦
	Gatorade™ 和 Powerade™
唇疱疹	用对氨基安息香酸唇香膏阻断，其他 UV 阻断剂
前驱症状	Abreva™ 或 Denavir™ 每 2h 用一次，全身药物对健康人通常不采用。Cytovene™、Valtrex™、Famvir™、Zovirax™ 和 Foscavir™ 对免疫抑制患者有效
热病疱疹/唇疱疹	干燥剂（乙醇、乙醚和氯仿），局部麻醉，对乙酰氨基酚，封闭敷料（Zilactin-L™），避免直接用指尖，健康人全身药效果最小
	Cytovene™、Valtrex™、Famvir™、Zovirax™、Foscavir™ 对免疫抑制患者有效
复发性口腔疱疹-1	局部麻醉，对乙酰氨基酚包衣剂（Kaopectate™、Magnesia™ 奶），封闭敷料（Orabase™、Zilactin-B™）
疱疹性瘭疽	全身用 Zovirax™ 或抗病毒药物同系物，通过使用屏障预防（手套）来避免
疱疹性结膜炎	见第 6 章附加信息

局部应用阿昔洛韦软膏进行治疗非常流行，尤其在前驱症状出现阶段进行治疗的效果最好[34~38]。被 FDA 批准用于治疗唇疱疹的阿昔洛韦药霜，其疗效比软膏更好，因为药霜更容易穿透皮肤和唇红部。Denavir™ 药霜（1% 喷阿昔洛韦）首次被 FDA 批准用于免疫

功能正常患者的复发性唇疱疹治疗[39, 40]。由于潜在的耐药性，抗病毒治疗药物在严重的原发性和复发性 HSV-1 病例的治疗中受到一定的限制[41~43]。

其他治疗药物包括环氧合酶抑制剂[44]、洗必泰[45]、疱疹净[46]、阿糖腺苷[47]和解螺旋酶引酶抑制剂[48]。对于很多感染病例来说，可以使用对氨基苯甲酸和其他能阻断紫外线的药物制成的唇膏或制剂来有效阻断唇疱疹[49]。

支持疗法和姑息疗法对原发性和复发性 HSV-1 感染的治疗也是必不可少的[50]。表 5.7 列出了在姑息疗法中使用的含有黏膜涂层剂和麻醉剂的口腔洗液，它们可以减轻复发性口内疱疹病变引起的不适感。

表 5.7　口腔溃疡治疗中使用的姑息漱口剂

局部麻醉剂	黏膜涂层剂
苯佐卡因（Ceatcaine™）液体	硫糖铝（Carafate™）悬液*
利多卡因（Xylocaine™）	氧化镁（Magnesia™）Phillips 液体奶
Dyclonine（Cyclone™）液体	氢氧化铅、氢氧化镁混合物（Maalox™）悬液
苯海拉明（Benadryl™）配剂**	白陶土和果胶制剂（kaopectate™）液体
苯海拉明（Benadryl™）糖浆**	氢氧化铝凝胶（Amphogel™）悬液
异丙嗪（Phenergan™）糖浆**	盖胃平（Gaviscon™）液体

特定的麻醉剂和黏膜涂层剂通常按 1:1 的体积比混合用于漱口。
*1.0g 片剂溶于 5ml H_2O 中配制。
** 抗组胺药与局部麻醉剂合用。

虽然在其他方面健康患者中，原发性 HSV-1 感染的预后是良好的，但是免疫抑制患者却更容易发生严重疾病[51, 52]。其他方面健康患者的损伤在第 10~14 天消退，并且不会以如此复杂的形式复发。然而，不幸的是，复发性 HSV-1 病变可能几个星期就要复发一次，这取决于患者的体格和其他个人因素。虽然病变具有一定的发病率，但是并发症却不常见。

在由于肿瘤[53]、癌症化疗[54~56]、放疗[57]或准备接受器官或组织移植[58~62]而引起的免疫抑制患者中，原发性和复发性 HSV-1 感染均有明显的并发症。在这些患者中，口内 HSV-1 病变更加严重且病程更长。在 HIV 阳性的免疫抑制个体中，复发性 HSV-1 感染非常广泛，就像 HSV-1 的原发性感染一样。在这些患者中，阿昔洛韦和相关的全身性抗病毒药物不仅常用于预防复发性感染，也用于治疗复发性感染[63]。

疱疹性瘭疽

在一些特定的个体中，疱疹性病变具有独特的表现。疱疹性瘭疽（herpetic whitlow）是常见的威胁牙科工作者的职业病危害[64~67]。这种情况是由于指垫或甲床周期性感染疱疹病毒引起的，与唇红部和口周皮肤的复发性 HSV-1 感染类似。在手指或指甲根部的外皮上会出现疼痛的疱疹样囊泡簇，随后囊泡会发生破裂、结痂和愈合（图 5.10）。阿昔洛韦对疱疹性瘭疽有治疗作用[68]。幸运的是，在广泛使用了保护装置后，这种职业危害几乎就消失了。但是疱疹性瘭疽仍然可以在手 - 生殖器接触后由 HSV-2 感染引发。

疱疹性结膜炎是牙科的另一种职业危害，但是在使用保护眼罩后，发病率显著下降（图 5.11）。虽然疱疹性结膜炎的发生频率低于疱疹性瘭疽，但是即使进行积极的治疗，仍然有可能导致失明[69, 70]。而且深度知觉的双眼视力在大多数牙科手术中都是必需的，因此疱疹性结膜炎的并发症可能会对受感染牙医的手术操作能力产生深远影响。

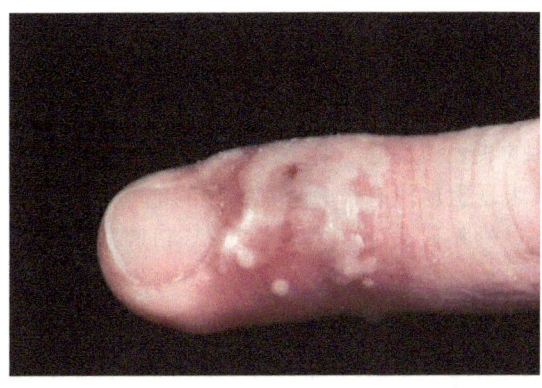 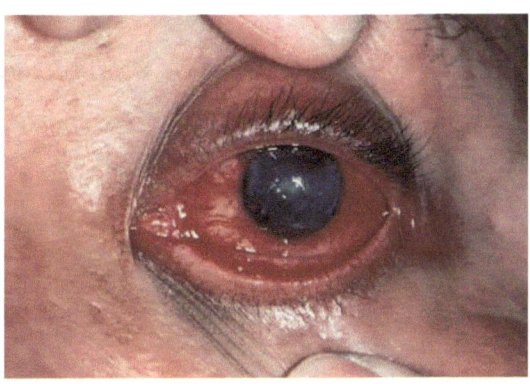

图 5.10 疱疹性瘭疽。在普遍预防之前，疱疹性瘭疽是牙科领域重要的职业危害。幸运的是，乳胶手套在所有牙科手术中的使用，使得这种感染几乎消除了。

图 5.11 疱疹性结膜炎。如果疱疹病毒感染眼睛后不进行处理，有可能导致失明。与疱疹性瘭疽一样，通过保护性眼罩的使用几乎消除了这种感染。

HSV-2

HSV-2 偶尔可作为口腔原发和复发疾病的病原体。由于 HSV-2 感染的诊断通常只是基于临床症状，而缺乏病毒培养或分型的辅助，所以 HSV-2 感染导致口腔病变的流行情况还不清楚。一种假设认为，口腔中 HSV-2 病变的增加是由口腔和生殖器接触频率的增加导致的，但也只是推测。

口腔 HSV-2 感染的临床表现与口腔 HSV-1 感染相同[71]（图 5.12），口腔 HSV-2 病变对相同治疗方法的反应也与 HSV-1 一致。

VZV 或 HHV-3

VZV 口腔病变与 HSV-1 具有很多相似之处[72]。两种病毒均导致原发性黏膜皮肤出疹和口腔内病变，表现为易破损的小疱、破裂后形成浅表溃疡[73]。

与 HSV-1 一样，VZV 原发性感染后潜伏于神经节中并可被激活。病毒激活后从神经元向轴突移行，沿着被感染神经的分布呈现特征性的疱疹。这种病变通常称为带状疱疹，被感染个体的年龄跨度较大，从儿童[74]

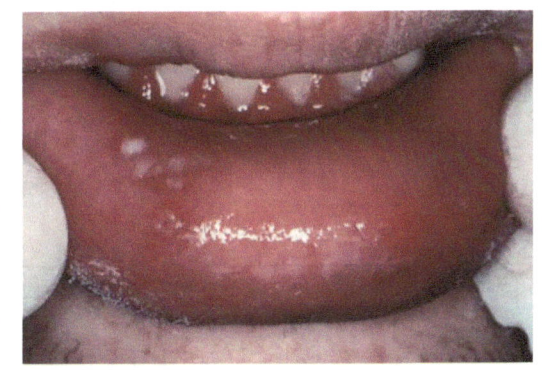

图 5.12 原发性 HSV-2 病变。这是口腔 - 生殖器接触而感染的病例，病变表现与 HSV-1 感染相同。

到老年人[75]均可发生。

虽然大多数成年人在儿童时代感染过VZV并发展为水痘，但是只有很少一部分人会复发。某些导致免疫抑制的因素更容易诱发带状疱疹。造血器官或淋巴系统恶性肿瘤、HIV阳性患者、化疗患者和器官移植患者复发的风险最高。有文献记载，神经根的物理外伤也是一种诱发因素。有一小部分患者发生特发性的VZV复发性感染，但是没有任何明显的诱发因素[76]。

口腔表现

虽然原发性VZV感染可以导致口腔病变，但表现不明显且容易被皮肤疾病所掩盖。完整的口腔内疱疹比较罕见，并且后期形成的浅表溃疡除了有不适感外，在数量或症状表现上也没有什么特别明显的地方。

相比之下，复发性VZV口腔病变则具有能确诊的病征[77]。通常会有疼痛或感觉异常的前驱症状，随后出现水疱疹，蔓延至中线处但不会跨越中线（图5.13）。小囊泡迅速破裂后形成浅表溃疡，并在两周内痊愈。疱疹后神经痛是常见的伴随症状，而且非麻醉性镇痛药经常起不到治疗效果[78-80]。虽然口腔并发症比较罕见，但是也有关于牙齿脱落和下颌骨坏死等并发症的报道[81, 82]。

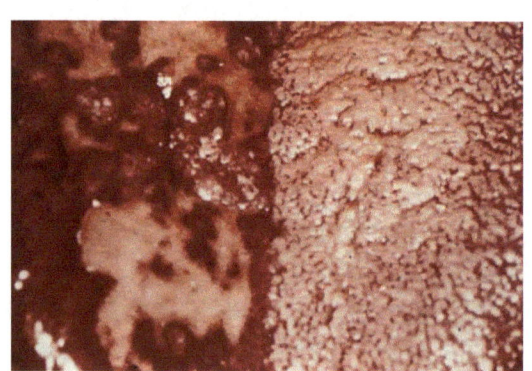

图5.13 复发性VZV感染。复发性VZV口腔感染的特征是损伤仅单侧分布且在中线处突然消失。

诊断

原发性VZV感染的诊断不依据口腔病变，原因有三个。第一，口内症状不显著；第二，原发性感染的初期症状不特异；第三，皮肤症状紧随口腔病变之后。

鉴别诊断

由于其独特的临床表现，复发性口内VZV感染几乎很少与其他病变混淆。但是，应考虑与其他的单侧疱疹囊泡病变进行鉴别诊断，如硬腭上复发性HSV-1感染。其他鉴别诊断见表5.8。

治疗和预后

对大多数个体来说，支持疗法可有效治疗原发性和复发性口内VZV感染，但是免疫

表5.8 VZV的鉴别诊断

HSV-1	原发病变影响口周皮肤、唇红部和所有口腔黏膜表面。复发口腔外病变表现为囊泡和前期的麻刺感、烧灼或悸动。所有损伤表现均发生在相同解剖位置。复发口腔内病变局限于角质化黏膜（如附着龈和硬腭）
原发水痘（水痘）	口腔损伤不常见，几乎没有临床意义
复发水痘 - 带状疱疹（带状疱疹）	口腔外和口腔内损伤均表现为单侧皮肤分布的疼痛性囊泡疹

抑制个体需要更积极的治疗。有报道称阿昔洛韦口服和静脉给药都是有效的，并且适用于免疫抑制患者[83~90]。但是在复发时必须尽可能早地用药才能收到比较好的效果。也有报道称，其他特异性抗病毒药物也是有效的，如伐昔洛韦、泛昔洛韦、阿糖腺苷[91]和疱疹净[92]。

与其他复发性病毒性口内病变（如HSV-1）相比，复发性VZV口内病变比较疼痛。虽然口腔内VZV病变具有很好的预后，但是在多次复发的个体中，口内病变的发病率明显升高。在面临对常规疗法没有反应的复发威胁时，免疫抑制个体更容易发生广泛的复发性病变。

虽然大多数牙科保健工作者在儿童时期曾经有过原发性水痘感染，但适当的感染控制措施可以预防牙科装置中这种病毒的未必会有的传播[93]。我们的后代人将会受益于针对病毒感染的疫苗接种，它从根本上清除了病毒的复发及其在牙科治疗环境中的传播[94]。

EBV

EBV或HHV-4也是一种疱疹病毒，它与多种感染和肿瘤进程相关[95~102]。很早之前，它就已经被认为是传染性单核细胞增多症的病原体，通常由分泌的感染性唾液传播。感染者在成年之前很少发展为典型的传染性单核细胞增多症[103]。过去10年间，最臭名昭著的是口腔毛状白斑和EBV的关系，在这之前口腔毛状白斑一直被认为只是HIV感染引起的独特的口腔黏膜病变。EBV也与非洲儿童的伯基特淋巴瘤和亚洲人的鼻咽癌有关联。表5.9列出了这些疾病的症状特点。

表5.9 EBV相关疾病（未包括传染性单核细胞增多症）

疾病	症状	治疗
伯基特淋巴瘤	常见于乌干达儿童	化疗
	下颌肿大	预后应慎重
	牙齿松动	
	疼痛和感觉异常	
鼻咽癌	种族倾向性（中国人）	放疗
	通常无症状	预后差
	粒状、绒状、红斑	
	未分化	
	常见颈部淋巴结转移	
口腔毛状白斑	主要发生于外侧舌	通常不治疗
	垂直波纹状，如毛状	鬼白树脂反应
		抗病毒药物反应
		停药后复发

口腔表现

传染性单核细胞增多症口腔病变的特征包括咽炎、软腭和口咽部血瘀点，在青壮年常伴有发热和颈部淋巴结病[104]（图5.14）。全身症状与病毒感染的全身表现相结合有助于传染性单核细胞增多症与相似口腔病变的鉴别诊断，如因口交和剧烈的咳嗽或喷嚏造成的口腔和咽部血瘀点（图5.15）。口腔并发症少见，但继发于传染性单核细胞增多症急性期的颅神经缺陷[105]、颈部脓肿[106]、腮腺肿大伴随面神经麻痹[107]和舌扁桃体炎[108]确有报道。

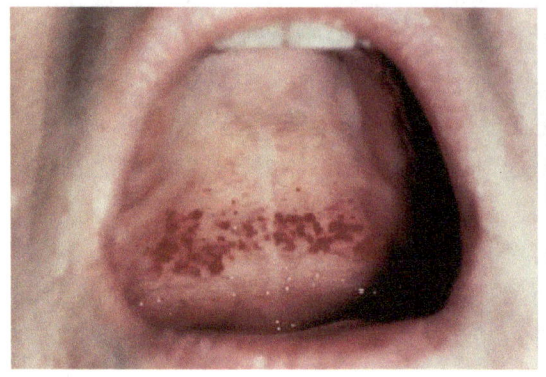

图 5.14 传染性单核细胞增多症。软腭和口咽部血瘀点，伴随低热、萎靡不振和颈部淋巴结病等全身症状是传染性单核细胞增多症的特征性病变（Source: Courtesy of J. Robert Newland, D.D.S., M.S., University of Texas, Houston Health Science Center, Dental Branch）。

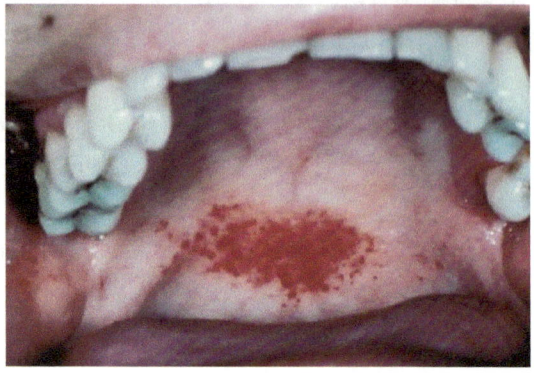

图 5.15 创伤性出血。软腭无症状的血瘀点是外伤的表现，图中所示为口交所致外伤（Source: Courtesy of J. Robert Newland, D.D.S., M.S., University of Texas, Houston Health Science Center, Dental Branch）。

伯基特淋巴瘤是一种高度分化的非霍奇金淋巴瘤，它是于1958年首次在乌干达儿童的地方性下颌肉瘤中发现的[109]。非洲伯基特淋巴瘤在比较年轻的人群中发生，男性占大多数，倾向于累及下巴[110~112]。检测数据明显表明，超过 90% 的非洲地方性伯基特淋巴瘤病例存在 EBV 感染[113, 114]，而不足 10% 的非地方性伯基特淋巴瘤病例存在 EBV 感染[115, 116]。EBV 阳性的伯基特淋巴瘤具有广泛累及下颌伴有下颌肿胀、牙齿松动和痛觉异常的特点[117~119]（图 5.16 和图 5.17），且在非洲和美洲的表现形式具有显著差异[120, 121]。

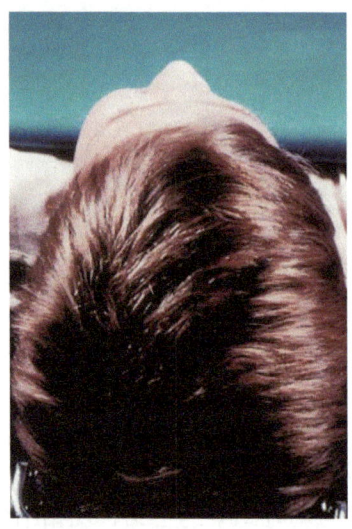

图 5.16 伯基特淋巴瘤。地方性伯基特淋巴瘤的特点是无症状、单侧面中部肿大和 X 射线下明显的骨质损坏。免疫组化实验证实了一种 B 细胞系和 EBV 有关。

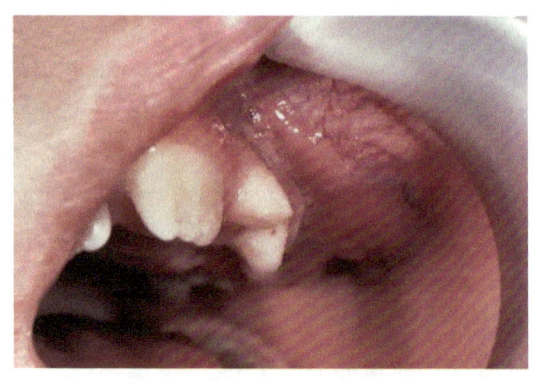

图 5.17 伯基特淋巴瘤。在口腔内伯基特淋巴瘤导致上颌前庭的闭塞和牙齿松动。

鼻咽癌是一种发生于咽隐窝的低分化、未分化和非角质化的癌症[122]，在中国人、爱斯基摩人、东南亚本土人及来自北非和科威特的阿拉伯人中常见[123]。EBV 常与该恶性肿瘤有关且似乎参与了癌症的致病过程[124,125]。鼻咽癌在中国大陆恶性肿瘤中几乎占到了 1/5，在东南亚为第三大肿瘤[126]。病变初期没有明显症状，颈部转移是主要的病症，然后出现鼻腔和听觉症状[127]，颅神经累及也有报道[128]。病变的临床表现为颗粒或绒毛状红斑。

口腔毛状白斑（oral hairy leukoplakia, OHL）是一种独特的 HIV 相关病变，表现为 EBV 诱导的、主要发生在外侧舌部位的上皮增生。这一病变将在"HIV 感染的口腔表现"这一章节进行详细讨论。

诊断

传染性单核细胞增多症的诊断很少完全依赖于口腔症状和体征。淋巴细胞增多和异型淋巴细胞的出现，结合其他相关的临床症状和体征可以高度提示为传染性单核细胞增多症。虽然快速血清学检测（如嗜异性抗体）可以方便地进行诊断，但是确诊仍然需要 EBV 特异性抗体的检测[129]。伯基特淋巴瘤和鼻咽癌的诊断都需要进行切口活检[130~136]。

治疗和预后

常规传染性单核细胞增多症的口咽部病变不需要治疗，因为它会随着感染的消退而自然愈合[137,138]，老年人的体征会更为严重[139]。虽然在大多数病例中，传染性单核细胞增多症是自限性的，但是发病率和 EBV 慢性感染的流行仍然是争论的根源[140]。在疾病早期治疗中建议使用阿昔洛韦。

CMV

传统意义上认为，CMV 与免疫功能正常宿主的唾液腺疾病相关[141,142]，也与被感染胚胎的出生缺陷有关[143~145]。CMV 还与一定数量的破坏性牙周疾病有关[146]。然而，近年来 CMV 被认为在 HIV 感染者继发免疫抑制个体中起到更加明显的作用。在 HIV 感染者中 CMV 感染的口腔表现将在"HIV 感染口腔表现"章节中进行讨论。

HHV-6

HHV-6 于 1986 年首次发现，1988 年确认为幼儿急疹或猝发疹的病原体。最近初步发现 HHV-6 与其他疾病也可能有关（如多发性硬化）[147~157]。目前还没有针对 HHV-6 感染的特异性抗病毒治疗方法[158]。

虽然似乎与 CMV 关系密切[159]，但是没有发现与 HHV-6 感染有关的特异性口腔表现。大多数成年人在婴儿时期接触过 HHV-6 并且唾液中带毒[160~162]。

HHV-7

虽然没有与 HHV-7 型相关的口腔病变的报道，但是在唾液中仍能检测到 HHV-7 病毒[163, 164]。

HHV-8

因为最近发现的 HHV-8 与 AIDS 患者中的卡波西肉瘤有关，所以又被称为卡波西肉瘤相关疱疹病毒（KSHV）。该病变将在"HIV 感染的口腔表现"章节中进行更为详尽的讨论。HHV-8 也与原发性渗出性淋巴瘤、多中心 Castleman 氏病、多发性骨髓瘤[166]和不同的淋巴增殖异常[167~169]有关，前两种病变在 HIV 感染个体中更加普遍[165]。

HPV

口腔上皮的乳头状和疣状增殖统称为口腔疣。鳞状细胞乳头状瘤是口腔乳头状病变的最大类型，约占所有口腔病变的 2.5%[170]。多种不同亚型的 HPV 与口腔鳞状细胞乳头状瘤和口腔寻常疣有关（HPV-2、HPV-6、HPV-11 和 HPV-57）。HPV-2 与皮肤寻常疣有关，HPV-6 和 HPV-11 与尖锐湿疣有关，HPV-11 也与喉乳头瘤和结膜乳头瘤有关。局灶性上皮增生症（Heck 氏病）中检测出 HPV-13 和 HPV-32 的存在。最有趣的是，在鳞状上皮不典型增生和肿瘤中检测到 HPV-16 和 HPV-18。在 HPV 的 100 多个亚型中，至少 13 个与鳞状上皮病变有关（表 5.10）。

表 5.10　HPV 的鉴别诊断

鳞状上皮乳头瘤	最常见的 HPV 相关的口腔病变；通常单独发生且带蒂；常发于唇、腭黏膜和悬雍垂
寻常疣	通常单独发生且无蒂；皮肤病变可能导致唇齿龈和前舌的自体感染
尖锐湿疣	通常发生于口腔-生殖器接触，社交史有助于确定高危行为；比其他 HPV 相关口腔病变更容易传播；通常发生于舌系带、前舌和软腭，并呈现多发、软质、无蒂、粉色的肉块
局部上皮增生（Heck 氏病）	多发的圆顶形或圆丘形、粉色软组织团，常发于唇、舌和颊黏膜；垂直传播特征可能与临床上类似的遗传性皮肤病相似

口腔疣

HPV 是乳头瘤病毒家族成员[171,172]，所有亚型均是 DNA 病毒。它们没有外壳但具有共同的抗原决定簇[173~175]。

虽然 HPV 在口腔黏膜上的感染被认为是直接接触引起的，但是大多数病例都很难确定感染的具体途径。垂直传播被认为是儿童感染的可能途径[176]。病毒在感染的上皮细胞核中复制，但是由于病毒拷贝数太低，所以在基底角质细胞中很难检测到[177]。HPV 也可以在正常的口腔鳞状上皮细胞中检测到[178~180]。

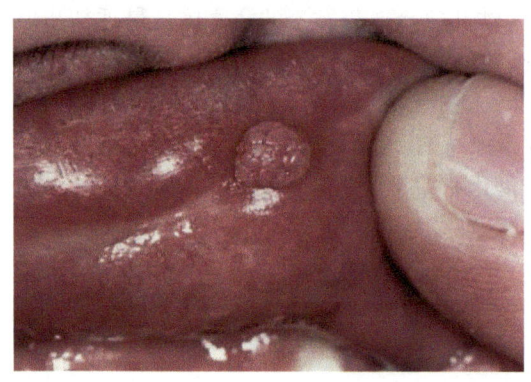

图 5.18　寻常疣。口腔黏膜寻常疣患者通常具有明显的手指损伤。咬伤后的自体传染导致唇黏膜病变。

口腔表现

口腔疣可发生于唇红部及口内黏膜的任何位置[181]（图 5.18）。口腔疣倾向于发生在硬腭、软腭和悬雍垂，超过 1/3 的口内病变发生于这些位置[182]。病变通常较小，最大直径小于 0.5cm。口内鳞状上皮乳头状瘤通常带蒂（图 5.19），而寻常疣通常不带蒂（图 5.20）。两种病变通常都比较独立且无症状，除非再次受到创伤。

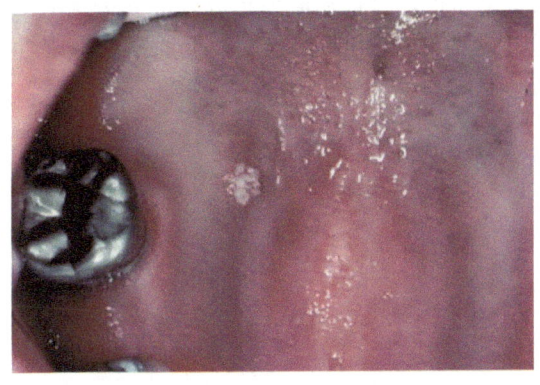 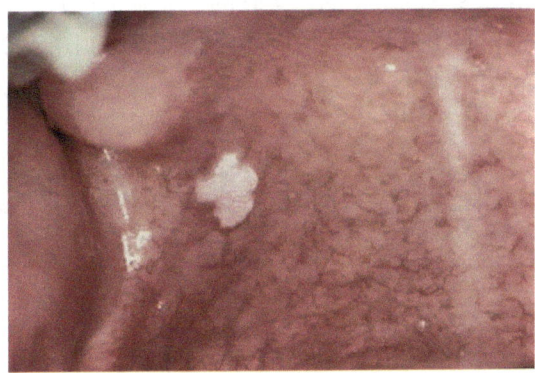

图 5.19　鳞状上皮细胞乳头状瘤。虽然有一些口腔鳞状上皮细胞乳头状瘤中 HPV 为阴性，但是通过 DNA 原位杂交技术在很多患者中检测到 HPV-2、HPV-6、HPV-11 或 HPV-57。

图 5.20　寻常疣。虽然口腔黏膜寻常疣病变通常无症状，但是患者可能会意识到它的存在，尤其当被感染组织可移动时。

诊断

除了很少例外，口腔鳞状上皮乳头状瘤和寻常疣病变具有相当明显的临床特征[183]。这两种病变均需要通过切口活检来诊断。常规苏木精伊红（HE）染色完全可用于诊断[184]，也可通过透射电镜来验证[185]。精确鉴定病毒的具体亚型需要利用分子诊断技术，如 DNA 原位杂交[186~193]。有趣的是，并不是所有染色阳性的鳞状上皮细胞乳头状瘤中都有 HPV 存在[194]。鉴别诊断见表 5.10。

治疗和预后

口腔疣最常用的治疗方法是保守性手术切除。电脱水和激光消融也已经成功应用于口腔疣的治疗。当病变发生于骨的正上方或牙齿附近时，不推荐使用冷冻或热消融技术进行治疗。虽然化学疗法和免疫疗法（如鬼臼树脂和 IFN）作为口腔疣的治疗方法没有经过广泛的评价，但是相对较轻的和较少发生的痛苦使得这种方法比手术切除更为可取。

因为 HPV 具有相对低的感染性，所以口腔疣有很好的预后。虽然手术切除的边缘界限不是特别精确，但是保守性切除手术后未见到明显的复发。很明显，如果感染源于皮肤病变，如指状疣，不管是被咬或咀嚼引起，均必须接受治疗。

尖锐湿疣

尖锐湿疣（condyloma acuminatum）或性病疣是主要与 HPV-6 和 HPV-11 感染相关的中等程度的病变[195]。病变几乎只发生在潮湿的鳞状上皮黏膜。在过去的 10 年间，口腔病变的发病率在异性恋和同性恋人群中明显增加[196~198]。儿童发生口腔病变则高度提示有性虐待[199]。虽然口腔 - 生殖器接触是口腔传染的主要机制，但是也存在自身传染的可能性。

口腔表现

与口腔鳞状上皮乳头状瘤和寻常疣不同的是，口腔尖锐湿疣的特点表现为感染数月后出现多发的、小的、柔软的、无蒂的团块。病变呈粉色，且最后融合形成外部乳头状增生并伴有不同程度的角质化（图 5.21 和图 5.22）。虽然病变可遍布口腔，但通常为自限性的[200~202]。

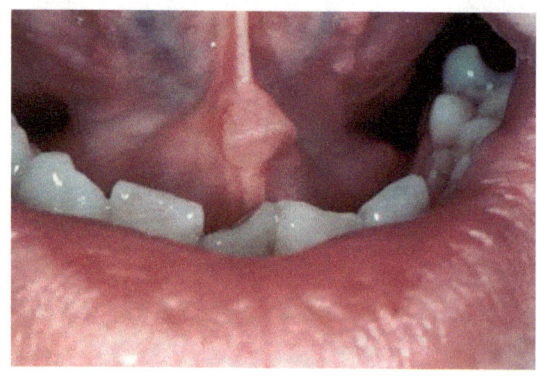 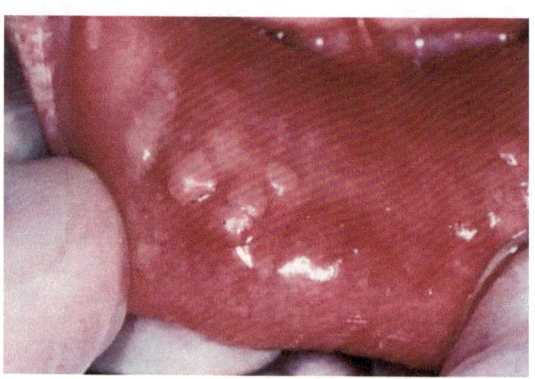

图 5.21　尖锐湿疣。由于同性恋和异性恋人群中口腔 - 生殖器接触的增加导致口腔内尖锐湿疣的发病率普遍升高。

图 5.22　尖锐湿疣。口腔内尖锐湿疣可以是多发，也可以单发（Source: Courtesy of J. Robert Newland, D.D.S., M.S., University of Texas, Houston Health Science Center, Dental Branch）。

诊断

口腔尖锐湿疣的确诊方法是切口活检。DNA 原位杂交可以确定具体的 HPV 型别，即 HPV-6 或 HPV-11。与其他口腔疣一样的是，在基底细胞一般检测不到病毒，因为病毒复制与角质细胞成熟平行发生。

治疗和预后

与其他口腔疣一样，外科手术是口腔尖锐湿疣的常规治疗方法，但是口腔尖锐湿疣的复发率更高，可能是由于病毒广泛感染了病灶周围的外观正常的细胞所致。因此，口腔尖锐湿疣的手术切除界限要更宽，以降低复发风险，通常要超出病变外几毫米。

虽然冷冻手术、激光消融术和电脱水法也已经成功用于治疗尖锐湿疣，但是这些方法在治疗骨上方和毗邻牙齿处的病变时要谨慎[203]。利用 IFN 和咪唑莫特对尖锐湿疣进行免疫治疗似乎是很有希望的，但是到目前为止，在口内病变治疗中的应用还极少[204,205]。

局灶性上皮增生症

局部上皮细胞增多症（focal epithelial hyperplasia，FEH），又称 Heck 氏病，于 1965 年在爱斯基摩和美洲印第安人中首次发现[206]，后来相继在南非、墨西哥和中美洲发现[207]。最初，关于这种疾病的病因有很多种解释，其中最常见的是遗传性皮肤病，因为它呈现连续感染几代的特征。现在普遍认为这种疾病是由 HPV-13 或 HPV-32 感染引起的，因其可被垂直传播，所以很像遗传缺陷[208,209]。虽然，在过去该病的报道只见于儿童，但是成年人也可被感染，且不论性别如何，感染率相当[210]。该病在一些民族中更为流行，但是也可见于其他民族。

口腔表现

局灶性上皮细胞增多症的临床特征为多发性、粉色、圆形顶或圆丘形的软组织块。虽然口腔黏膜任何位置均可被感染，但是常好发于颊黏膜、舌头和唇黏膜[211~213]（图5.23~图5.25）。

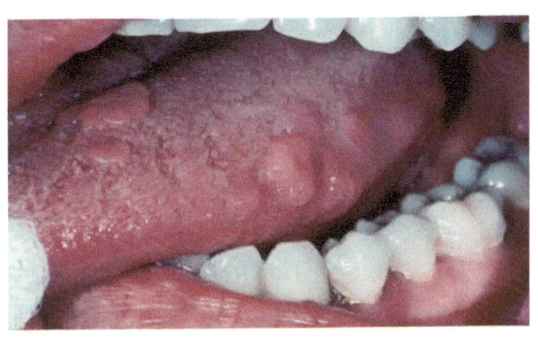

图 5.23　局灶性上皮细胞增生症（Heck 氏病）。局灶性上皮细胞增生症的口内病变和其他 HPV 黏膜感染相似，包括尖锐湿疣。

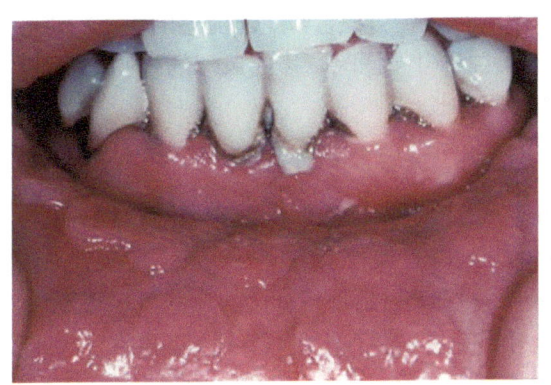

图 5.24　局灶性上皮细胞增生症（Heck 氏病）。由于受累黏膜广泛，局灶性上皮细胞增生症引起的病变很难明确治疗。

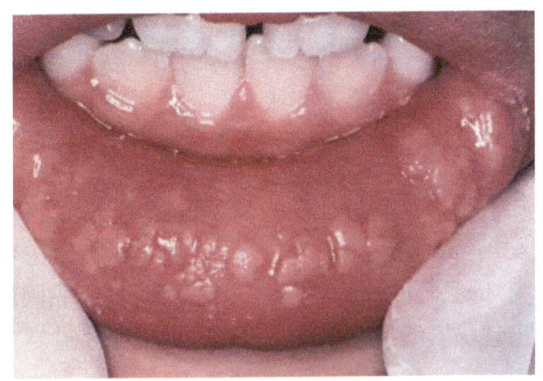

图 5.25　局灶性上皮细胞增生症（Heck 氏病）。局灶性上皮细胞增生症可表现为病毒的垂直传播。图中的患者是由母亲垂直传播而来，母亲的病变见图 5.23 和图 5.24。患者的两个亲兄妹和祖母也同样被感染。

诊断

FEH 的临床表现差异显著，可从不易察觉到显著的病变。明显的病例很少，可能与多发性未成熟纤维增生或口腔尖锐湿疣混淆。常规组织病理学检查提示病毒感染引起上皮细胞增生，分子生物学诊断技术，如 DNA 原位杂交用来确定 HPV 的亚型，如 HPV-13 和 HPV-32[214~217]。

治疗和预后

虽然 FEH 病变是病毒引起的，但是传染性相对较低。单独的病变在妨碍功能或美观时可以切除[218]，但是该病正常的扩散特性不利于所有病变的手术切除。需要特别注意是，一些未经任何治疗干预的患者发生明显的病变自发消退[219]。有一种推测认为，这种消退表示发生了病毒识别延迟和随之而来的细胞介导的免疫活化。

HPV 与口腔疣的关系

如同 EBV，HPV 和黏膜癌变也有一定的关系[220~236]。虽然 HPV 与口腔恶性肿瘤[237~241]

和假定的癌前病变条件[242]有关,但是它在口腔癌症发生中起到的确切作用依然未知[243~247]。近期发表的 94 篇文章表明,与正常口腔黏膜相比,HPV 在口腔恶性肿瘤和癌前病变中检出率明显增加[248]。

副黏病毒

副黏病毒是由不同 RNA 病毒组成的一个家族,包括麻疹病毒、腮腺炎病毒、副流感病毒、人呼吸道合胞病毒及其他几种只对动物致病的病毒。但是该家族中只有麻疹和腮腺炎两种病毒引起明显的口腔病变。

麻疹

麻疹是一种由具有高度传染性的麻疹病毒感染所致疾病,它与引起流感的正黏病毒相似,都是经污染的空气飞沫通过呼吸道传播的。它与引起德国麻疹或风疹的披膜病毒[249]虽然有共同的临床症状,但是后者症状持续的时间更长。

口腔表现

麻疹具有特征性的临床过程,首先是 7~10 天的潜伏期,然后出现典型的前期征兆:发热、不适、结膜炎、畏光和咳嗽[250]。在 48h 内,口腔黏膜上出现小红斑,中央伴有白色坏死斑(Koplik 氏斑,又称麻疹口腔黏膜斑),1~2 天后出现特征性的皮肤斑丘疹[251]。出现黏膜溃疡、牙龈炎和冠周炎也有报道[252]。有趣的是,感染具有季节性,以冬春季为主。

诊断

即使麻疹伴发口腔病变,它的诊断也极少以最初的口腔病变为依据。前期的临床症状和体征虽可提示原发性病毒感染,但都是非特异性的。在唾液中可以检测到抗麻疹抗体[253]。虽然 Koplik 氏斑与其他溃疡性口炎没有什么区别,但是当未免疫者出现麻疹临床征兆时,应高度怀疑。

治疗和预后

除了支持疗法外,麻疹没有特异性治疗方法。虽然 Koplik 氏斑的症状具有多变性,但是保守的口腔冲洗可以有效地控制任何口腔不适感。在其他方面健康的个体中发生诸如脑炎、血小板减少性紫癜和继发感染等并发症是非常少见的。

腮腺炎

腮腺炎的病原体为腮腺炎病毒。腮腺炎是人类最常见的唾液腺疾病,多发于冬春季,但全年均可发生。病毒通过直接接触感染的气溶胶唾液飞沫的方式传播。

虽然腮腺炎的概念来源于腮腺感染,但实际上腮腺炎是一种全身性病毒感染,累及了其他腺体组织和肝脏、肾脏、胰脏及神经系统[254]。

口腔表现

儿童感染后通常表现为非特异性的发热、寒战、不适和头痛等前兆。最初的耳前疼痛可高度怀疑为腮腺炎，而随后的腮腺肿大是确诊所必需的。约有 3/4 的感染者表现为双侧腮腺肿大。腮腺肿大需要 7 ~ 10 天以上才能消退，症状也就随之减轻[198~256]。

由于基质水肿的原因，唾液腺导管，尤其是腮腺的 Stensen 氏导管会受到压迫，所以这种感染的特点是任何刺激唾液腺分泌的活动，如进食均可导致急性不适感。

其他病毒感染偶尔也会出现类似于腮腺炎的临床症状和体征，如 A 组柯萨奇病毒、埃柯病毒和 CMV。腮腺炎的急性发作特征和患者的典型年龄可以有效地排除唾液腺肿大是因为罹患肿瘤的可能性。单侧发病的腮腺也很像涎腺增大症，尤其是当水肿围绕 Stensen 氏管而限制涎腺流动时。对于没有接种过疫苗及伴有单侧和双侧腮腺肿大儿童，应首先考虑是腮腺炎[257]。

治疗和预后

腮腺炎主要是对症治疗，辅以卧床休息和镇痛药[258]。严重病例的治疗偶尔使用皮质激素。儿童患者可出现脑炎、心肌炎和肾炎等并发症，而成年人腮腺炎最严重的并发症是睾丸炎和偶发的卵巢炎。

柯萨奇病毒

柯萨奇病毒是小核糖核酸病毒家族的成员，最初在纽约柯萨奇小镇发现。由柯萨奇病毒引起的具有明显口腔表现的两种疾病是手足口病和疱疹性咽峡炎，通常经由唾液飞沫传播。

手足口病

手足口病（Hand, foot and mouth disease，HFMD）具有高度传染性，一般通过感染性唾液传播，粪-口途径传播也有报道[259~261]。手足口病最常见的病原体是 A-16 型柯萨奇病毒，其他亚型也有引发手足口病的报道[262~265]。该病毒主要感染 5 岁以下儿童并引起流行[266]，偶尔会发生死亡病例。有趣的是，手足口死亡病例不具有口腔溃疡的特点[267]。

口腔表现

感染者在短暂的潜伏期后出现低热、萎靡不振、淋巴腺肿大和口腔痛等症状[268]。黏膜病变最初表现为小囊泡，然后迅速破裂形成浅表溃疡，浅表溃疡被假膜覆盖并被红斑晕包围，与复发性口腔溃疡相似[269, 270]（图 5.26）。

虽然病毒易感部位为腭、舌和口腔黏膜，但在口腔黏膜的所有部位均有病变发生的报道。手和足部皮肤病变与口腔病变同时发生或稍晚于口腔病变发生，表现为红色斑丘疹（图 5.27）。皮肤病变最终转归为小囊泡破裂形成浅表溃疡后结痂[271]。

诊断

虽然手足口病的诊断主要依据临床症状和体征，但是抗体滴度也有助于临床疑似患者的确诊，也可从完整小囊泡收集病毒进行培养鉴定，随后在特定位置出现的皮肤病变也有助于缩小鉴别诊断的范围[272]。

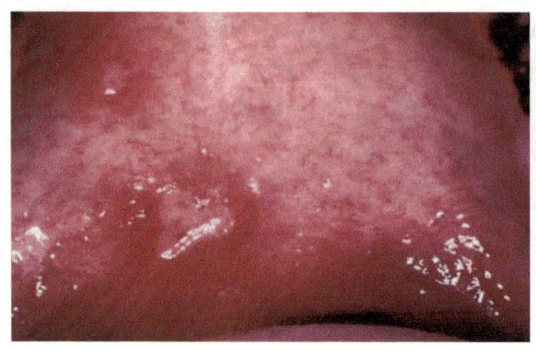

图 5.26 手足口病。虽然手足口病的口腔病变与口腔溃疡相似，但是手足口病伴随有手部和足部的非特异性的斑丘疹和水泡样疹。

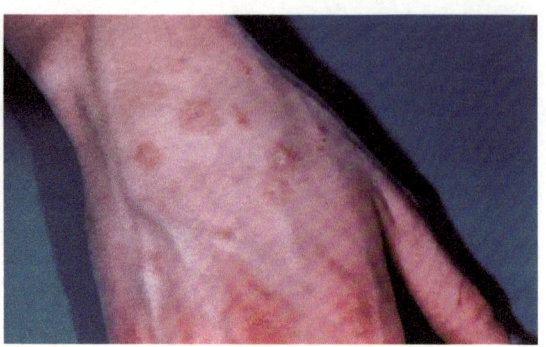

图 5.27 手足口病。手足口病的皮肤病变可以与复发性口腔溃疡进行鉴别诊断（Source: Courtesy of J. Robert Newland, D.D.S., M.S., University of Texas, Houston Health Science Center, Dental Branch）。

治疗和预后

因为手足口病属于自限性疾病，所以手足口病的治疗通常是对症治疗。止痛药适用于发热治疗，保守性口腔冲洗可明显减少伴发症状。低强度激光疗法也可有效去除手足口病所致的口腔溃疡[273]。但是，对再次感染是否仍具有免疫力，知之甚少。

疱疹性咽峡炎

疱疹性咽峡炎是一种急性病毒感染，可由多种不同型别的 A 组柯萨奇病毒引起（包括 A1~A6、A8、A10 和 A22 型）。疱疹性咽峡炎和手足口病同样经感染性唾液飞沫传播，但粪-口途径传播也有报道。其特点是，病毒感染呈地方性且高发于夏秋季，且儿童比成人易感[274~277]。

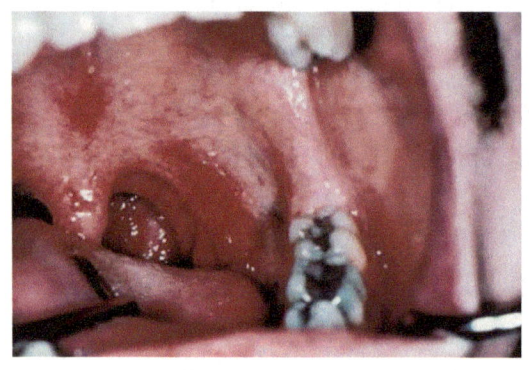

图 5.28 疱疹性咽峡炎。疱疹性咽峡炎通常影响口腔后部和口咽部，而颊、舌和唇黏膜没有明显的受累（Source: Courtesy of J. Robert Newland, D.D.S., M.S., University of Texas, Houston Health Science Center, Dental Branch）。

口腔表现

暴露于病毒后，感染者会有短暂性和非特异性的前驱症状，如发热和萎靡不振，然后发生红斑咽炎和吞咽困难，再集中大量出现累及软腭、扁桃弓和咽喉的斑片状水泡疹（图 5.28）。其余口腔黏膜不受影响是该病的特点。小囊泡迅速破裂形成被伪膜覆盖及红斑晕环绕的浅表溃疡，与复发性口腔溃疡表现相似。该病变在 1 周内消退，没有任何其他明显的症状[278]。

诊断

疱疹性咽峡炎通常以临床症状和体征为基础作出诊断。用血清抗体检测和从完整囊泡中培养病毒的方法来确诊。

疱疹性咽峡炎的口腔病变可能会与复发性口腔溃疡和原发性 HSV-1 口腔感染混淆。复发性口腔溃疡不会主要局限于口腔后部和咽喉，也没有伴随损伤的全身症状。原发性 HSV-1 病变虽然会表现出发热和不适，但不会累及牙龈和唇。

治疗和预后

由于轻微感染的本质且缺少特异性抗病毒治疗，所以疱疹性咽峡炎的治疗采用支持性治疗和对症治疗的方法，患者对保守性口腔冲洗和含漱反应良好。要避免使用含有类固醇的药物制剂。虽然可能存在针对再感染的免疫力，但是因为有很多不同型别的病毒都可以导致疱疹性咽峡炎，所以仍然有可能发生由大体相近但免疫原性不同的柯萨奇病毒引起的再次感染。

人类免疫缺陷病毒

自从 1981 年首例卡波西肉瘤报道以来，HIV 感染和 AIDS 的口腔表现在 HIV/AIDS 流行中扮演了重要的角色（表 5.11）[279, 280]。所有的口腔病变并不是由 HIV 感染本身直接导致的，而是由随后的免疫抑制所引发的[281]。这种免疫抑制不仅导致抗感染能力下降，而且可能在抑制病毒能力的下降和致瘤性转化作用的增强中起到一定的作用。

表 5.11 HIV 感染相关口腔病变分类（修订版）

组 1：与 HIV 感染密切相关的病变	黑色素沉着
念珠菌病	坏死性（溃疡性）口炎
红斑念珠菌	血小板减少性紫癜
伪膜念珠菌	非特异性溃疡
病毒性疾病	组 3：HIV 感染相关的其他病变
毛状白斑	细菌性感染
牙周疾病	衣氏放线菌
线状牙龈红斑	大肠埃希杆菌
坏死性溃疡性牙龈炎	克雷伯杆菌肺炎
坏死性溃疡性牙周炎	上皮（杆菌性）血管瘤
卡波西肉瘤	猫抓病
非霍奇金淋巴瘤	药物反应
组 2：不常见的 HIV 感染相关的病变	溃疡
细菌性感染	多形性红斑
鸟分枝杆菌	苔癣样病变
结核分枝杆菌	中毒性表皮松弛
病毒感染	真菌感染
HSV	新型隐球菌
人乳头状瘤病毒	念珠地丝菌
尖锐湿疣	夹膜组织胞浆菌
局灶性上皮增生症	毛霉菌（毛霉菌病/接合菌病）
寻常疣	黄曲霉菌
VZV	神经系统失调
带状疱疹	面神经麻痹
水痘	三叉神经痛
唾液腺疾病	复发性阿弗他溃疡
唾液分泌减少导致的口干症	病毒感染
单侧或双侧主要唾液腺肿大	CMV
其他	传染性软疣

因为 HIV 相关口腔病变主要不是由病毒引起的，所以本部分的内容是 HIV 阳性感染者中发生的细菌、真菌和病毒性口腔疾病[282~289]。这些患者是根据与 HIV 感染的相关性及欧共体（European Community，EC）信息交流中心关于 HIV 感染相关口腔问题、世界卫生组织（WHO）合作中心关于免疫缺陷病毒相关口腔表现和 1992 年 9 月美国 HIV 感染相关口腔表现研讨会采用的共同标准而分组的[290]。

一些关于 HIV 感染和 AIDS 相关口腔表现的优秀综述[291~320]及大量发生在高危人群包括同性恋和双性恋男性[321,322]、注射毒品使用者[323]、血友病[324]以及其他特殊人群包括妇女[325]、儿童[326~332]、非洲人[333,334]和其他族裔群体[335~339]中的 HIV 感染及 AIDS 相关口腔表现病例均已发表和报道。

第 1 组：与 HIV 感染密切相关的病变

念珠菌病

口腔念珠菌感染是人类最常见的口腔真菌感染[340~344]，也是 HIV 阳性的男性和女性中最常表现出来的口腔感染[345~350]。绝大部分病例是由白色念珠菌引起[351]，也有其他口腔分离物的报道[352~355]。虽然某些病例可能最初并没有症状，但是患者最终会主诉为非特异性的口腔烧灼感，并且常伴有口腔痛和吞咽困难[356,357]。在 HIV 病例中，口腔念珠菌病，尤其是发展成食道念珠菌病是一种不良预后的表现[358~360]。幸运的是，在高效抗逆转录病毒治疗（highly active antiretroviral therapy，HAART）的措施下，包括口腔念珠菌病在内的很多 HIV 相关疾病的发病率显著下降[361]。

许多 HIV 阳性患者潜伏有白色念珠菌，但其他方面正常[362~364]。多种宿主因素，主要是免疫抑制破坏了正常口腔生态微生物平衡而经常导致念珠菌病[365~368]。

口腔念珠菌病的传统表现为急性假膜，呈特征性白色、凝乳样的可移动斑块，斑块移除后可见红斑基底，偶尔有出血现象（图 5.29 和图 5.30）。但 HIV 感染者经常会表现出红斑念珠菌病，这种病变除了可见的浅表真菌菌落或斑块外，与急性假膜型的临床表现完

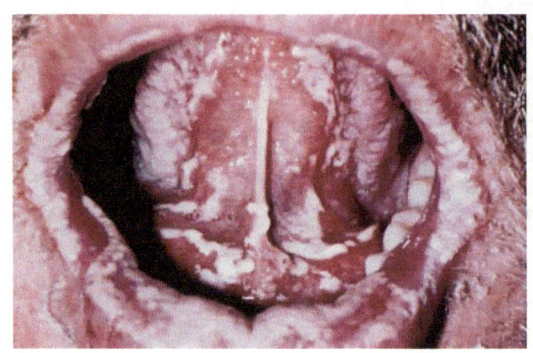

图 5.29　假膜型念珠菌病。严重的假膜型念珠菌病病例可能具有明显的口腔外症状。表面真菌集落移除后表现出侵蚀性红斑黏膜基底（Source: Courtesy of J. Robert Newland, D.D.S., M.S., University of Texas, Houston Health Science Center, Dental Branch）。

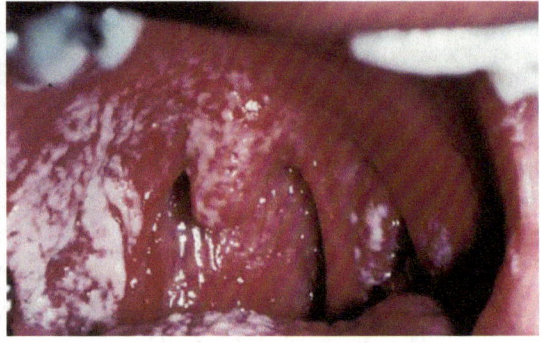

图 5.30　假膜型念珠菌病。口腔后部和口咽部的假膜型念珠菌病常引起吞咽困难。

全一样[369]（图5.31和图5.32）。这种弥漫性口腔红斑通常由于缺乏明显真菌感染的特点，有时就会掩盖真正的临床表现。正中菱形舌炎是白色念珠菌感染特有的表现，在没有任何其他口腔念珠菌相关病变时也会出现（图5.33）。

口腔念珠菌病的诊断相对比较简单，氢氧化钾试剂通常足以诊断。但是其他快速诊断方法也已经应用于疾病诊断，如利用CandidaSure™进行的乳胶凝集法（Life Sign First Care, Somerset, NJ）或利用荧光染料Calcofluor White进行的免疫荧光染色法[370]。虽然采集菌落进行培养可鉴别菌落，但是念球菌相对缓慢的生长速度可能会影响到适当的治疗措施的介入。于是，一种简化的、适宜操作的口腔念珠菌便捷培养系统被开发出来，即Oricult-N™, Orion Diagnostica Espoo, Finland[371]。

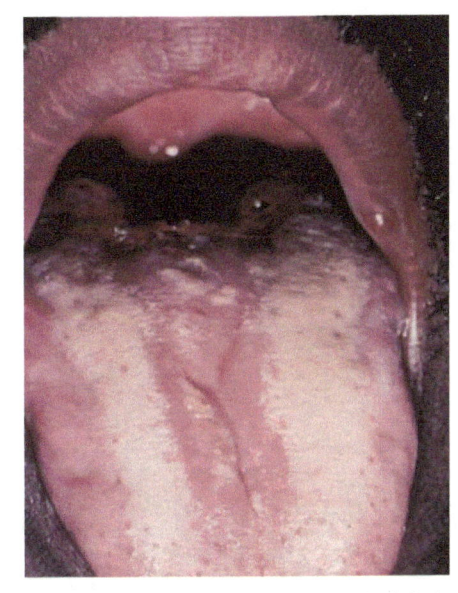

图5.31 红斑念珠菌病。与假膜型念珠菌病不同的是，红斑念珠菌病没有任何表面菌落，临床上也不表现为片状黏膜红斑。当该病发生在舌头上时，舌背面经常发生乳头状病变。

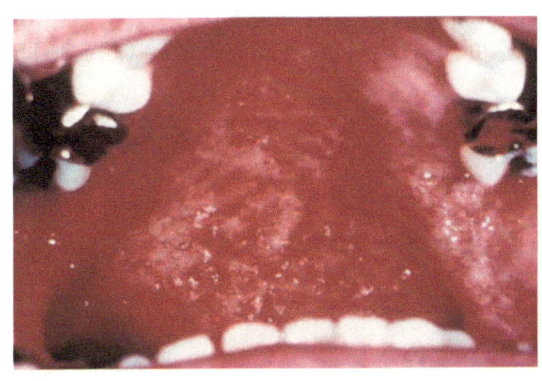

图5.32 红斑念珠菌病。腭部红斑念珠菌病常表现为弥漫性红斑，伴有口腔痛和吞咽困难，有时可见分散的浅表真菌菌落（Source: Courtesy of J. Robert Newland, D.D.S., M.S., University of Texas, Houston Health Science Center, Dental Branch）。

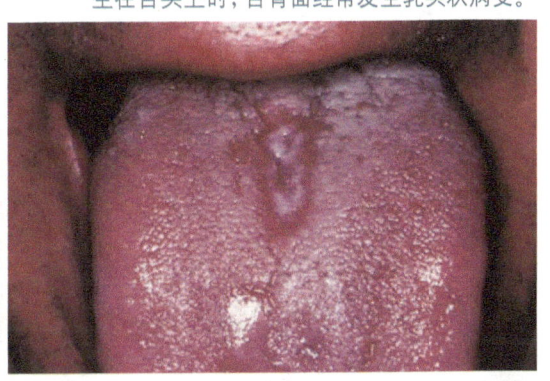

图5.33 正中菱形舌炎。正中菱形舌炎具有典型的临床表现，即使口腔内致病微生物已经消除，其菱形的乳头状病变区域有时仍会持续存在。

HIV阳性患者口腔念珠菌病的治疗效果在一定程度上与其免疫抑制程度成正比[372]，并且不同个体治疗的效果也不一样[373,374]。口服片剂，如克霉唑或制霉菌素和抗真菌口腔冲洗剂，常对具有一定免疫功能的患者有效[375~378]。全身抗真菌治疗，如酮康唑、氟康唑和伊曲康唑，对更加严重或顽固性病例及对每天口服5次糖锭剂的治疗方法依从性不好的病例有效[379~385]。各种抗菌和抗真菌剂也被用来预防口腔念珠菌病[386~389]。其他含抗真菌药的药物制剂如静脉注射液、口服悬浮液、霜剂和膏剂在处理特殊的临床情况时也是很有帮助的，如重症感染、儿童患者、口周感染和活动的牙科手术设备的组织支撑面。

据报道，一些白色念珠菌对唑类抗真菌药物具有耐药性[390~396]，这种耐药性可能是由于多种菌株共同感染造成的[397,398]，尽管有证据表明在单个患者体内仅存在单一类型的白色念珠菌[399,400]。

在 HIV 阳性病例中，口腔念珠菌病的发生是体现其免疫抑制程度的较好指标[401,402]。除了最严重的免疫抑制患者，其他所有患者的口腔念珠菌感染都具有良好的预后[403~405]。但是由于念珠菌普遍存在，所以复发的频率非常高。不幸的是，由于缺乏念珠菌预防措施，复发很普遍无一例外。

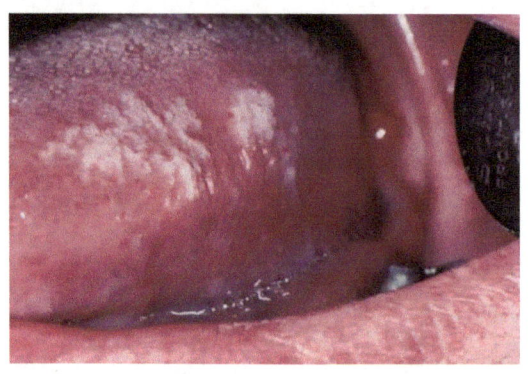

图 5.34 口腔毛状白斑。在临床表现上，口腔毛状白斑可能与继发于使用烟草、舌头咀嚼或其他功能失常性习惯的白斑相似。它的确诊需要进行针对 EBV 的 DNA 原位杂交。

毛状白斑

20 世纪 80 年代初期，Greenspan 及其同事首次报道了在旧金山男同性恋中发生的口腔毛状白斑（oral hairy lenkoplakia，OHL）[406~408]，后来在其他 HIV 感染危险人群中也有发现，如血友病患者和受血者[409~412]。最初报道的 OHL 病例的病变发生于舌背侧，累及丝状乳头，使病变呈现"毛状"外观。大多数病变发生在舌侧面，呈皱褶状，且可延伸至口咽部（图 5.34 和图 5.35）[413]。舌腹侧的 OHL 更多的表现为斑块状（图 5.36）。

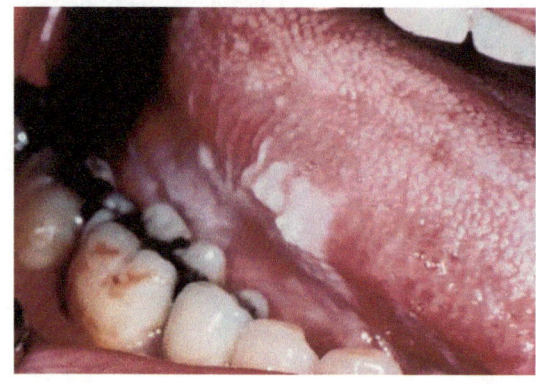

图 5.35 口腔毛状白斑。口腔毛状白斑常发生于舌侧边缘，呈皱褶状（Source: Courtesy of J. Robert Newland, D.D.S., M.S., University of Texas, Houston Health Science Center, Dental Branch）。

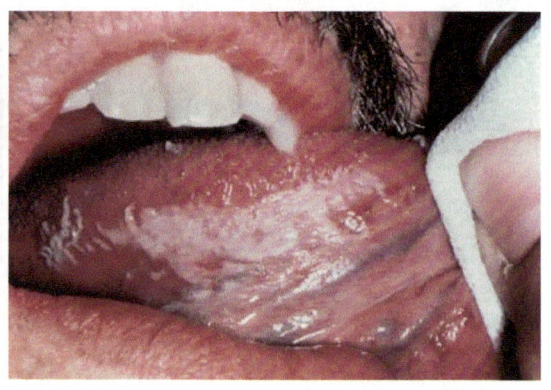

图 5.36 口腔毛状白斑。舌背侧受累的丝状乳头呈现"毛状"外观，而舌腹侧病变多呈现斑片状。

口腔毛状白斑不是 HIV 感染的特异性症状，而是广泛免疫抑制的表现[414, 415]。目前，已在 HIV 阴性但接受过骨髓[416~420]、肾[421~423]、肝[424]和心脏[425]器官移植的患者及 HIV 阴性但患有骨髓增生异常综合征的患者[426]中发现了相同的病变。在 HIV 阴性且免疫力正常个体中发生 OHL 病例是非常罕见的[427,428]。

口腔毛状白斑的特点是继发于 EBV 复制的上皮细胞增生[429~431]。EBV 倾向于感染口腔角质形成细胞[432]，可以在 HIV 阳性和阴性个体的口腔组织中检测到[433~435]。HPV 也会在一些 OHL 样本检测到，但其意义还是有待商榷的[436]。根据临床表现来判断 OHL 时，可能会和一些其他疾病混淆，尤其当 HIV 血清阳性确定时，因为摩擦导致的过度角化、烟草相关白斑、增生型念珠菌和斑块型扁平苔藓等疾病都与 OHL 的表现相似[437~439]。

在 HIV 阳性个体中，利用活组织切片和 HE 染色可观察到空泡样及其他特征性上皮变化，通常足以用于 OHL 的诊断。但是在其他口腔黏膜疾病中这种变化也可发生，因此在 HIV 感染者中，OHL 的确诊必须借助于 DNA 原位杂交[440,441]。EBV 的超微结构特征如被感染上皮细胞也非常有特点[442,443]。脱落细胞学的免疫诊断染色技术检查[444,445]和一种无创性的毛刷活检技术[446]也被用于 OHL 的诊断。

除非在一定程度上涉及功能或美观问题，口腔毛状白斑并不需要任何明确的干预措施[447]。虽然口服抗病毒药物可使疾病消退，如阿昔洛韦[448,449]、脱氧无环鸟苷[450]、二羟基-丙氧基甲基-鸟嘌呤（DHPG）[451]、齐多夫定[452~454]和万乃洛韦[455]，但是一旦停药，疾病就会复发。维生素 A 也被用于 OHL 的局部治疗[456]，鬼臼树脂[457,458]和外科手术[459]也被成功地用于 OHL 的治疗。虽然 OHL 的预后是良好的，但 OHL 是 HIV 整体进展不良预后的标志，也就是 OHL 的发生预示着免疫系统功能将更加低下[460~462]。

牙周疾病

HIV 感染的牙龈和牙周表现依然是异性恋和同性恋 HIV 感染的口腔标志[463~468]。以前称为 HIV 相关牙龈炎的线形牙龈红斑的特点为红斑边缘性牙龈炎，偶尔伴发齿槽龈红斑和前庭黏膜红斑[467]（图 5.37 和图 5.38）。与 HIV 阴性的边缘性牙龈炎不同的是，红斑不会因采取口腔卫生保健措施而消失，如刷牙和使用牙线。

HIV 阳性感染者中患有线形牙龈红斑的群体将发展为坏死性牙龈炎和牙周炎，以前分别称为 HIV 相关牙龈炎和 HIV 相关牙周炎[468,469]。这些患者病情进展迅速，牙周组织很快被损坏，包括牙周附着的丧失和底层牙槽骨的吸收（图 5.39）。有时，这些破坏性进展延伸到牙周外引起起始于牙周的坏死性口腔炎（图 5.40）。这种感染导致邻近黏膜和底层骨

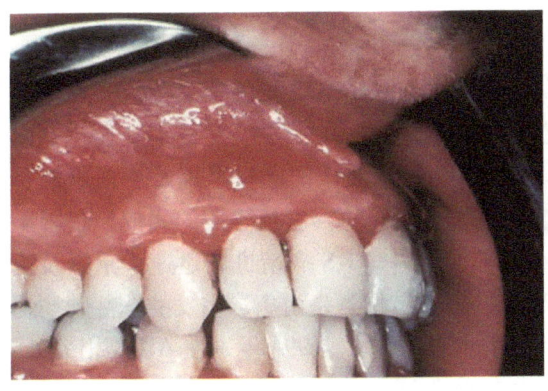

图 5.37 线形牙龈红斑。线形牙龈红斑的特点是亮红色边缘性牙龈炎，普通的口腔卫生保健措施不能使其消除。与健康个体相比，患者的口腔微生物菌群没有明显差异。

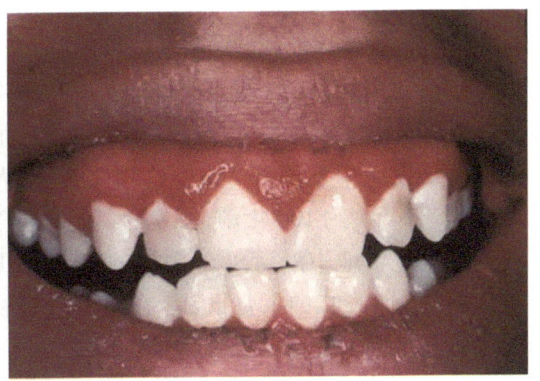

图 5.38 线形牙龈红斑。HIV 阳性的儿童患者和成人患者具有相同的牙龈表现（Source: Courtesy of J. Robert Newland, D.D.S., M.S., University of Texas, Houston Health Science Center, Dental Branch）。

组织的大范围破坏，并可能危及生命。

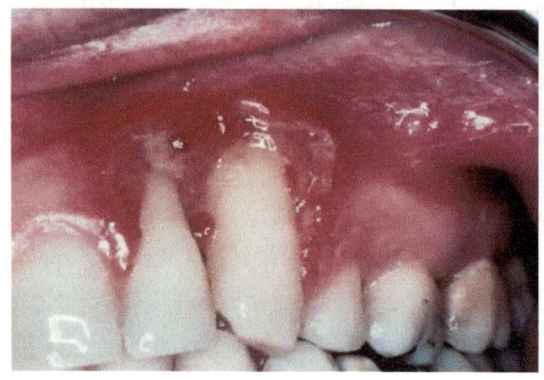 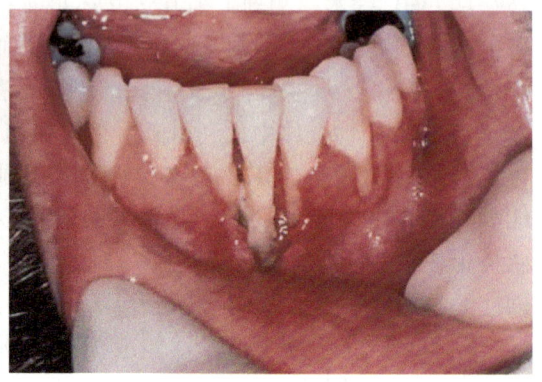

图 5.39 坏死性牙周炎。坏死性牙周炎的表现是以牙周附着和底层骨吸收为特点的快速根尖迁移。

图 5.40 坏死性口腔炎。坏死性口腔炎患者表现为软组织的坏死性破坏，伴随着自发性出血、齿槽骨外露、死骨形成和急性剧烈疼痛（Source: Courtesy of J. Robert Newland, D.D.S., M.S., University of Texas, Houston Health Science Center, Dental Branch）。

一般情况下，引起 HIV 阳性和阴性的牙周疾病患者的病原体没有明显区别[470-474]，这意味着牙周疾病的发生是一个持续衰退的过程，从健康的牙周到线形牙龈红斑再到坏死性牙龈炎和牙周炎[475]。

一旦 HIV 血清阳性得到确认，HIV 相关牙周病的诊断完全依靠临床表现。所有这类疾病特征性地对常规治疗措施均具有耐受性，如增加口腔卫生措施。除了局部清创外，局部和全身抗生素治疗如洗必泰和甲硝唑、即时跟进护理和长期保健是控制病情所必需的[476~479]。

如能及时控制病情的恶化，HIV 相关牙周病的预后是良好的，虽然之前的牙周破坏是不可逆的，但是感染者也必须一丝不苟地呵护个人口腔卫生并坚持专业的牙科护理。

卡波西肉瘤

卡波西肉瘤（kaposi's sarcoma，KS）是第一种被界定的 AIDS 相关疾病，从开始出现就一直是 AIDS 并发的最普遍的恶性肿瘤，尤其是在男同性恋中[480,481]。尽管血管内皮在肉瘤的组织发生中发挥着一定的作用[483]，但人们一般认为卡波西肉瘤只是累及小血管的恶性肿瘤[482]。大约 100 年前，KS 的典型病变被描述为顽固性的、生长缓慢的病变，仅限于皮肤，常见于地中海后裔男子的下肢。在 HIV 阳性患者中，KS 病情进展迅速，常累及内脏，是感染者死亡的主要原因。在 HIV 流行初期，KS 就被推测是由病毒诱发的恶性肿瘤，因为它在美国的传播与其他传染性疾病的流行非常相似[484,485]。1994 年，在 AIDS 相关 KS 中鉴定出了疱疹类病毒序列[486]。第二年，在没有感染 HIV 的 KS 病例中也检出了相同的 DNA 序列[487]。几位学者在唾液[488~491]、口腔 KS[492] 和未患 KS 的口腔组织[493,494] 中都鉴定出了 HHV-8 型。从结果可以看出，HHV-8 是 KS 患者的必要而非充分条件[495~498]。据估计，HHV-8 在全世界具有 10%~25% 的感染率，但是在其他方面健康的个体中，它似乎是受到了免疫控制[499,500]。

在 HIV 患者中，1/3 的可见性 KS 发生在口腔或头颈部皮肤，这一点对牙科保健工作者特别重要。此外，虽然在过去 10 年里，由于 HAART 的问世和 KS 对免疫缺陷的敏感性导致 AIDS 患者的 KS 相对发病率一直在下降，但是 KS 仍然是 AIDS 最常见的口腔恶性肿瘤[501~503]。腭部虽然是 KS 的好发部位，但所有口内黏膜表面及骨内均有 KS 报道[504]。早期病变在外观上表现为斑点状外观，由浅红色变为紫色（图 5.41～图 5.43）；而晚期病变更多的表现出结节状特点（图 5.44～图 5.48），并可能引起下方骨组织的破坏[505]。

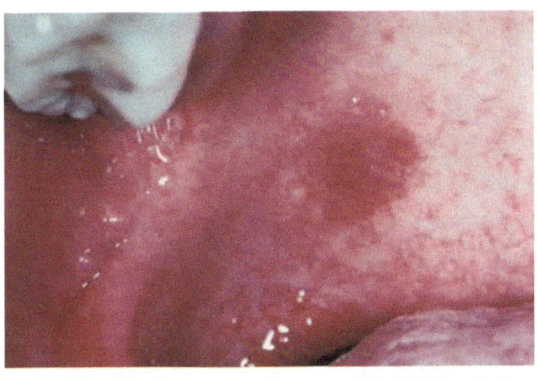

图 5.41 卡波西肉瘤。卡波西肉瘤早期常无症状，病变呈现扁平状，发生由红色到紫色的颜色改变，临床表现与黏膜瘀斑相似（Source: Courtesy of J. Robert Newland, D.D.S., M.S., University of Texas, Houston Health Science Center, Dental Branch）。

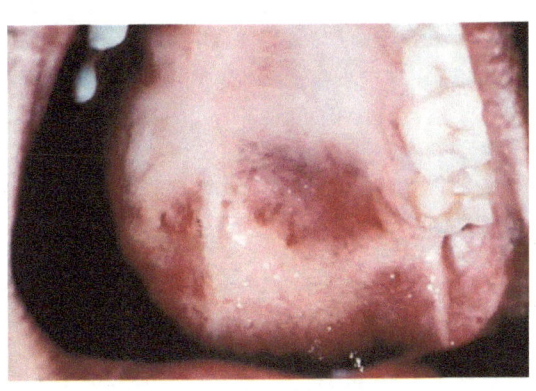

图 5.42 卡波西肉瘤。腭部是口腔卡波西肉瘤的最好发部位。

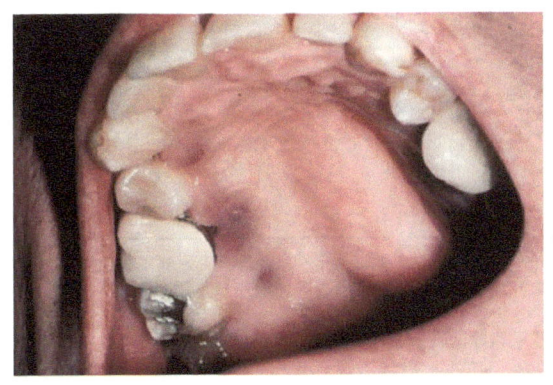

图 5.43 卡波西肉瘤。在有些情况下，腭部卡波西肉瘤与牙科手术导致的创伤表现相似。

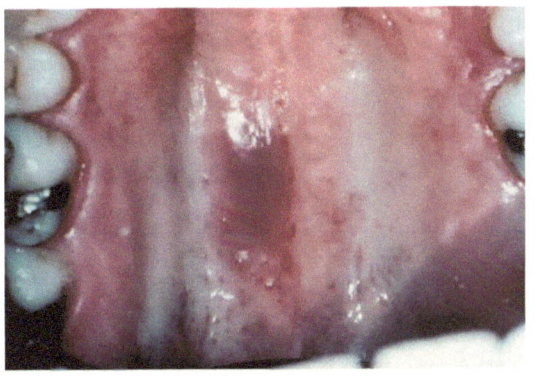

图 5.44 卡波西肉瘤。卡波西肉瘤进一步发展后表现为结节状外观，并且更容易被患者注意到（Source: Courtesy of J. Robert Newland, D.D.S., M.S., University of Texas, Houston Health Science Center, Dental Branch）。

由于 KS 和上皮（杆菌性）血管瘤病在组织病理学上具有相似性，所以即使 KS 发生在经过血清学确诊的 HIV 患者中，也需要通过活组织切片检查来确诊[506, 507]。另外，虽然 CMV 在 KS 发病中的作用还不清楚，但是在口腔 KS 病变中也有 CMV 存在的报道[508]（表 5.12）。

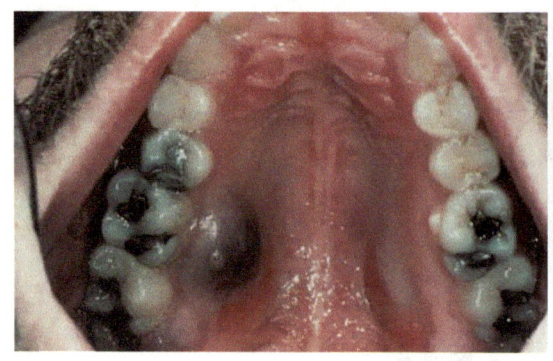

图 5.45　卡波西肉瘤。腭部结节状病变可能会扩大到影响说话和吞咽功能。

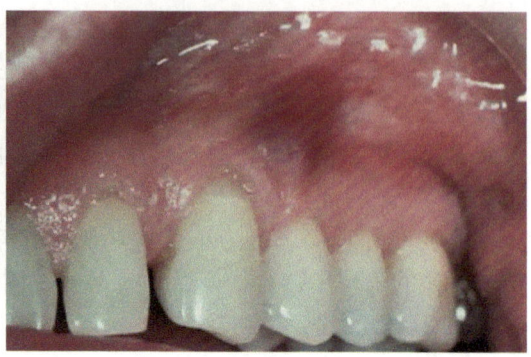

图 5.46　卡波西肉瘤。卡波西肉瘤在牙龈上的早期病变也能会被误认为是牙龈囊肿（Source: Courtesy of J. Robert Newland, D.D.S., M.S., University of Texas, Houston Health Science Center, Dental Branch）。

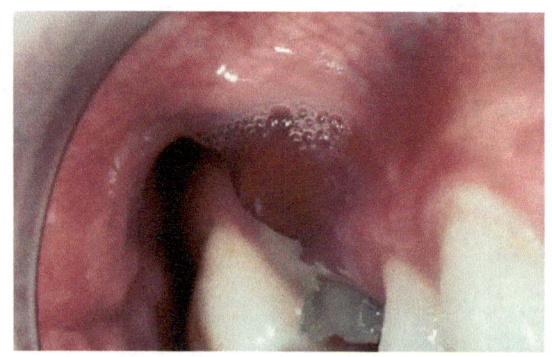

图 5.47　卡波西肉瘤。牙龈是卡波西肉瘤在口腔的第二好发部位（Source: Courtesy of J. Robert Newland, D.D.S., M.S., University of Texas, Houston Health Science Center, Dental Branch）。

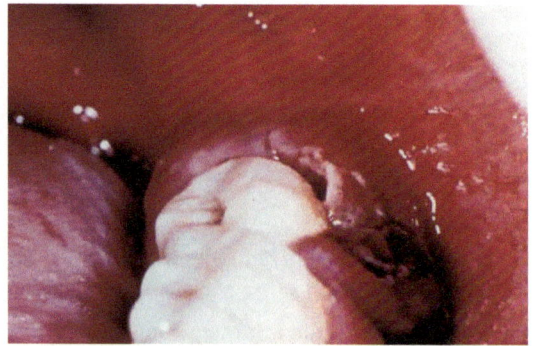

图 5.48　卡波西肉瘤。卡波西肉瘤的牙龈病变继续发展会导致明显的牙周破坏（Source: Courtesy of J. Robert Newland, D.D.S., M.S., University of Texas, Houston Health Science Center, Dental Branch）。

表 5.12　卡波西肉瘤的鉴别诊断

卡波西肉瘤	最好发于牙龈和硬腭，也可累及任何部位的口腔黏膜；1/3 的口腔 KS 患者具有头颈部皮肤病变；早期病变常表现为红色斑点状，也可为紫色结节状；大多数病变无症状，除非继发创伤
杆菌性血管瘤病	红褐色的黏膜皮肤丘疹和结节，与口腔卡波西肉瘤的临床表现相似；源于巴尔通体的病灶性感染；病原体为特定菌株；病变对抗生素敏感
非霍奇金淋巴瘤	最好发于腭部和牙槽嵴，可能局限于软组织；常累及下颌，发生牙齿松动、疼痛和感觉异常现象；颜色多变，由粉红色到紫色

只有当口腔内 KS 病变影响到功能或美观时通常才进行治疗，但不包括其他的全身性治疗。放疗最初是用来缩小肿瘤体积的[509]，但是由于放射毒性和随后的黏膜炎等并发症限制了它的应用。虽然大面积切除肿瘤组织能暂时地缓解功能障碍，但是病变面积还会再次扩大。光动力疗法由于几乎没有副作用，所以是比较成功的治疗方法[510]。虽然对于一些患者来说，全身抗病毒治疗（齐多夫定）合并免疫治疗（α-IFN）是有效的[511,512]，但是

贫血和全身症状限制了它的广泛应用。最近，在病变内部注射长春碱进行治疗已经成功用于诱导肿瘤硬化和缓解（图 5.49 和图 5.50）[513,514]。十四烷基硫酸钠（Sotradecol™）也被用作局部口腔 KS 病变的硬化剂[515]。治疗口腔 KS 时，也应配合治疗其他 HIV 相关口腔症状[516,517]。

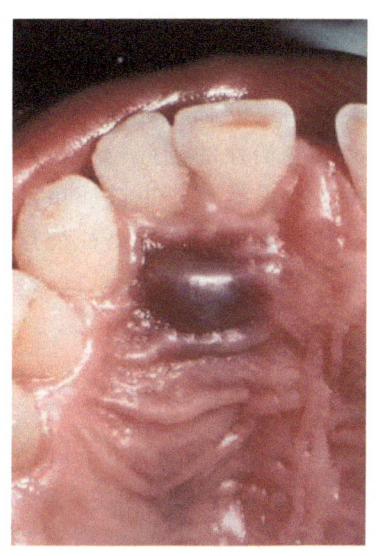

图 5.49 卡波西肉瘤（治疗前）。发生在硬腭前部的卡波西肉瘤同下颌前部牙齿的创伤一样发生功能性障碍（Source: Courtesy of J. Robert Newland, D.D.S., M.S., University of Texas, Houston Health Science Center, Dental Branch）。

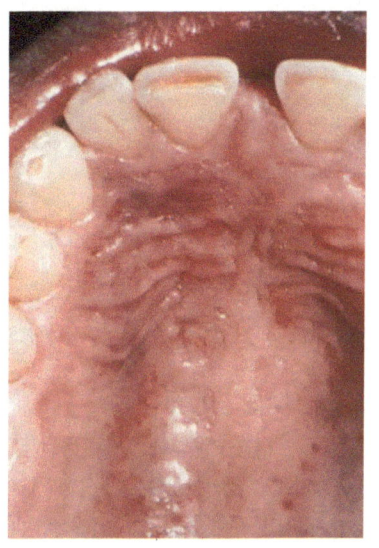

图 5.50 卡波西肉瘤（治疗后）。图 5.49 中的病变经过 6 周时间的长春碱病变内注射治疗后的效果（Source: Courtesy of J. Robert Newland, D.D.S., M.S., University of Texas, Houston Health Science Center, Dental Branch）。

由于口腔 KS 发病率远远高于最终病死率，因此，与机会性感染相比，它的预后要相对较好。事实上，部分由于 HAART 的使用增加，AIDS 相关 KS 总体病死率似乎在降低[518]。虽然在 KS 消退患者中检出了针对 HHV-8 的 IgG 和 IgA 抗体，但是它的意义仍不明确[519]。不幸的是，口腔 KS 病变很难获得长期缓解，且随着时间的推移病变可复发，也可出现新的病变。

非霍奇金淋巴瘤

非霍奇金淋巴瘤（Non-Hodgkin's lymphoma，NHL）是 AIDS 患者第二大常见的恶性肿瘤[520~526]。绝大部分患者具有结外受累现象，其中，中枢神经系统、骨髓、肠道和黏膜皮肤位点最常受累。大约有 5% 的 AIDS 伴发 NHL 者具有明显的口腔病变[527]。口腔 NHL 属于 B 细胞型，大部分为高分化瘤，且许多肿瘤组织中含有 EBV 的 DNA[528~530]。

据报道，口腔 NHL 主要累及腭部和牙槽嵴，也可由于肿瘤扩张而累及口腔内其他部位[531~533]（图 5.51）。病变可呈现不同的临床表现，从坏死性溃疡性牙龈炎到巨大的肿瘤块，而且病变呈现独立性和多病灶性[534~538]。患者最初可无症状，但当发生骨累及时，会发生牙齿松动和感觉异常等表现。早期病变可能会与非瘤性牙龈病变混淆，而当病情进展后又与转移癌、黑色素瘤或恶性组织细胞增生症具有相同的临床表现。

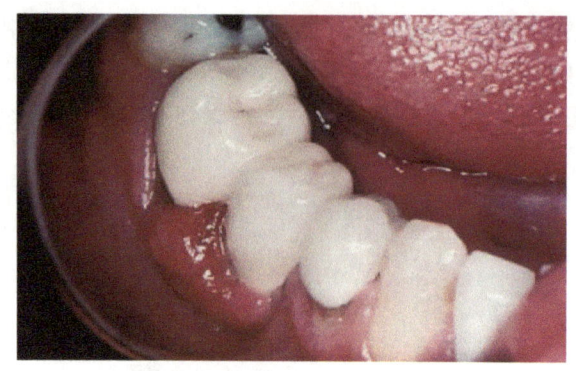

图 5.51 非霍奇金淋巴瘤。非霍奇金淋巴瘤（NHL）是 AIDS 患者第二大常见的恶性肿瘤，疾病早期症状与牙龈的良性反应性病变相似，如化脓性肉芽肿

NHL 的诊断既需要常规组织病理学对肿瘤进行分级，又需要特殊的免疫组化技术对肿瘤进行定性和再分类，如 EBV、B 细胞和 T 细胞标志物的检测。

伴发 NHL 的患者病情有一个迅速进展和消退的临床过程。传统化疗对早期病变治疗的反应较好，但效果并不持久。虽然放疗也被应用，但是在没有化疗辅助的情况下往往疗效不够理想[539]。

第 2 组：不常见的与 HIV 感染相关的病变

细菌性感染

在 HIV 阳性个体中，结核分枝杆菌胞内复合体（*Mycobacterium Avium*-intercellulare complex，MAC）和结核分枝杆菌（*Mycobacterim Tuberculosis*，TB）的检出率越来越高[540,541]，包括儿童在内[542,543]。大约 50% 的 HIV 阳性者至少有过一次的结核菌感染经历[544,545]。

MAC 感染需要通过肺暴露途径，被认为是免疫抑制患者不可避免的环境暴露[546~549]。微生物迅速寄居于肺和胃肠道黏膜[550~554]，并且具有多种药物抗性的特点[555~563]。MAC 感染的表现包括 HIV 感染者的口腔溃疡，并应考虑该病变的鉴别诊断。

虽然总体上来说，MAC 较常见，但是在特定高危人群中 TB 发生频率比 MAC 更高，如海地人和注射吸毒者[564]。TB 在美国的总体感染率是 2.5%，在美国出生的 AIDS 患者中的感染率低于 3%，而在海地生 AIDS 患者中的感染率为 13%[565]。在美国，大约 1/4 的肺外 TB 病例发生在 HIV 阳性个体中[566,567]。

在多数病例的 HIV 感染过程中，TB 发生早于 MAC[568]，并且对没有使用保护措施和合适的感染控制措施的牙科及其他健康护理工作者造成明显的威胁[569]。正如 MAC 一样，TB 一般通过污染的唾液气溶胶传播[570,571]。不幸的是，虽然结核病可防可治[572,573]，但是防治方法在高风险感染患者中很难实施，而且治疗依从性较低[574]。近几年最令人关注的是多耐药性 TB 的出现，它们导致免疫抑制和免疫功能正常个体的 TB 相关死亡率升高[575]。

TB 的口腔病变是非特异性的，最常见的临床表现为伴有不同症状的无痛溃疡[576]（图 5.52～图 5.54）。组织病理学

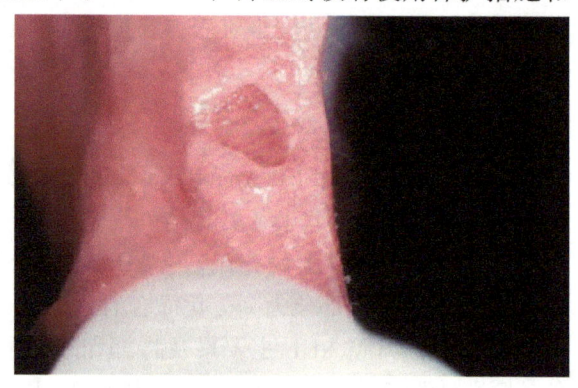

图 5.52 肺结核。肺结核的口腔症状可表现为未痊愈的溃疡，与鳞状细胞癌相似（Source: Courtesy of J. Robert Newland, D.D.S., M.S., University of Texas, Houston Health Science Center, Dental Branch）。

检查特征性的肉芽肿时可能并不明显，口腔结核分枝杆菌的培养也不可靠。对表现出非吸收性口腔溃疡的免疫抑制个体，应重点考虑 TB 黏膜表现的可能性。

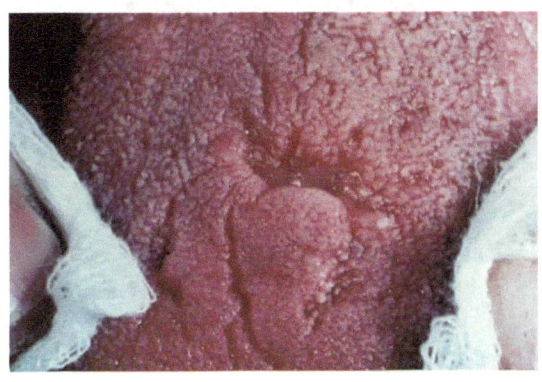

图 5.53　肺结核。发生在舌头上的结核性溃疡是硬结性的、具有不规则的边界（Source: Courtesy of J. Robert Newland, D.D.S., M.S., University of Texas, Houston Health Science Center, Dental Branch）。

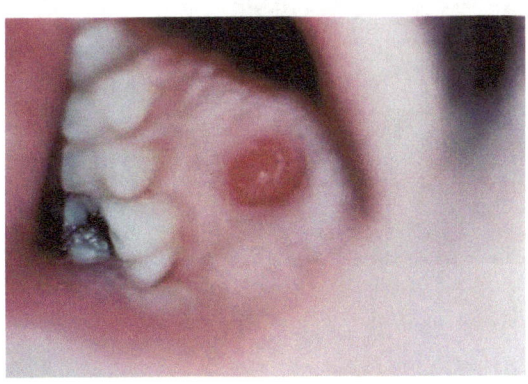

图 5.54　肺结核。肺结核也可感染腭部，临床表现与恶性唾液腺肿瘤相似（Source: Courtesy of J. Robert Newland, D.D.S., M.S., University of Texas, Houston Health Science Center, Dental Branch）。

黑色素沉着

HIV 阳性个体有时表现出病因不明的弥漫性口腔色素沉着斑块，这种现象与内分泌异常或色素紊乱的临床表现类似[577,578]。在长达 24 个月的随访中，6.4% 的 HIV 阳性个体的颊黏膜、嘴唇、牙龈和腭部发生棕黑色斑，而阴性对照为 3.6%[579]（图 5.55）。皮肤和指甲的色素沉着也有见报道[580]。

虽然某些治疗药物如酮康唑、氯法齐明和叠氮胸苷有时能加重口腔色素沉着[581]，但是在没有使用这些药物的 HIV 阳性个体的口腔黏膜黑色素细胞仍然能被激活[582]。然而，由于在 HIV 阴性个体中有时也会发生口腔色素沉着，所以这些发现的意义尚存在争议[583]。尽管如此，当有口腔黏膜色素沉着同时具有其他提示性发现时，应增加对 HIV 感染的怀疑[584]。

坏死性（溃疡性）口腔炎

坏死性（溃疡性）口腔炎虽然不常见，但它是坏死性（溃疡性）牙周炎的更严重的蔓延表现[585]。在临床表现上让人联想到坏疽性口腔炎，在解剖位置上又区别于坏死性（溃疡性）牙周炎[586]。它的特点是破坏性病变会蔓延至非牙周软组织和骨组织，伴有大量的上皮细胞和结缔组织坏死及骨组织塌陷[587,588]（图 5.56），有时可危及生命。坏死性口腔炎最好的治疗方法是局部清创、牙科预防、止痛和抗菌治疗，如洗必泰和甲硝唑[589]。

唾液腺疾病

HIV 阳性和 AIDS 患者的唾液腺疾病表现为口干症和唾液腺肿大[590~594]，儿童比成人多见。临床特点和组织病理学表现与良性淋巴上皮疾病相似，如干燥综合征[595~604]。大多数感染患者表现为双侧腮腺肿大、唾液分泌量减少[605~607]。全唾液中的 HIV 检出水平较低[608~614]、唾液蛋白降低、sIgA 增加[615]。唾液传播 HIV 的危险性极低[616,617]。最近，

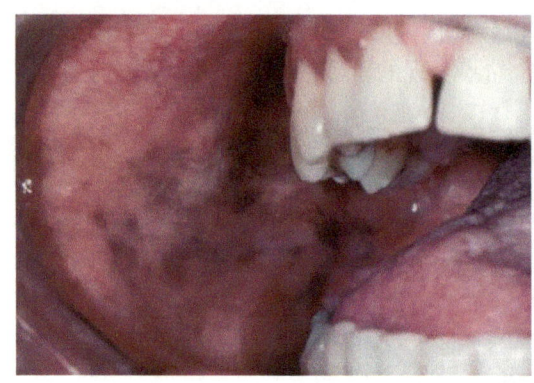 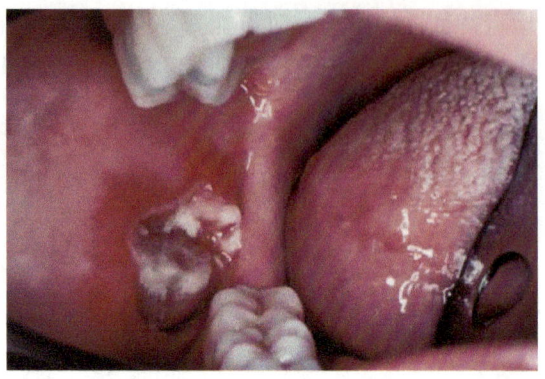

图 5.55　色素沉着。在 HIV 阳性个体中，口腔黏膜色素沉着的发生有多种诱因，但是自发性色素沉着的意义尚属未知。

图 5.56　坏死性口腔炎。虽然没有鉴别出病原体，但是坏死性口腔炎具有极大的破坏性。

FDA 批准了一项基于口腔液体的 HIV 快检方法，即 OraQuick™（OraSure Technologies，Bethlehem，PA）[618,619]。

HIV 感染患者的唾液腺疾病应该与口腔干燥综合征进行平行治疗。为了预防龋齿发病率的升高，口腔卫生必须格外注意[620,621]。催涎剂如口香糖对刺激残留的功能性唾液腺实质是非常有帮助的[622]，而毛果芸香碱能够以最小的副作用取得同样的效果。新批准的胆碱能受体激动剂 Evoxac™（西维美林）（Daiichi Pharmaceutical Corp.，Tokyo，Japan）能够结合于毒蕈碱受体，对受损的唾液腺起到相同的作用[623,624]。

血小板减少性紫癜

血小板减少性紫癜（thrombocytopenic purpura，TP）是由于血小板破坏的增加引起的，在 HIV 阳性和 AIDS 患者中并不常见[625~627]，但是 TP 的口腔病变可以作为显著的早期临床症状[628,629]（图 5.57）。此外，HIV 阳性者的口腔黏膜血管病变需要非常准确地与其他临床症状相似的病变进行鉴别诊断，如卡波西肉瘤和上皮多发性血管瘤[630,631]。牙龈活检一直是 TP 诊断的有用工具[632]。治疗方法包括泼尼松、免疫球蛋白治疗和脾切除[633]。

非特异性溃疡

因为 HIV 阳性患者具有病因不明的各种口腔溃疡[634]，所以没有任何理由怀疑 HIV 阳性患者表现出的口腔溃疡病因比一般人群少。然而，关键是要在抗炎或专业的姑息治疗前排除感染性溃疡。糖皮质激素[635] 和沙利度胺[636] 已成功地用于治疗难治性溃疡。

HSV

发生在 HIV 阳性儿童和成人的 HSV 感染的诊断和治疗面临着困难[637~640]。HSV 常单独感染或与其他口腔微生物共同感染 HIV 阳性患者[641,642]，大多为 HSV-1 型且复发性感染，也有 HSV-2 型和原发性感染的报道[643]。不幸的是，在免疫抑制个体中复发性 HSV-1 感染常引起广泛的、严重的且长期累及非角质化和角质化黏膜的疾病，与免疫功能正常个体的原发性 HSV-1 感染相似[644,645]（图 5.58）。此类患者在发病人群中占有很大比例。

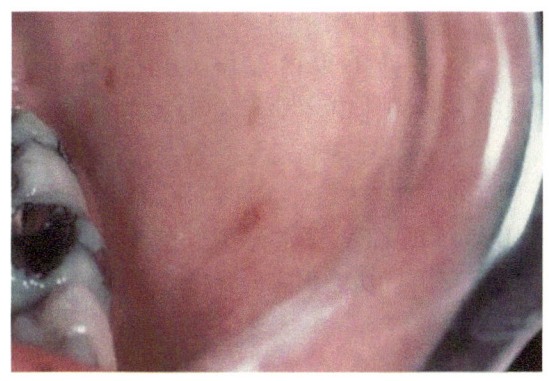
图 5.57 血小板减少性紫癜。口腔黏膜瘀斑可能是血小板减少性紫癜的最早发病迹象。

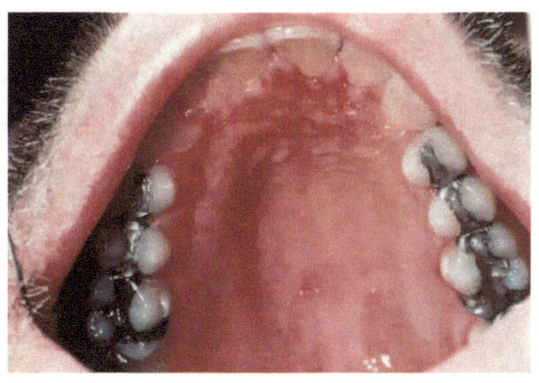
图 5.58 HSV-1 型。AIDS 患者的复发性口腔 HSV-1 病变与原发性 HSV-1 感染相似,主要发生在角质化黏膜,如硬腭和附着龈,且病程漫长。

HSV-1 病变的诊断方法有脱落细胞法（察内克试验）[646]、直接免疫荧光法[647]、免疫过氧化物酶法[648]、放射免疫分析法[649]和病毒培养[650]。各种抗病毒药物已用于疾病的预防和治疗，包括阿昔洛韦、伐昔洛韦、泛昔洛韦、更昔洛韦和膦甲酸[651~660]。不幸的是，有报道称在 HIV 阳性个体中出现了阿昔洛韦和膦甲酸抗性的 HSV-1 感染[661~663]。

尖锐湿疣

大概是由于口腔-生殖器接触的原因，在 HIV 阳性个体中，口腔尖锐湿疣（condyloma acuminatum，CA）或性病疣常见于舌头、舌系带、牙龈和嘴唇[664,665]。DNA 原位杂交能够检出常规的 HPV-6 和 HPV-11 感染[666,667]。

病变通常为无症状、粉红色、肥厚的软组织肿块，肿块表面光滑且有圆突（图 5.59 和图 5.60）。由于病毒比较容易传播，所以病变应该清除。虽然手术切除可以最快地清除病变，但激光手术和冷冻手术也是有效的[668]。鬼臼树脂和 IFN 已用于非口腔尖锐湿疣的治疗，但是对于口腔黏膜尖锐湿疣的疗效仍有待观察。

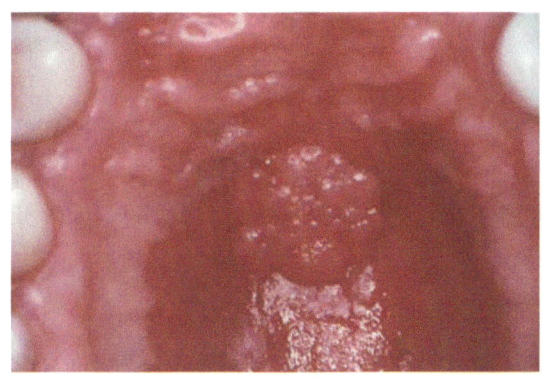
图 5.59 尖锐湿疣。口腔尖锐湿疣常见于 HIV 阳性和 AIDS 患者。

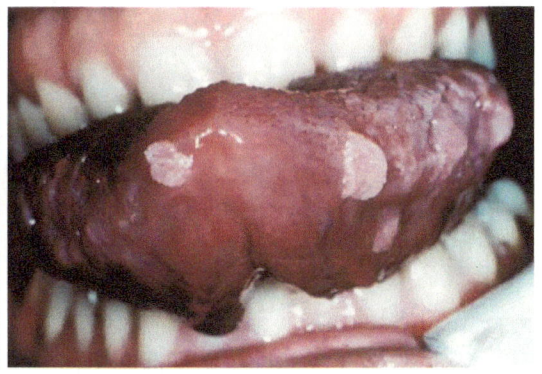
图 5.60 尖锐湿疣。由于黏膜受累面积较大，多发性口腔尖锐湿疣比较难治（Source: Courtesy of J. Robert Newland, D.D.S., M.S., University of Texas, Houston Health Science Center, Dental Branch）。

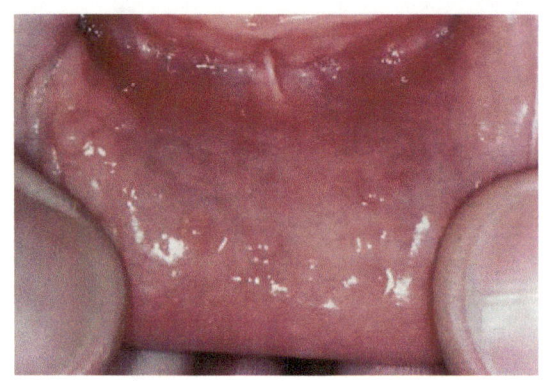

图5.61 局灶性上皮增生症（Heck氏病）。局灶性上皮增生症由HPV-13和HPV-32引起，也见于HIV阳性和AIDS患者。

局灶性上皮增生症

局灶性上皮增生症（FEH）可见于HIV阳性个体中[669]。病变为多发性、无症状、肉色的丘疹和斑块，累及全部口腔黏膜表面（图5.61）。DNA原位杂交证明为HPV-13或HPV-32的感染。在不影响美观或没有出现功能损害时，FEH是不需要考虑治疗的。

口腔疣

在HIV阳性和AIDS患者中可发生口腔寻常疣、鳞状上皮乳头状瘤及不同于尖锐湿疣以外的其他疣[670~672]（图5.62和图5.63）。同样在免疫功能正常的患者中，这些病变中均检出不同亚型的HPV，且出现中空细胞和其他口腔疣特征性的组织病理学特点[673]。偶有不常见HPV亚型的报道，如屠夫疣的病原体HPV-7[674]。

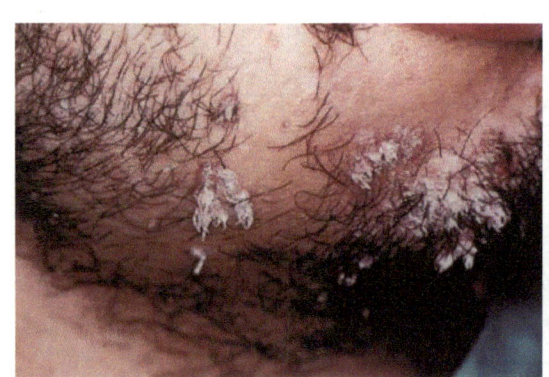

图5.62 寻常疣。口周皮肤上的多发性寻常疣病变。

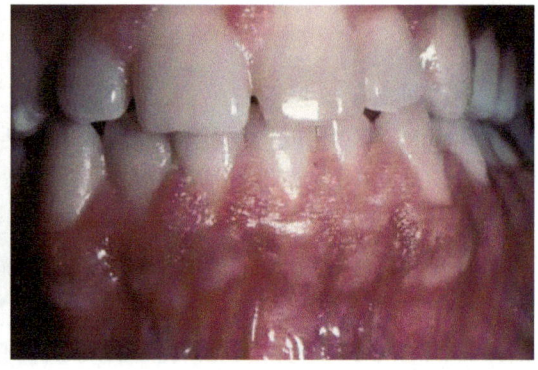

图5.63 寻常疣。当发生在牙龈上、由不同HPV亚型引起的寻常疣病变广泛时，治疗常带来并发症。

与尖锐湿疣不同的是，这些口腔疣似乎是不太可能蔓延或传播。单个的或局灶性病变集落应当清除，但如果多发灶病变不能清除，快速、大面积蔓延的可能性也很小。据报道，外用西多福韦，一种胞嘧啶的嘌呤类似物，也能有效地治疗HIV阳性个体中的顽固性牙龈疣[675]。

带状疱疹

VZV感染（水痘）在免疫抑制个体中可导致死亡[676~678]。复发性口腔VZV感染（带状疱疹）是引发严重疾病的病因[679~686]。虽然在HIV阳性和AIDS患者中，原发性VZV的口腔表现与免疫功能正常个体相似[687]，但是它的临床表现往往被其他共存感染所掩盖[688~690]。复发性口腔VZV病变具有特征性的、沿被感染神经的单侧分布特点，多条神经可能受累（图5.64）。

阿昔洛韦、伐昔洛韦和泛昔洛韦通常替代旧的抗病毒药如阿糖腺苷用于 VZV 感染的治疗[691~697]。溴乙烯脱氧尿苷、膦甲酸、更昔洛韦和其他阿昔洛韦同系物也被提倡用于治疗 VZV 感染[698,699]。由于与其他疱疹病毒的共同感染，在免疫抑制个体中发现了对阿昔洛韦耐药性的 VZV 感染[700~703]。多种口腔清洗剂配合镇痛药使用也非常有助于缓解 VZV 感染导致的口腔不适。

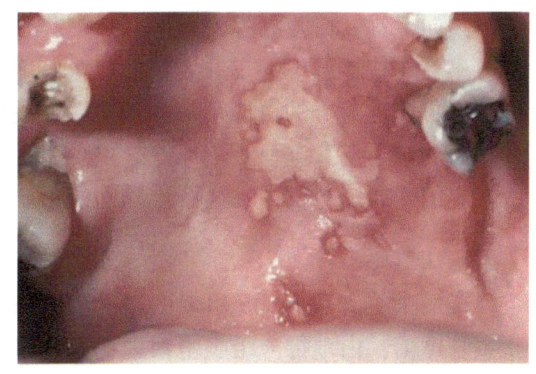

图 5.64 复发性 VZV 感染。口腔带状疱疹的特点为沿被感染神经的单侧分布。

第 3 组：与 HIV 感染相关的其他病变

细菌性感染

在 HIV 感染个体中存在着大量的非典型口腔细菌的感染，包括放线菌、大肠杆菌和肺炎克雷伯菌[704,705]。虽然这些感染的临床表现并非独一无二，但是必须强调适当的诊断方法包括细菌培养的重要性，因为它们可以确保及时给予适当的治疗。

上皮（杆菌性）血管瘤和猫抓病

上皮（杆菌性）血管瘤 [epithelioid (bacillary) angiomatosis, EA] 是一种假瘤性的传染性疾病，以皮肤黏膜褐色丘疹和血管源性结节为特点[706~708]。EA 的病原体是属于革兰氏阴性杆菌的巴尔通体（旧称罗卡利马体），与猫抓病的病原体相似但略有不同，用 Warthin-Starry 银染法可以明确地进行鉴定[709~718]。

在临床和组织病理学特征上，HIV 阳性和 AIDS 患者的病变与卡波西肉瘤相似[719~725]。作为一种传染性疾病，EA 对红霉素和其他抗生素的治疗反应良好[726~730]。

病变的准确诊断是非常重要的，原因有以下三点。首先，误诊会导致对 AIDS 患者的分期不当。其次，误诊会使卡波西肉瘤患者遭受不必要的、有害的治疗。最后，误诊可导致免疫抑制个体中潜在的致命性机会性感染的增强。

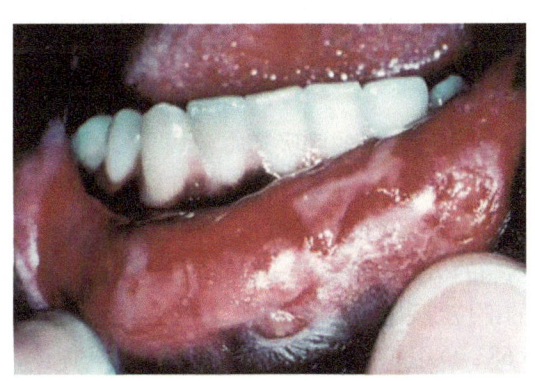

图 5.65 药物反应。同时使用多种药物治疗的患者发生药物反应和相互作用的风险更高，而且很多药物反应都有口腔黏膜表现（Source: Courtesy of J. Robert Newland, D.D.S., M.S., University of Texas, Houston Health Science Center, Dental Branch）。

药物反应

免疫抑制个体对不同药物治疗的反应也不同，包括弥漫性口腔溃疡、多形性红斑、苔藓样反应和毒性表皮坏死[731~734]（图 5.65）。在 HIV 阳性个体中，由于同时使用多种治疗药物，往往包括实验性药物，这使药物反应发生的可能性大大增加[735~778]。所有这些情况都倾向于累及口腔黏膜，而不累及皮肤，可能会与感染性的口腔溃疡混淆[739,740]。

虽然这些情况下的皮肤表现简化了临床鉴别诊断，但是如果没有皮肤表现，就必须要排除病毒源性疱疹的可能性，如HSV-1。皮质类固醇治疗、抗菌口腔冲洗剂及免疫调节剂如左旋咪唑可对某些患者有效[741~744]。病原体的确定是预防复发的关键。但不幸的是，某些特定的病原体可发生逃逸而难以确定。

真菌感染

HIV感染者或AIDS患者的口腔中有许多机会性真菌感染的报道[745~747]。病原体包括新生隐球菌、白地霉、组织胞浆菌、毛霉菌（毛霉菌病/接合菌病）和黄曲霉菌。

对免疫抑制个体来说，隐球菌感染是非常严重的，会危及生命，即使进行积极的抗真菌治疗，也常常会引发脑膜炎并导致患者迅速死亡[748,749]。在AIDS患者中，这是第四大最常见的机会性感染。虽然最初的感染途径是肺，但是病原体很快扩散到各种器官，包括皮肤和口腔黏膜。

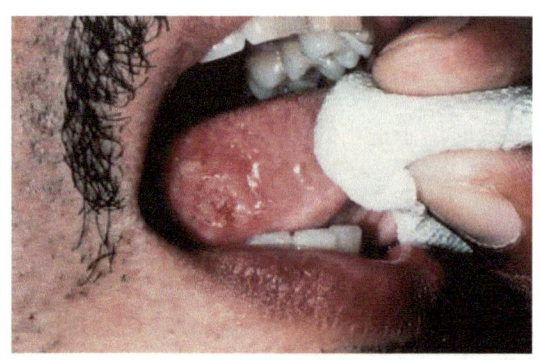

图5.66 隐球菌病。AIDS患者中口腔黏膜的新型隐球菌感染表现为硬结、非愈合性溃疡，边界突起成卷，与其他炎症和肿瘤的黏膜表现类似（Source: Lynch and Naftolin[755]，©1987 with permission from Elsevier）。

全身症状往往不明确，可能包括肺功能障碍、不明原因发热和头痛。虽然疾病的假设诊断以脑脊液的组织病理学检查或印度墨水染色的结果为基础，但是适当地进行确诊性真菌培养对诊断也是有帮助的。治疗方法包括强效唑类抗真菌药物治疗、氟胞嘧啶和两性霉素B[750~754]。几例口腔隐球菌病累及舌头和上颚[755~758]（图5.66），病变通常表现为侵蚀性的软组织肿块。

在免疫抑制个体中，口腔地霉菌病是一种罕见的机会性霉菌病[759]。在HIV感染者中，大多数口腔白地霉菌感染的主要表现为非特异性牙龈炎，在接受局部制霉素治疗后消退。

组织胞浆菌病是由组织胞浆菌引起的，在美国是最常见的呼吸道霉菌病[760]。它是密西西比和俄亥俄河谷的地方病，可引起典型的肺部症状和体征[761]。原发性肺部组织胞浆菌病的口腔病变是不常见的[762]，但HIV阳性和AIDS患者的口腔病变病例已见于许多报道中[763~767]。多达50%的伴发播散性组织胞浆菌病的AIDS患者存在口腔病变[653]。

播散性组织胞浆菌病的口腔病变最常累及的部位是舌、颚和颊黏膜。病变表现为边界不清的溃疡性软组织肿胀[768,769]（图5.67和图5.68）。组织病理学检查可见明显的病原体，真菌培养可以确诊[770,771]。特异性荧光抗体染色也可用于确诊。使用唑类同系物和两性霉素B进行强效抗真菌药物治疗对感染相当有疗效[772~776]。

毛霉菌病（藻菌病或接合菌病）是一种由不同来源，如土壤、发霉面包和腐烂的果蔬的腐生真菌引起的机会性真菌感染[777]。病原体倾向于侵染血管，引起广泛的梗死和大面积的组织坏死[778,779]。虽然在过去这种情况主要发生在控制很差的糖尿病和血液肿瘤患者

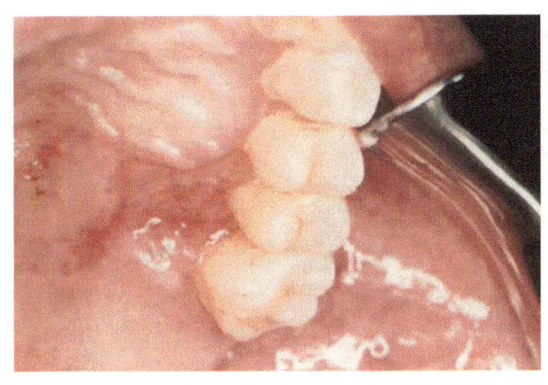

图 5.67 组织胞浆菌病。组织胞浆菌是密西西比山谷的地方病,在 AIDS 患者中可见这种真菌感染引起的无痛性口腔溃疡。

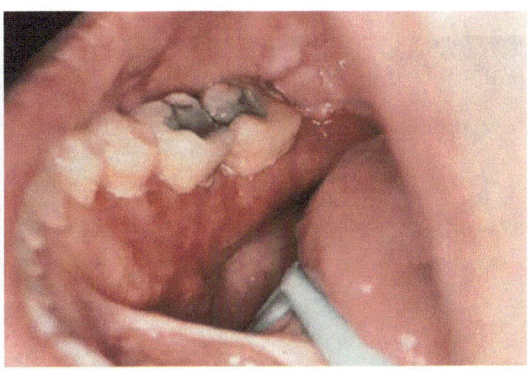

图 5.68 组织胞浆菌病。组织胞浆菌病的口腔黏膜感染也表现为牙龈的非特异性肿大和浅表溃疡。

身上,但是在 HIV 阳性和 AIDS 患者中也有此类病例的报道[780,781]。口腔病变在早期可能会出现组织肿大,但在后期或控制情况很差时,病变出现特征性的恶性组织坏死和死骨组织塌陷。两性霉素 B 是传统的治疗药物,而唑类抗真菌药物也被证明是有效的[782]。

在 HIV 阳性和 AIDS 患者中,曲霉菌是一种不常见的真菌感染[783,784]。黄曲霉是环境中流行的最常见的致病菌,倾向于在免疫抑制患者的鼻腔和呼吸系统繁殖[785]。从免疫抑制患者的上颌骨窦中分离到的病原体已经被培养出来[786]。感染一旦发生,病原体的菌丝形式会产生破坏上皮组织的外毒素。此外,黄曲霉倾向于侵染血管组织,从而导致血栓和周围组织的血管性坏死。两性霉素 B 和伊曲康唑都能有效治疗此类感染,尤其是在感染早期[787]。

神经紊乱

HIV 感染者可发生面部麻痹、三叉神经痛和面瘫[788~792]。虽然在 HIV 感染和 AIDS 患者中周围神经病变较为常见,但是却很少累及颅神经。第 5 对和第 7 对颅神经是最容易被感染的,但目前还不清楚这些临床症状和体征是否由 HIV 感染直接或间接机制如血管痉挛引起[793]。

复发性阿弗他口炎

复发性阿弗他口炎(recurrent aphthous stomatitis,RAS)又称口腔溃疡,它不是 HIV 感染特有的,但给相当多的美国人带来了痛苦[794,795]。虽然许多复发性口腔溃疡是由病毒感染口腔黏膜引起的,但发生在 HIV 阳性个体中的口腔溃疡无非就是阿弗他溃疡。从临床表现、病变发生位置、病因缺乏和对治疗的反应情况可以判断出,在 HIV 阳性个体中 RAS 具有一定的发病率,尽管疱疹样溃疡更为普遍[796~798](图 5.69)。重型阿弗他溃疡发病率的上升提示免疫状况的恶化[799~801](图 5.70)。

局部皮质激素治疗轻型阿弗他溃疡十分有效[802]。全身使用皮质激素对重型阿弗他溃疡进行治疗时要慎重[803]。抗菌性口腔冲洗剂可以有效减少细菌在阿弗他溃疡假膜上定殖,如四环素口服混悬液[804]。治疗阿弗他溃疡建议使用沙立度胺[805~807]、秋水仙素[808]和 IFN[809]。

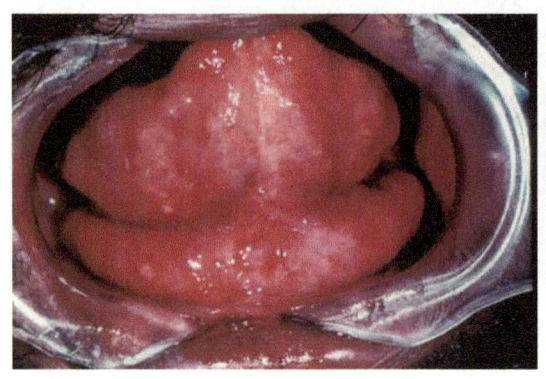

图 5.69 轻型阿弗他溃疡。轻型阿弗他溃疡是 HIV 阳性和 AIDS 患者常见的并发症。

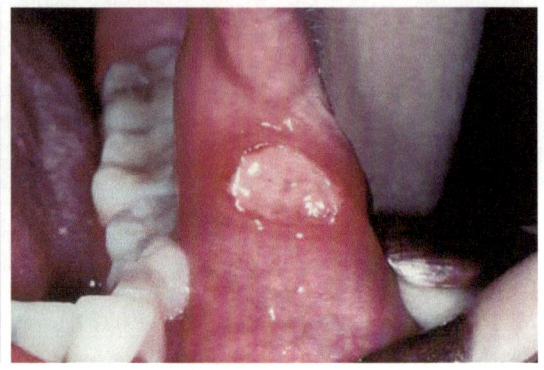

图 5.70 重型阿弗他溃疡。重型阿弗他溃疡给 HIV 阳性和 AIDS 患者带来明显不适感，即使给予积极的治疗，也需要数周甚至数月才能痊愈。

病毒感染

在 HIV 阳性个体唾液中可检测到 CMV[810,811]，并被认为是某些 AIDS 患者发生口腔溃疡的病原体[812]。虽然 CMV 口腔感染的表现远不及眼部表现和其他表现明显，但它是免疫抑制个体全身性病毒感染的独特口腔表现[813]。CMV 和坏死性牙龈炎及卡波西肉瘤之间的关系已有报道[814]。

口腔 CMV 感染通常表现为突起的非硬结性溃疡，被可变红斑围绕[815~822]（图 5.71 和图 5.72）。据报道，口腔 CMV 感染病例与 HIV 相关牙周疾病[823] 及一些累及下颌骨的疾病相似[824]。通过口腔涂片的免疫组化检测可对 CMV 进行确诊[825]。作为疱疹病毒，CMV 对阿昔洛韦治疗的反应良好，IFN、阿糖腺苷、更昔洛韦和膦甲酸也能有效预防和治疗 CMV 感染[826~830]。皮质激素能够增加 HIV 阳性个体患 CMV 的风险，如果可能应尽量避免使用[831]。

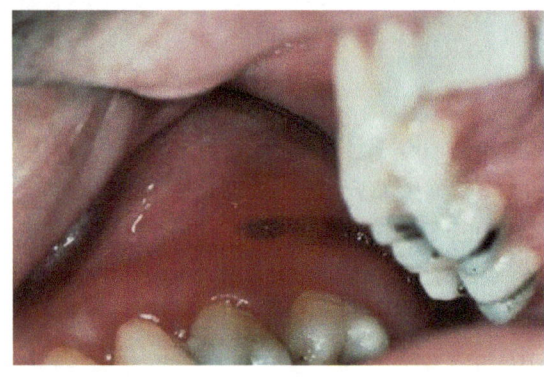

图 5.71 CMV。CMV 性溃疡与复发性阿弗他溃疡相似，表现为被假膜覆盖、被红斑晕围绕的比较浅的病变基底。

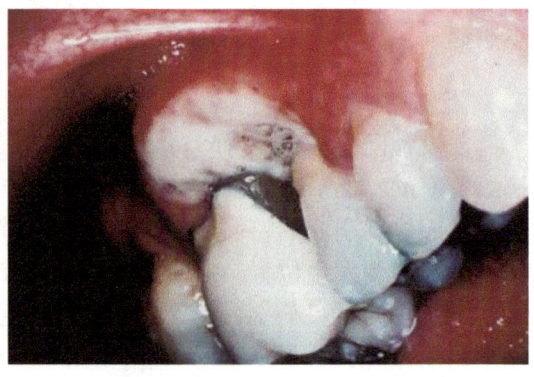

图 5.72 CMV。发生在牙龈的 CMV 性溃疡可能与明显的牙周破坏有关。

传染性软疣

众所周知，传染性软疣（molluscum contagiosum）是由痘病毒引起的特点鲜明的皮肤病变[832~834]。在 HIV 阳性和 AIDS 患者中也有皮肤受累的报道[835~843]。HIV 阳性的传染性软疣患者虽然能引起口周皮肤病变[844~847]，但是口内病变极为罕见[848~850]。在此类皮肤感染的治疗中，有效的治疗方法包括抗病毒治疗和感染皮肤的化学脱皮[851,852]。

参 考 文 献

[1] Laskaris G. Oral manifestations of infectious diseases.Dent Clin North Am 1996;40:395–423.

[2] Spruance S, Overall J Jr, Kern E, et al. The natural history of recurrent herpes simplex labialis. N Engl J Med 1977;297:69–74.

[3] Spruance SL. The natural history of recurrent oralfacial herpes simplex virus infection. Semin Dermatol 1992;11:200–206.

[4] Scully C, Bagg J. Viral infections in dentistry. Curr Opin Dent 1992;2:102–115.

[5] Waggoner-Fountain LA, Grossman LB. Herpes simplex virus. Pediatr Rev 2004;25:86–93.

[6] Miller CS, Jacob RJ, Hiser DG. UV-enhanced replication of herpes simplex virus in DNA-repair competent and deficient fibroblasts. Oral Surg Oral Med Oral Pathol 1993;75:602–609.

[7] Hebert A, Berg J. Oral mucous membrane diseases of childhood. Semin Dermatol 1992;11:80–87.

[8] Scully C. Ulcerative stomatitis, gingivitis, and skin lesions. An unusual case of primary herpes simplex infection. Oral Surg Oral Med Oral Pathol 1985;59:261–263.

[9] Fenton SJ, Unkel JH. Viral infections of the oral mucosa in children: a clinical review. Pract Periodontics Aesthet Dent 1997;9:683–690.

[10] Axell T, Liedholm R. Occurrence of recurrent herpes labialis in an adult Swedish population. Acta Odontol Scand 1990;48:119–123.

[11] Griffin JW. Recurrent intraoral herpes simplex virus infection. Oral Surg 1965;19:209–213.

[12] Sheridan PJ, Hermann EC. Intraoral lesions of adults associated with herpes simplex virus. Oral Surg 1971;32:390–397.

[13] Oranje AP, Folkers E. The Tzanck smear: old, but still of inestimable value. Pediatr Dermatol 1988;5:127–129.

[14] Burns JC. Diagnostic methods for herpes simplex infection: a review. Oral Surg 1980;50:346–349.

[15] Kimura H, Shibata M, Kuzushima K, Nishikawa K, Nishiyama Y, Morishima T. Detection and direct typing of herpes simplex virus by polymerase chain reaction.Med Microbiol Immunol 1990;179:177–184.

[16] Silverman S Jr, Beumer J. Primary herpetic gingivostomatitis of adult onset. Oral Surg 1973;36:496–503.

[17] Stoopler ET, Pinto A, DeRossi SS, et al.Herpes simplex and varicella-zoster infections: clinical and laboratory diagnosis. Gen Dent 2003;51:281–286.

[18] Weathers DR, Griffin JW. Intraoral ulcerations of recurrent herpes simplex and recurrent aphthae: two distinct clinical entities. J Am Dent Assoc 1970;81: 81–87.

[19] Sciubba JJ. Herpes simplex and aphthous ulcerations: presentation, diagnosis and management-an update. Gen Dent 2003;51:510–516.

[20] Hirsch M, Schooley R. Treatment of herpesvirus infections. N Engl J Med 1983;309:963–970.

[21] Villarreal EC. Current and potential therapies for the treatment of herpes-virus infections. Prog Drug Res 1996;60:263–307.

[22] De Clercq E. Antiviral drugs in current clinical use. J Clin Virol 2004;30:115–113.

[23] Griffiths PD. Tomorrow's challenges for herpesvirus management: potential applications for valacyclovir. J Infect Dis 2002;186(suppl 1):S131–S137.

[24] Wu JJ, Brentjens MH, Torres G, et al. Valacyclovir in the treatment of herpes simplex, herpes zoster, and other viral infections. J Cutan Med Surg 2003;7:372–381.

[25] Raborn GW, Grace MG. Recurrent herpes simplex labialis: selected therapeutic options. J Can Dent Assoc 2003;69:498–503.

[26] Huber MA. Herpes simplex type-1 virus infection. Quintessence Int 2003;34:453–467.

[27] Brady RC, Bernstein DI. Treatment of herpes simplex virus infections. Antiviral Res 2004;61:73–81.

[28] Kleymann G. Novel agents and strategies to treat herpes simplex virus infections. Expert Opin Invest Drugs 2003;12:165–183.

[29] Habbema L, DeBoulle K, Roders GA, Katz DH. NDocosanol 10% cream in the treatment of recurrent herpes labialis: a randomized, double-blind, placebocontrolled study. Acta Derm Venerecol 1996;76:479–481.

[30] Sasadeusz JJ, Sacks SL. Systemic antivirals in herpesvirus infections. Dermatol Clin 1993;11:171–185.

[31] Jensen LA, Hoehns JD, Squires CL. Oral antivirals for the acute treatment of recurrent herpes labialis. Ann Pharmacother 2004;38:705–709.

[32] Malmstrom J, Ruokonen H, Konttinen YT, et al. Herpes simplex virus antigens and inflammatory cells in oral lesions in recurrent erythema multiforme. Immunoperoxidase and autoradiographic studies. Acta Derm Venereol 1990;70:405–410.

[33] Chilukuri S, Rosen T. Management of acyclovirresistant herpes simplex virus. Dermatol Clin 2003;21:311–320.

[34] Spruance S, Schnipper L, Overall J Jr, et al. Treatment of herpes simplex labialis with topical acyclovir in polyethylene glycol. J Infect Dis 1982;146:85–90.

[35] Fiddian A, Ivanyi L. Topical acyclovir in the management of recurrent herpes labialis. Br J Dermatol 1983;109:321–326.

[36] Perna JJ, Eskinazi DP. Treatment of oro-facial herpes simplex infections with acyclovir: a review. Oral Surg Oral Med Oral Pathol 1988;65:689–692.

[37] Spruance S, Stewart JC, Rowe NH, McKeough MB, Wenerstrom G, Freeman DJ. Treatment of recurrent herpes simplex labialis with oral acyclovir. J Infect Dis 1990;161:185–190.

[38] Lavelle CL. Acyclovir: is it an effective virostatic agent for orofacial infections? J Oral Pathol Med 1993;22:391–401.

[39] Spruance SL, Rea TL, Thoming C, Tucker R, Saltzman R, Boon R. Penciclovir cream for the treatment of herpes simplex labialis. A randomized, multicenter, double-blind, placebo-controlled trial. Topical Penciclovir Collaborative Study Group. JAMA 1997;277(17):1374–1379.

[40] Boon R, Goodman JJ, Martinez J, Marks GL, Gamble M, Welch C. Penciclovir cream for the treatment of sunlight-induced herpes simplex labialis: a randomized, double-blind, placebo-controlled trial. Penciclovir Cream Herpes Labialis Study Group. Clin Ther 2000;22:76–90.

[41] Epstein JB, Scully C. Herpes simplex virus in immunocompromised patients: growing evidence of drug resistance. Oral Surg Oral Med Oral Pathol 1991;72:47–50.

[42] Bacon TH, Levin MJ, Leary JJ, et al. Herpes simplex virus resistance to acyclovir and penciclovir after two decades of antiviral therapy. Clin Microbiol Rev 2003;16:114–128.

[43] Morfin F, Thouvenot D. Herpes simplex virus resistance to antiviral drugs. J Clin Virol 2003;26:29–37.

[44] Wachsman M, Aurelian L, Burnett JW. The prophylactic use of cyclooxygenase inhibitors in recurrent herpes simplex infections. Br J Dermatol 1990;123: 375–380.

[45] Park JB, Park NH. Effect of chlorhexidine on the in vitro and in vivo herpes simplex virus infection. Oral Surg Oral Med Oral Pathol 1989;67:149–153.

[46] Spruance S, Stewart J, Freeman D. Early application of topical 15% idoxuridine in dimethyl sulfoxide shortens the course of herpes simplex labialis: a multicenter placebo-controlled trial. J Infect Dis 1990;161: 191–197.

[47] Rowe NH, Brooks SL, Young SK, et al. A clinical trial of topically applied 3 per cent vidarabine against recurrent herpes labialis. Oral Surg 1979;47:142–147.

[48] Kleymann G. New antiviral drugs that target herpesvirus helicase primase enzymes. Herpes 2003;10: 46–52.

[49] Rooney J, Bryson Y, Mannia O, et al. Prevention of ultraviolet light-induced herpes labialis by sunscreen. Lancet 1991;338:1419–1422.

[50] Miller CS, Redding SW. Diagnosis and management of orofacial herpes simplex virus infections. Dent Clin North Am 1992; 36:879–895.

[51] Birek C, Patterson B, Maximiw WC, Minden MD. EBV and HSV infections in a patient who had undergone bone marrow transplantation: oral manifestations and diagnosis by in situ nucleic acid hybridization. Oral Surg Oral Med Oral Pathol 1989;68:612–617.

[52] Barrett AP. Chronic indolent orofacial herpes simplex virus infection in chronic leukemia: a report of three cases. Oral Surg Oral Med Oral Pathol 1988;66:387–390.

[53] Epstein JB, Sherlock C, Page JL, Spinelli J, Phillips G. Clinical study of herpes simplex virus infection in leukemia. Oral Surg Oral Med Oral Pathol 1990;70: 38–43.

[54] Wingard JR. Oral complications of cancer therapies. Infectious and noninfectious systemic consequences. NCI Monogr 1990;9:21–26.

[55] Redding SW. Role of herpes simplex virus reactivation in chemotherapy-induced oral mucositis. NCI Monogr 1990; 9:103–105.

[56] Fleming P. Dental management of the pediatric oncology patient. Curr Opin Dent 1991;1:577–582.

[57] Redding SW, Luce EB, Boren MW. Oral herpes simplex virus infection in patients receiving head and neck radiation. Oral Surg Oral Med Oral Pathol 1990;69: 578–580.

[58] Heimdahl A, Mattsson T, Dahllof G, Lonnquist B, Ringden O. The oral cavity as a port of entry for early infections in patients treated with bone marrow transplantation. Oral Surg Oral Med Oral Pathol 1989;68: 711–716.

[59] Woo SB, Sonis ST, Sonis AL. The role of herpes simplex virus in the development of oral mucositis in bone marrow transplant recipients. Cancer 1990;66:2375–2379.

[60] Schubert MM, Peterson DE, Flournoy N, Meyers JC, Truelove EL. Oral and pharyngeal herpes simplex virus infection after allogeneic bone marrow transplantation: analysis of factors associated with infection. Oral Surg Oral Med Oral Pathol 1990;70:286–293.

[61] Campton CM. Oral care for the renal transplant patient. ANNA J 1991;18:39–41.

[62] Arnow PM. Infections following orthotopic liver transplantation. HPB Surg 1991;3:221–232.

[63] Saral R. Oral complications of cancer therapies. Management of acute viral infections. NCI Monogr 1990;9:107–110.

[64] Rowe NH, Heine CS, Kowalski CJ. Herpetic whitlow: an occupational disease of practicing dentists. J Am Dent Assoc 1982;105:471–473.

[65] Walker LG, Simmons BP, Lovallo JL. Pediatric herpetic hand infections. J Hand Surg 1990;15:176–180.

[66] Gunbay T, Gunbay S, Kandemir S. Herpetic whitlow. Quintessence Int 1993;24:363–364.

[67] Lewis MA. Herpes simplex virus: an occupational hazard in dentistry. Int Dent J 2004;54:103–111.

[68] Schwandt NW, Mjos DP, Lubow RM. Acyclovir and the treatment of herpetic whitlow. Oral Surg Oral Med Oral Pathol 1987;64:255–258.

[69] Wander AH. Herpes simplex and recurrent corneal disease. Int Ophthalmol Clin 1984;24:27–38.

[70] Mader TH, Stulting RD. Viral keratitis. Infect Dis Clin North Am 1992;6:831–849.

[71] Nahmias AJ, Roizman B. Infection with herpes simplex viruses 1 and 2. N Engl J Med 1973;289:781–289.

[72] Weller T. Varicella and herpes zoster. N Engl J Med 1983;309:1362–1368.

[73] Badger GR. Oral signs of chickenpox (varicella): report of two cases. J Dent Child 1980;47:349–531.

[74] Rogers RS 3rd, Tindall JP. Herpes zoster in children. Arch Derm 1972;106:204–207.

[75] Beck JD, Watkins C. Epidemiology of nondental oral disease in the elderly. Clin Geriatr Med 1992;8: 461–482.

[76] McKenzie CD, Gobetti JP. Diagnosis and treatment of orofacial herpes zoster: report of cases. J Am Dent Assoc 1990;120:679–681.

[77] Nally FF, Ross IH. Herpes zoster of the oral and facial structures. Report of five cases and discussion. Oral Surg 1971;32:221–234.

[78] Johnson RW, Whitton TL. Management of herpes zoster (shingles) and postherpetic neuralgia. Expert Opin Pharmacother 2004;5:551–559.

[79] Johnson RW. Herpes zoster in the immunocompetent patient: management of post-herpetic neuralgia. Herpes 2003;10:38–45.

[80] Singh D, Kennedy DH. The use of gabapentin for the treatment of postherpetic neuralgia. Clin Ther 2003; 25:852–889.

[81] Muto T, Tsuchiya H, Sato K, Kanazawa M. Tooth exfoliation and necrosis of the mandible—a rare complication following trigeminal herpes zoster: report of a case. J Oral Maxillofac Surg 1990;48:1000–1003.

[82] Lin JR, Huang CC. Oral complications following a herpes zoster infection of trigeminal nerve. Chang Keng I Hsueh 1993;16:75–80.

[83] Serota F, Starr S, Bryan C, et al. Acyclovir treatment of herpes zoster infections. JAMA 1982;247:2132–2135.

[84] Nicholson KG. Antiviral therapy. Varicella-zoster virus infections, herpes labialis and mucocutaneous herpes, and cytomegalovirus infections. Lancet 1984; 2:677–681.

[85] Huff J, Bean B, Balfour H, et al. Therapy of herpes zoster with oral acyclovir. Am J Med 1988;85:84–89.

[86] Morton P, Thompson A. Oral acyclovir in the treatment of herpes zoster in general practice. N Z Med J 1989;102:93–95.

[87] Harding SP, Porter SM. Oral acyclovir in herpes zoster ophthalmicus. Curr Eye Res 1991; 10(suppl):177–182.

[88] Wallace MR, Bowler WA, Oldfield 3rd EC. Treatment of varicella in the immunocompetent adult. J Med Virol Suppl 1993;1:90–92.

[89] Suga S, Yoshikawa T, Ozaki T, Asano Y. Effect of oral acyclovir against primary and secondary viraemia in incubation period of varicella. Arch Dis Child 1993;69:639–642.

[90] Wagstaff AJ, Faulds D, Goa KL. Aciclovir. A reappraisal of its antiviral activity, pharmacokinetic properties and therapeutic efficacy. Drugs 1994;47:153–205.

[91] Whitley R, Soong S, Dolin R, et al. Early vidarabine therapy to control the complications of herpes zoster in immunosuppressed patients. N Engl J Med 1982; 307:971–975.

[92] De Clercq E. Antivirals for the treatment of herpesvirus infections. J Antimicrob Chemother 1993; 32(suppl A):121–132.

[93] Porter SR. Infection control in dentistry. Curr Opin Dent 1991;1:429–435.

[94] Brentjens MH, Yeung-Yue KA, Lee PC, et al. Vaccines for viral diseases with dermatologic manifestations. Dermatol Clin 2003;21:349–369.

[95] Straus SE, Cohen JI, Tosato G, Meier J. NIH conference. Epstein-Barr virus infections: biology, pathogenesis, and management. Ann Intern Med 1993;118:45–58.

[96] Mao EJ, Smith CJ. Detection of Epstein-Barr virus (EBV) DNA by the polymerase chain reaction (PCR) in oral smears from health individuals and patients with squamous cell carcinoma. J Oral Pathol Med 1993;22:12–17.

[97] Cruchley AT, Williams DM, Niedobitek G, et al. Epstein-Barr virus: biology and disease. Oral Dis 1997;3(suppl 1):S156–S163.

[98] Solomides CC, Miller AS, Christman RA, et al. Lymphomas of the oral cavity: histology, immunologic type, and incidence of Epstein-Barr virus infection. Hum Pathol 2002;33:153–157.

[99] Ikediobi NI, Tyring SK. Cutaneous manifestations of Epstein-Barr infection. Dermatol Clin 2002;20:283–289.

[100] Spano JP, Busson P, Atlan D, et al. Nasopharyngeal carcinomas: an update. Eur J Cancer 2003;39:2121–2135.

[101] Ambinder RF. Epstein-Barr virus-associated lymphoproliferative disorders. Rev Clin Exp Hematol 2003; 7:362–374.

[102] Shimakage M, Horii K, Tempaku A, et al. Association of Epstein-Barr virus with oral cancers. Hum Pathol 2002;33:608–614.

[103] Macsween KF, Crawford DH. Epstein-Barr virusrecent advances. Lancet Infect Dis 2003;3:131–140.

[104] Lambore S, McSherry J, Kraus AS. Acute and chronic symptoms of mononucleosis. J Fam Pract 1991;33:33–37.

[105] Maddern BR, Werkhaven J, Wessel HB, Yunis E. Infectious mononucleosis with airway obstruction and multiple cranial nerve paresis. Otolaryngol Head Neck Surg 1991;104:529–532.

[106] Westmore GA. Cervical abscess: a life-threatening complication of infectious mononucleosis. J Laryngol Otol 1990;104:358–359.

[107] Johnson PA, Avery C. Infectious mononucleosis presenting as a parotid mass with associated facial nerve palsy. Int J Oral Maxillofac Surg 1991;20:193–195.

[108] Har-El G, Josephson JS. Infectious mononucleosis complicated by lingual tonsillitis. J Laryngol Otol 1990;104:651–653.

[109] Magrath IT. African Burkitt's lymphoma. History, biology, clinical features, and treatment. Am J Pediatr Hematol Oncol 1991;13:222–246.

[110] Jacobs P. The malignant lymphomas in Africa. Hematol Oncol Clin North Am 1991;5:953–982.

[111] Walter PR, Klotz F, Alfy-Gattas T, Minko-Mi-Etoua D, Nguembi-Mbina C. Malignant lymphomas in Gabon (equatorial Africa): a morphologic study of 72 cases. Hum Pathol 1991;22:1040–1043.

[112] Okpala IE, Akang EE, Okpala UJ. Lymphomas in University College Hospital, Ibadan, Nigeria. Cancer 1991;68:1356–1360.

[113] Syrjanen S, Kallio P, Sainio P, Fuju C, Syrjanen K. Epstein-Barr virus (EBV) genomes and c-myc

oncogene in oral Burkitt's lymphomas. Scand J Dent Res 1992;100:176–180.

[114] Joske D, Knecht H. Epstein-Barr virus in lymphomas: a review. Blood Rev 1993;7:215–222.

[115] Shih LY, Liang DC.Non-Hodgkin's lymphomas in Asia. Hematol Oncol Clin North Am 1991;5:983–1001.

[116] Prevot S, Hamilton-Dutoit S, Audouin J, Walter P, Pallesen G, Diebold J. Analysis of African Burkitt's and high-grade B cell non-Burkitt's lymphoma for Epstein-Barr virus genomes using *in situ* hybridization. Br J Haematol 1992;80:27–32.

[117] Soderholdm AL, Lindqvist C, Heikinheimo K, Forssell K,Happonen RP.Non-Hodgkin's lymphomas presenting through oral symptoms. Int J Oral Maxillofac Surg 1990;19:131–134.

[118] Anavi Y, Kaplinsky C, Calderon S, Zaizov R. Head, neck, and maxillofacial childhood Burkitt's lymphoma: a retrospective analysis of 31 patients. J Oral Maxillofac Surg 1990;48:708–713.

[119] Svoboda WE, Aaron GR, Albano EA. North American Burkitt's lymphoma presenting with intraoral symptoms. Pediatr Dent 1991;13:52–58.

[120] Stiller CA, Parkin DM. International variations in the incidence of childhood lymphomas. Paediatr Perinat Epidemiol 1990;4:303–324.

[121] Ahmed M, Khan AH, Mansoor A, Khan MA, Saeed S. Burkitt's lymphoma–a study of 50 consecutive cases. J Pak Med Assoc 1993;43:151–153.

[122] Loh LE, Chee TS, John AB. The anatomy of the fossa of Rosenmuller—its possible influence on the detection of occult nasopharyngeal carcinoma. Singapore Med J 1991;32:154–155.

[123] Cvitkovic E, Bachouchi M, Armand JP. Nasopharyngeal carcinoma. Biology, natural history, and therapeutic implications. Hematol Oncol Clin North Am 1991;5:821–838.

[124] Niedobitek G, Herbst H, Young LS. Epstein-Barr virus and carcinomas. Int J Clin Lab Res 1993;23:17–24.

[125] Dickens P, Srivastava G, Loke SL, Chan CW, Liu YT. Epstein-Barr virus DNA in nasopharyngeal carcinomas from Chinese patients in Hong Kong. J Clin Pathol 1992;45:396–397.

[126] Neel HB 3rd. Nasopharyngeal carcinoma: diagnosis, staging, and management. Oncology 1992;6:87–95.

[127] Van Hasselt CA, Skinner DW. Nasopharyngeal carcinoma. An analysis of 100 Chinese patients. S Afr J Surg 1990;28:92–94.

[128] Sham JS, Cheung YK, Choy D, Chan FL, Leong L. Cranial nerve involvement and base of the skull erosion in nasopharyngeal carcinoma. Cancer 1991; 68:422–426.

[129] Bailey RE. Diagnosis and treatment of infectious mononucleosis. Am Fam Physician 1994;49:879–888.

[130] Stein JE, Schwenn MR, Jacir NN, Harris BH. Surgical restraint in Burkitt's lymphoma in children. J Pediatr Surg 1991;26:1273–1275.

[131] McGuire LJ, Lee JC. The histopathologic diagnosis of nasopharyngeal carcinoma. Ear Nose Throat J 1990;69:229–236.

[132] Hawkins EP, Krischer JP, Smith BE, Hawkins HK, Finegold MJ.Nasopharyngeal carcinoma in children—a retrospective review and demonstration of Epstein-Barr viral genomes in tumor cell cytoplasm: a report of the Pediatric Oncology Group. Hum Pathol 1990;21: 805–810.

[133] Akao I, Sato Y, Mukai K, et al. Detection of Epstein-Barr virus DNA in formalin-fixed paraffin-embedded tissue of nasopharyngeal carcinoma using polymerase chain reaction and *in situ* hybridization. Laryngoscope 1991;101:279–283.

[134] Littler E, Baylis SA, Zeng Y, Conway MJ, Mackett M, Arrand JR. Diagnosis of nasopharyngeal carcinoma by means of recombinant Epstein-Barr virus proteins. Lancet 1991;337:685–689.

[135] Ohshima K, Kikuchi M, Masuda Y, et al. Epstein-Barr viral genomes in carcinoma metastasis to lymph

nodes. Association with nasopharyngeal carcinoma. Acta Pathol Jpn 1991;41:437–443.

[136] Pearson GR. Epstein-Barr virus and nasopharyngeal carcinoma. J Cell Biochem Suppl 1993;17F:150–154.

[137] Andersson JP. Clinical aspects on Epstein-Barr virus infection. Scand J Infect Dis Suppl 1991;80:94–104.

[138] Chetham MM, Roberts KB. Infectious mononucleosis in adolescents. Pediatr Ann 1991;20:206–213.

[139] Axelrod P, Finestone AJ. Infectious mononucleosis in older adults. Am Fam Physician 1990;42:1599–1606.

[140] Fark AR. Infectious mononucleosis, Epstein-Barr virus, and chronic fatigue syndrome: a prospective case series. J Fam Pract 1991;32:202–209.

[141] Daley TD, Lovas LG. Diseases of the salivary glands: a review. J Can Dent Assoc 1991;57:411–414.

[142] Lucin P, Pavic I, Polic B, Jonjic S, Koszinowski UH. Gamma interferon-dependent clearance of cytomegalovirus infection in salivary glands. J Virol 1992; 66:1977–1984.

[143] Marx JL. Cytomegalovirus: a major cause of birth defects. Science 1975;190:1184–1186.

[144] Glick M, Goldman HS. Viral infections in the dental setting: potential effects on pregnant HCWs. J Am Dent Assoc 1993;124:79–86.

[145] Landolfo S, Gariglio M, Gribaudo G, et al. The human cytomegalovirus. Pharmacol Ther 2003;98:269–297.

[146] Slots J.Update on human cytomegalovirus in destructive periodontal disease. Oral Microbiol Immunol 2004;19:217–223.

[147] Peterslund NA. Herpesvirus infection: an overview of the clinical manifestations. Scand J Infect Dis Suppl 1991;80:15–20.

[148] Wahren B, Linde A.Virological and clinical characteristics of human herpesvirus 6. Scand J Infect Dis Suppl 1991;80:105–109.

[149] Oren I, Sobel JD. Human herpesvirus type 6: review. Clin Infect Dis 1992;14:741–746.

[150] Okada K, Ueda K, Kusuhara K, et al. Exanthema subitum and human herpesvirus 6 infection: clinical observations in fifty-seven cases. Pediatr Infect Dis J 1993;12:204–208.

[151] Caserta MT, Hall CB.Human herpesvirus-6.Annu Rev Med 1993;44:377–383.

[152] Asano Y,Yoshikawa T, Suga S, et al. Clinical features of infants with primary human herpesvirus 6 infection (exanthem subitum, roseola infantum). Pediatrics 1994;93:104–108.

[153] Dewhurst S, Skrincosky D, van Loon N. Human Herpesvirus 6. Expert Rev Mol Med 1997;1:1–17.

[154] Clark DA. Human herpesvirus 6. Rev Med Virol 2000;10:155–173.

[155] Caserta MT, Mock DJ, Dewhurst S.Human herpesvirus 6. Clin Infect Dis 2001;33:829–833.

[156] Dockerell DH. Human herpesvirus 6: molecular biology and clinical features. J Med Microbiol 2003; 52(pt 1):5–18.

[157] Abdel-Haq NM, Asmar BI. Human herpesvirus 6 (HHV6) infection. Indian J Pediatr 2004;71:89–96.

[158] Rathore MH. Human herpesvirus 6. South Med J 1993;86:1197–1201.

[159] Lawrence GL, Chee M, Craxton MA, Gompels UA, Honess RW, Barrell BG. Human herpesvirus 6 is closely related to human cytomegalovirus. J Virol 1990;64:287–299.

[160] Fox JD, Briggs M, Ward PA, Tedder RS. Human herpesvirus 6 in salivary glands. Lancet 1990;336: 590–593.

[161] Bagg J.Human herpesvirus-6: the latest human herpes virus. J Oral Pathol Med 1991;20:465–468.

[162] Saito I, Nishimura S, Kudo I, Fox RI, Moro I. Detection of Epstein-Barr virus and human herpes virus type 6 in saliva from patients with lymphoproliferative diseases by the polymerase chain reaction.Arch Oral Biol 1991;36:779–784.

[163] Dewhurst S, Skrincosky D, van Loon N. Human herpesvirus 7. Expert Rev Mol Med 1997;1:1–10. 138 Mucosal Immunology and Virology

[164] De Araujo T, Berman B, Weinstein A. Human herpesviruses 6 and 7. Dermatol Clin 2002;20:301–306.

[165] Cannon M, Cesarman E. Kaposi's sarcoma-associated herpes virus and acquired immunodeficiency syndrome-related malignancy. Semin Oncol 2000;27: 409–419.

[166] Cathomas G. Human herpes virus 8: a new virus discloses its face.Virchows Arch 2000;436:195–206.

[167] Malnati MS, Dagna L, Ponzoni M, et al. Human Herpesvirus 8 (HHV-8/KSHV) and hematologic malignancies. Rev Clin Exp Hematol 2003;7:374–405.

[168] Cioc AM, Allen C, Kalmar JR, et al. Oral plasmablastic lymphomas in AIDS patients are associated with human herpesvirus 8. Am J Surg Pathol 2004;28:41–46.

[169] Flaitz CM, Nichols CM, Walling DM, et al. Plasmablastic lymphoma: an HIV-associated entity with primary oral manifestations. Oral Oncol 2002;38:96–102.

[170] Eversole LR. Papillary lesions of the oral cavity: relationship to human papillomaviruses. J Calif Dent Assoc 2000;28:922–927.

[171] Howley PM. The human papillomaviruses. Arch Pathol Lab Med 1982;106:429–432.

[172] Scully C, Cox MF, Prime SS, Maitland NJ. Papillomaviruses: the current status in relation to oral disease. Oral Surg Oral Med Oral Pathol 1988;65: 526–532.

[173] Lutzner M, Kuffer R, Blanchet-Bardon C, Blanchet-Bardon C, Croissant O. Different papillomaviruses as causes of oral warts. Arch Dermatol 1982;188:393–397.

[174] de Villiers EM, Hirsch-Benham A, von-Knebel-Doeberitz C, Neumann C, zur Hausen H. Two newly identified human papillomavirus types (HPV 40 and 57) isolated from oral mucosal lesions. Virology 1989;171:248–253.

[175] von Knebel Doeberitz M. Papillomaviruses in human disease: Part I. Pathogenesis and epidemiology of human papillomavirus infections. Eur J Med 1992;1: 415–423.

[176] Syrjanen S, Puranen M. Human papillomavirus in fections in children: the potential role of maternal transmission. Crit Rev Oral Biol Med 2000;11:259–274.

[177] Steinberg BM, Auborn KJ. Papillomaviruses in head and neck disease: pathophysiology and possible regulation. J Cell Biochem Suppl 1993;17F:155–164.

[178] Jalal H, Sanders CM, Prime SS, Scully C, Maitland NJ. Detection of human papilloma virus type 16 DNA in oral squames from normal young adults. J Oral Pathol Med 1992;21:465–470.

[179] Kellokoski JK, Syrjanen SM, Chang F, Yliskoski M, Syrjanen KJ. Southern blot hybridization and PCR in detection of oral human papillomavirus (HPV) infections in women with genital HPV infections. J Oral Pathol Med 1992;21:459–464.

[180] Lawton G, Thomas S, Schonrock J, Monsour F, Frazer I. Human papillomaviruses in normal oral mucosa: a comparison of methods for sample collection. J Oral Pathol Med 1992;21:265–269.

[181] Garlick JA, Taichman LB. Human papillomavirus infection of the oral mucosa. Am J Dermatopathol 1991;13:386–395.

[182] Scully C, Epstein J, Porter S, Cox M. Viruses and chronic disorders involving the human oral mucosa. Oral Surg Oral Med Oral Pathol 1991;72:537–544.

[183] Premoli-de-Percoco G, Christensen R. Human papillomavirus in oral verrucal-papillary lesions. A comparative histological, clinical and immunohistochemical study. Pathologica 1992;84:383–392.

[184] Green TL, Eversole LR, Leider AS. Oral and labial verruca vulgaris: clinical, histological, and immunohistochemical evaluation. Oral Surg Oral Med Oral Pathol 1986;62:410–416.

[185] Broich G, Sasaki T. Electron microscopic demonstration of HPV in oral warts. Microbiologica 1990;13: 27–34.

[186] Eversole LR, Laipis PJ, Green TL. Human papillomavirus type 2 DNA in oral and labial verruca vulgaris. J Cutan Pathol 1987;14:319–325.

[187] Eversole LR, Laipis PJ. Oral squamous papillomas: detection of HPV DNA by *in situ* hybridization. Oral Surg Oral Med Oral Pathol 1988;65:545–550.

[188] Greer RO Jr, Douglas JM Jr, Breese P, Crosby KL. Evaluation of oral and laryngeal specimens for human papillomavirus (HPV) DNA by dot blot hybridization. J Oral Pathol Med 1990;19:35–38.

[189] Zeuss MS, Miller CS, White DK. *In situ* hybridization analysis of human papillomavirus DNA in oral mucosal lesions. Oral Surg Oral Med Oral Pathol 1991; 71:714–720.

[190] Miller CS, Zeuss MS, White DK. *In situ* detection of HPV DNA in oral mucosal lesions. A comparison of two hybridization kits. J Oral Pathol Med 1991;20: 403–408.

[191] Miller CS, White DK, Royse DD. *In situ* hybridization analysis of human papillomavirus in orofacial lesions using a consensus biotinylated probe. Am J Dermatopathol 1993;15:256–259.

[192] Rodu B. New approaches to the diagnosis of oral softtissue disease of viral origin. Adv Dent Res 1993;7: 207–212.

[193] Premoli-de-Percoco G, Galindo I, Ramirez JL, Perrone M, Rivera H. Detection of human papillomavirusrelated oral verruca vulgaris among Venezuelans. J Oral Pathol Med 1993;22:113–116.

[194] Welch TB, Barker BF, Williams C. Peroxidaseantiperoxidase evaluation of human oral squamous cell papillomas. Oral Surg Oral Med Oral Pathol 1986; 61:603–606.

[195] Kellokoski J, Syrjanen S, Syrjanen K, Yliskoski M. Oral mucosal changes in women with genital HPV infection. J Oral Pathol Med 1990;19:142–148.

[196] Summers L, Booth DR. Intraoral condyloma acuminatum. Oral Surg 1974;38:273–278.

[197] Emmanouil DE, Post AC. Oral condyloma acuminatum in a child: case report. Pediatr Dent 1987;9:232–235.

[198] Panici PB, Scambia G, Perrone L, et al. Oral condyloma lesions in patients with extensive genital human papillomavirus infection. Am J Obstet Gynecol 1992;167: 451–458.

[199] Kui LL, Xiu HZ, Ning LY. Condyloma acuminatum and human papillomavirus infection in the oral mucosa of children. Pediatr Dent 2003;25:149–153.

[200] Knapp MJ, Uohara GI. Oral condyloma acuminatum. Oral Surg 1967;23:538–545.

[201] Doyle JL, Grodjesk JE, Manhold JH Jr. Condyloma acuminatum occurring in the oral cavity. Oral Surg 1968;26:434–440.

[202] Swan RH, McDaniel RK, Dreiman BB, Rome WC. Condyloma acuminatum involving the oral mucosa. Oral Surg 1981;51:503–508.

[203] Marquard JV, Racey GL. Combined medical and surgical management of intraoral condyloma acuminatum. J Oral Surg 1981;39:459–461.

[204] Eron L, Judson F, Tucker S, et al. Interferon therapy for condyloma acuminata. N Engl J Med 1986;315: 1059–1064.

[205] Browder JF, Araujo OE, Myer NA, Flowers FP. The interferons and their use in condyloma acuminata. Ann Pharmacother 1992;26:42–45.

[206] Archard HO, Heck JW, Stanley HR. Focal epithelial hyperplasia: an unusual and mucosal lesion found in Indian children. Oral Surg Oral Med Oral Pathol 1965;20:201–212.

[207] Lamey PJ, Lewis MA, Rennie JS, Beattie AD. Heck's disease. Br Dent J 1990;168:251–252.

[208] Ficarra G, Adler-Storthz K, Galeotti F, Shillitoe E. Focal epithelial hyperplasia (Heck's disease): the first reported case from Italy. Tumori 1991;77:83–85.

[209] Premoli-de-Percoco G, Cisternas JP, Ramirez JL, Galindo I. Focal epithelial hyperplasia: humanpapillomavirus-induced disease with a genetic predisposition in a Venezuelan family. Hum Genet 1993; 91:386–388.

[210] Cohen PR, Hebert AA, Adler-Storthz K. Focal epithelial hyperplasia: Heck disease. Pediatr Dermatol 1993;10:245–251.

[211] Jaramillo F, Rodriquez G. Multiple oral papules in a native South American girl. Focal epithelial hyperplasia (Heck's disease).Arch Dermatol 1991;127:888–892.

[212] Morrow DJ, Sandhu HS, Daley TD. Focal epithelial hyperplasia (Heck's disease) with generalized lesions of the gingiva. A case report. J Periodontol 1993;64:63–65.

[213] Harris AM, van Wyk CW. Heck's disease (focal epithelial hyperplasia): a longitudinal study. Community Dent Oral Epidemiol 1993;21:82–85.

[214] Henke RP, Guerin-Reverchon I, Milde-Langosch K, Koppang HS, Loning T. *In situ* detection of human papillomavirus types 13 and 32 in focal epithelial hyperplasia of the oral mucosa. J Oral Pathol Med 1989;18:419–421.

[215] Garlick JA, Calderon S, Buchner A, Mitrani-Rosenbaum S. Detection of human papillomavirus (HPV) DNA in focal epithelial hyperplasia. J Oral Pathol Med 1989;18:172–177.

[216] Padayachee A, van Wyk CW. Human papillomavirus (HPV) DNA in focal epithelial hyperplasia by *in situ* hybridization. J Oral Pathol Med 1991;20:210–214.

[217] Premoli-de-Percoco G, Galindo I, Ramirez JL. *In situ h*ybridization with digoxigenin-labelled DNA probes for the detection of human papillomavirus-induced focal epithelial hyperplasia among Venezuelans. Virchows Arch A Pathol Anat Histopathol 1992;420: 295–300.

[218] Luomanen M. Oral focal epithelial hyperplasia removed with CO_2 laser. Int J Oral Maxillofac Surg 1990;19:205–207.

[219] Obalek S, Janniger C, Jablonska S, Favre M, Orth G. Sporadic cases of Heck disease in two Polish girls: association with human papillomavirus type 13. Pediatr Dermatol 1993;10:240–244.

[220] Scully C, Prime S, Maitland N. Papillomaviruses: their possible role in oral disease. Oral Surg Oral Med Oral Pathol 1985;60:166–174.

[221] Evans AS, Mueller NE.Viruses and cancer.Causal associations. Ann Epidemiol 1990;1:71–92.

[222] Shillitoe EJ. Relationship of viral infection to malignancies. Curr Opin Dent 1991;1:398–403.

[223] Chang F, Syrjanen S, Kellokoski J, Syrjanen K. Human papillomavirus (HPV) infections and their associations with oral disease. J Oral Pathol Med 1991;20: 305–307.

[224] Shroyer KR, Greer RO Jr. Detection of human papillomavirus DNA by *in situ* DNA hybridization and polymerase chain reaction in premalignant and malignant oral lesions. Oral Surg Oral Med Oral Pathol 1991;71: 708–713.

[225] Shillitoe EJ, Steele C. Inhibition of the transformed phenotype of carcinoma cells that contain human papillomavirus. Ann N Y Acad Sci 1992;660:286–287.

[226] Steele C, Sacks PG, Adler-Storthz K, Shillitoe EJ. Effect on cancer cells of plasmids that express antisense RNA of human papillomavirus type 18. Can Res 1992;52:4706–4711.

[227] Steele C, Cowsert LM, Shillitoe EJ. Effects of human papillomavirus type 18–specific antisense oligonucleotides on the transformed phenotype of human carcinoma cell lines. Cancer Res 1993;53(suppl 10):2330–2337.

[228] Shillitoe EJ, Schantz SP, Spitz MR, Hecht SS. Environmental carcinogenesis and its prevention: the head and neck cancer model. Cancer Res 1993;53:2189–2191.

[229] Woods KV, Shillitoe EJ, Spitz MR, Schantz SP, Adler-Storthz K. Analysis of human papillomavirus DNA in oral squamous cell carcinomas. J Oral Pathol Med 1993;22:101–108.

[230] Masucci MG. Viral immunology of human tumors. Curr Opin Immunol 1993;5:693–700.

[231] Sugerman PB, Shilitoe EJ. The high risk human papillomaviruses and oral cancer: evidence for and against a causal relationship. Oral Dis 1997;3:130–147.

[232] Leigh IM, Buchanan JA, Harwood CA, et al. Role of human papillomaviruses in cutaneous and oral manifestations of immunosuppression. J Acquir Immune Defic 1999;21(suppl 1):S49–S57.

[233] Hafcamp HC, Manni JJ, Speel EJ. Role of human papillomavirus in the development of head and neck squamous cell carcinomas. Acta Otolaryngol 2004;124: 520–526.

[234] Syrjanen S. Human papillomavirus infections and oral tumors. Med Microbiol Immunol (Berl) 2003;192: 123–128.

[235] Herrero R. Human papillomavirus and cancer of the upper aerodigestive tract. J Natl Cancer Inst Monogr 2003;31:47–51.

[236] Scully C. Oral squamous cell carcinoma; from an hypothesis about a virus to concern about sexual transmission. Oral Oncol 2002;38:227–234.

[237] Watts SL, Brewer EE, Fry TL. Human papillomavirus DNA types in squamous cell carcinomas of the head and neck. Oral Surg Oral Med Oral Pathol 1991;71: 701–707.

[238] Tsuchiya H, Tomita Y, Shirasawa H, Tanzawa H, Sato K, Simizu B. Detection of human papillomavirus in head and neck tumors with DNA hybridization and immunohistochemical analysis. Oral Surg Oral Med Oral Pathol 1991;71:721–725.

[239] Howell RE, Gallant L. Human papillomavirus type 16 in an oral squamous carcinoma and its metastasis. Oral Surg Oral Med Oral Pathol 1992;74:620–626.

[240] Cannon CR, Hayne ST. Concurrent verrucous carcinomas of the lip and buccal mucosa. South Med J 1993;86:691–693.

[241] Huang ES, Gutsch D, Tzung KW, Lin CT. Detection of low level of human papilloma virus type 16 DNA sequences in cancer cell lines derived from two welldifferentiated nasopharyngeal cancers. J Med Virol 1993;40:244–250.

[242] Jontell M, Watts S, Wallstrom M, Levin L, Sloberg K. Human papilloma virus in erosive oral lichen planus. J Oral Pathol Med 1990;19:273–277.

[243] Young SK, Min KW. *In situ* DNA hybridization analysis of oral papillomas, leukoplakias, and carcinomas for human papillomavirus. Oral Surg Oral Med Oral Pathol 1991;71:726–729.

[244] Eversole R. The human papillomaviruses and oral mucosal disease. Oral Surg Oral Med Oral Pathol 1991;71:700.

[245] Maden C, Beckmann AM, Thomas DB, et al. Human papillomaviruses, herpes simplex viruses, and the risk of oral cancer in men. Am J Epidemiol 1992;135: 1093–1102.

[246] McKaig RG, Baric RS, Olshan AF. Human papillomavirus and head and neck cancer: epidemiology and molecular biology. Head Neck 1998;20:250–265.

[247] Vasudevan DM, Vijayakumar T. Viruses in human oral cancers. J Exp Clin Cancer Res 1998;17:27–31.

[248] Miller CS, Johnstone BM. Human papillomavirus as a risk factor for oral squamous cell carcinoma: a metaanalysis, 1982–1997. Oral Surg Oral Med Oral Pathol Oral Radiol Endod 2001;91:622–635.

[249] Grahnen H. Maternal rubella and dental defects. Odontologisk Revy 1958;9:181–192.

[250] Perry RT, Halsey NA. The clinical significance of measles: a review. J Infect Dis 2004;189(suppl 1):S4–S16.

[251] Cunha BA. Smallpox and measles: historical aspects and clinical differentiation. Infect Dis Clin North Am 2004;18:79–100.

[252] Katz J,Guelmann M, Stavropolous F, et al. Gingival and other oral manifestations in measles virus infection. J Clin Periodontol 2003;30:665–668.

[253] Perry KR, Brown DW, Parry JV, Panday S, Pipkin C, Richards A. Detection of measles,mumps, and rubella antibodies in saliva using antibody capture radioimmunoassay. J Med Virol 1993;40:235–240.

[254] Ito M, Go T, Okuno T, Mikawa H. Chronic mumps virus encephalitis. Pediatr Neurol 1991;7:467–470.

[255] Zou ZJ,Wang SL, Zhu JR,Yu SF, Ma DQ,Wu YT. Recurrent parotitis in children. A report of 102 cases. Chin Med J 1990;103:576–582.

[256] McQuone SJ.Acute viral and bacterial infections of the salivary glands. Otolaryngol Clin North Am 1999;32: 793–811.

[257] Waldman HB. Have your young pediatric patients been immuized properly ASDC. J Dent Child 1998;65: 107–110.

[258] Brook I.Diagnosis and management of parotitis.Arch Otolaryngol Head Neck Surg 1992;118:469–471.

[259] Ferson MJ, Bell SM. Outbreak of Coxsackievirus A16 hand, foot, and mouth disease in a child day-care center. Am J Public Health 1991;81:1675–1676.

[260] Thomas I, Janniger CK.Hand, foot,and mouth disease. Cutis 1993;52:265–266.

[261] Frydenberg A, Starr M.Hand, foot and mouth disease. Aust Fam Physician 2003;32:594–595.

[262] Enterovirus surveillance—United States, 1997–1999. MMWR 2000;49:913–916.

[263] Hooi PS, Chua BH, Lee CS, et al.Hand, foot and mouth disease: University of Malaya Medical Center experience. Med J Malaysia 2002;57:88–91.

[264] McMinn PC. An overview of the evolution of enterovirus 71 and its clinical and public health significance. FEMS Microbiol Rev 2002;26:91–107.

[265] Chan KP, Goh KT, Chong CY, et al. Epidemic hand, foot and mouth disease caused by human enterovirus 71, Singapore. Emerg Infect Dis 2003;9:78–85.

[266] Adler JL, Mostow SR, Mellin H, Janney JH, Joseph JM. Epidemiologic investigation of hand, foot, and mouth disease. Am J Dis Child 1970;120:309–313.

[267] Chong CY, Chan KP, Shah VA, et al. Hand, foot and mouth disease in Singapore: a comparison of fatal and non-fatal cases. Acta Paediatr 2003;92:1163–1169.

[268] Shah VA, Chong CY, Chan KP, et al. Clinical characteristics of an outbreak of hand, foot and mouth disease in Singapore. Ann Acad Med Singapore 2003;32: 381–387.

[269] McKinney RV. Hand, foot, and mouth disease: a viral disease of importance to dentists. J Am Dent Assoc 1975;91:122–127.

[270] Lopez-Sanchez A, Guijarro Guijarro B, Vallejo Hernanez G.Human repercussions of foot and mouth disease and other similar viral diseases. Med Oral 2003;8:26–32.

[271] Toida M,Watanabe F, Goto K, et al. Usefulness of lowlevel laser for control of painful stomatitis in patients with hand-foot-and-mouth disease. J Clin Laser Med Surg 2003;21:363–367.

[272] McCourt JW. Hand-foot-and-mouth disease: report of a case in Texas. Tex Dent J 1991;108:13–16.

[273] Buchner A. Hand, foot, and mouth disease. Oral Surg 1976;41:333–337.

[274] Zahorsky J. Herpetic sore throat. South Med J 1920;13:871–872.

[275] Zahorsky J. Herpangina (a specific disease). Arch Pediatr 1924;41:181–184.

[276] Robinson CR, Doane FW, Rhodes AJ. Report of an outbreak of febrile illness with pharyngeal lesions and exanthem: Toronto, 1957, isolation of group A Coxsackie virus. Can Med Assoc J 1958;79:615–621.

[277] Yamadera S, Yamashita K, Kato N, Akatsuka M, Miyamura K, Yamazaki S. Herpangina surveillance in Japan, 1982–1989. A report of the national epidemiological surveillance of infectious agents in Japan. Jpn J Med Sci Biol 1991;44:29–39.

[278] Lang SD, Singh K. The sore throat.When to investigate and when to prescribe. Drugs 1990;40:854–862.

[279] Edwards P, Wodak A, Cooper DA, Thompson IL, Penny R. The gastrointestinal manifestations of AIDS. Aust N Z J Med 1990; 20:141–148.

[280] Royce RA, Luckmann RS, Fusaro RE,Winkelstein W Jr. The natural history of HIV-1 infection: staging classifications of disease. AIDS 1991;5:355–364.

[281] Mbopi-Keou FX, Belec L, Teo CG, et al. Synergism between HIV and other viruses in the mouth. Lancet Infect Dis 2002;2:416–424.

[282] Greenspan D, Greenspan JS. Oral manifestations of HIV infection. AIDS Clin Care 1997;9:29–33.

[283] Grbic JT, Lamster IB.Oral manifestations of HIV infection. AIDS Patient Care STDS 1997;11:18–24.

[284] Patton LL, Phelan JA, Ramos-Gomez FJ, et al. Prevalence and classification of HIV-associated oral lesions. Oral Dis 2002;8(suppl 2):98–109.

[285] Shirlaw PJ, Chikte U, MacPhail L, et al. Oral and dental care and treatment protocols for the management of HIV-infected patients. Oral Dis 2002;8(suppl 2):136–143.

[286] Ramos-Gomez FJ, Flaitz C, Catapano P, et al. Classification, diagnostic criteria, and treatment recommendations for orofacial manifestations in HIVinfected pediatric patients. Collaborative Workgroup on Oral Manifestations of Pediatric HIV Infection. J Clin Pediatr Dent 1999;23:85–96.

[287] Ramos-Gomez FJ, Petru A, Hilton JF, et al. Oral manifestations and dental status in paediatric HIV infection. Int J Paediatr Dent 2000;10:3–11.

[288] Kozinetz CA, Carter AB, Simon C, et al. Oral manifestations of pediatric vertical HIV infection. AIDS Patient Care STDS 2000;14:89–94.

[289] Magalhaes MG, Bueno DF, Serra E, et al. Oral manifestations of HIV positive children. J Clin Pediatr Dent 2001;25:103–106.

[290] Classification and diagnostic criteria for oral lesions in HIV infection. EC-Clearinghouse on Oral Problems Related to HIV Infection and WHO Collaborating Centre on Oral Manifestations of the Immunodeficiency Virus. J Oral Pathol Med 1993;22:289–291.

[291] Rosenberg RA, Schneider KL, Cohen NL. Head and neck presentations of the acquired immunodeficiency syndrome. Laryngoscope 1984;94:642–646.

[292] Wofford DT, Miller RI. Acquired immune deficiency syndrome (AIDS): disease characteristics and oral manifestations. J Am Dent Assoc 1985;111:258–261.

[293] Marcusen DC, Sooy CD. Otolaryngologic and head and neck manifestations of acquired immunodeficiency syndrome (AIDS). Laryngoscope 1985;95:401–405.

[294] Barr CE, Torosian JP, Quinones-Whitmore GD. Oral manifestations of AIDS: the dentist's responsibility in diagnosis and treatment. Quintessence Int 1986;17: 711–717.

[295] Schiodt M, Pindborg JJ. AIDS and the oral cavity. Epidemiology and clinical oral manifestations of human immune deficiency virus infection: a review. Int J Oral Maxillofac Surg 1987;16:1–14.

[296] Reichart PA, Gelderblom HR, Becker J, Kuntz A. AIDS and the oral cavity. The HIV-infection: virology, etiology, origin, immunology, precautions and clinical observations in 110 patients. Int J Oral Maxillofac Surg 1987;16:129–153.

[297] Greenspan D, Greenspan JS. Oral mucosal manifestations of AIDS? Dermatol Clin 1987;5:733–737.

[298] Silverman S Jr. AIDS update: oral findings, diagnosis, and precautions. J Am Dent Assoc 1987;115:559–563.

[299] Roberts MW, Brahim JS, Rinne NF. Oral manifestations of AIDS: a study of 84 patients. J Am Dent Assoc 1988;116:863–866.

[300] Greenspan D, Greenspan JS. The oral clinical features of HIV infection. Gastroenterol Clin North Am 1988; 17:535–543.

[301] Greenspan JS, Greenspan D, Winkler JR. Diagnosis and management of the oral manifestations of HIV infection and AIDS. Infect Dis Clin North Am 1988;2: 373–385.

[302] Alessi E, Cusini M, Zerboni R. Mucocutaneous manifestations in patients with human immunodeficiency virus. J Am Acad Dermatol 1990;22:1260–1269.

[303] Brahim JS, Roberts MW. Oral manifestations of human immunodeficiency virus infection. Ear Nose Throat J 1990;69:464–474.

[304] van der Waal I, Schulten EA, Pindborg JJ. Oral manifestations of AIDS: an overview. Int Dent J 1991;41:3–8.

[305] Scully C, Laskaris G, Pindborg J, Porter SR, Reichart P. Oral manifestations of HIV infection and their management. I. More common lesions. Oral Surg Oral Med Oral Pathol 1991;71:158–166.

[306] Kelly M, Siegel MA, Balciunas BA, Konzelman JL. Oral manifestations of human immunodeficiency virus infection. Cutis 1991;47:44–49.

[307] Silverman S Jr. AIDS update. Oral manifestations and management. Dent Clin North Am 1991;35:259–267.

[308] Sciubba JJ. Recognizing the oral manifestations of AIDS. Oncology 1992;6:64–75.

[309] Barr CE. Oral diseases in HIV-1 infection. Dysphagia 1992;7:126–137.

[310] Greenspan D, Greenspan JS. Oral lesions of HIV infection: features and therapy. AIDS Clin Rev 1992; 225–239.

[311] Greenspan JS, Barr CE, Sciubba JJ, Winkler JR. Oral manifestations of HIV infection. Definitions, diagnostic criteria, and principles of therapy. The U.S.A. Oral AIDS Collaborative Group. Oral Surg Oral Med Oral Pathol 1992;73:142–144.

[312] Pindborg JJ. Global aspects of the AIDS epidemic. Oral Surg Oral Med Oral Pathol 1992;73:138–141.

[313] Ficarra G, Shillitoe EJ. HIV-related infections of the oral cavity. Crit Rev Oral Biol Med 1992;3:207–231.

[314] Scully C. Oral infections in the immunocompromised patient. Br Dent J 1992;172:401–407.

[315] Greenspan D, Greenspan JS. Oral manifestations of human immunodeficiency virus infection. Dent Clin North Am 1993;37:21–32.

[316] Itin PH, Lautenschlager S, Fluckiger R, Rufli T. Oral manifestations in HIV-infected patients: diagnosis and management. J Am Acad Dermatol 1993;29: 749–760.

[317] Barzan L, Tavio M, Tirelli U, Comoretto R. Head and neck manifestations during HIV infection. J Laryngol Otol 1993;107:133–136.

[318] Oral manifestations of HIV infection. In: JS Greenspan, D Greenspan, eds. Proceedings of the Second International Workshop. Chicago: Quintessence, 1994.

[319] Itin PH, Lautenschlager S. Viral lesions of the mouth in HIV-infected patients. Dermatology 1997;194:1–7.

[320] Samonis G, Mantadakis E, Maraki S. Orofacial viral infections in the immunocompromised host. Oncol Rep 2000;7:1389–1394.

[321] Silverman S Jr, Migliorati CA, Lozada-Nur F, Greenspan D,Conant MA. Oral findings in people with or at high risk for AIDS: a study of 375 homosexual males. J Am Dent Assoc 1986;11:187–192.

[322] Feigal DW, Katz MH, Greenspan D, et al. The prevalence of oral lesions in HIV-infected homosexual and bisexual men: three San Francisco epidemiological cohorts. AIDS 1991;5:519–525.

[323] Barone R, Ficarra G, Gaglioti D, Orsi A, Mazzotta F. Prevalence of oral lesions among HIV-infected intravenous drug abusers and other risk groups. Oral Surg Oral Med Oral Pathol 1990;69:169–173.

[324] Bolski E, Hunt RJ. The prevalence of AIDS-associated oral lesions in a cohort of patients with hemophilia. Oral Surg Oral Med Oral Pathol 1988;65:406–410.

[325] Hankins CA, Handley MA. HIV disease and AIDS in women: current knowledge and a research agenda. J Acquir Immune Defic Syndr 1992;5:957–971.

[326] Silverman S Jr, Wara D. Oral manifestations of pediatric AIDS. Pediatrician 1989;16:185–187.

[327] Ketchem L, Berkowitz RJ, McIlveen L, Forrester D, Rakusan T. Oral findings in HIV-seropositive children. Pediatr Dent 1990;12:143–146.

[328] Davis MJ. Oral health care in pediatric AIDS. N Y State Dent J 1990;56:25–27.

[329] Moniaci D, Cavallari M, Greco D, et al. Oral lesions in children born to HIV-1 positive women. J Oral Pathol Med 1993;22:8–11.

[330] Asher RS, McDowell J, Acs G, Belanger G. Pediatric infection with the human immunodeficiency virus (HIV): head, neck, and oral manifestations. Spec Care Dentist. 1993;13:113–116.

[331] Fine DH, Tofsky N, Nelson EM, et al. Clinical implications of the oral manifestations of HIV infection in children. Dent Clin North Am 2003;47:159–174.

[332] Ramos-Gomez F. Dental considerations for the paediatric AIDS/HIV patient. Oral Dis 2002;8(suppl 2): 49–54.

[333] Tukutuku K, Muyembe-Tamfum L, Kayembe K, Odio W, Kandi K, Ntumba M. Oral manifestations of AIDS in heterosexual population in a Zaire hospital. J Oral Pathol Med 1990;19:232–234.

[334] Tukutuku K, Muyembe-Tamfum L, Kayembe K, Mavuemba T, Sangua N, Sekele I. Prevalence of dental caries, gingivitis, and oral hygiene in hospitalized AIDS cases in Kinshasa, Zaire. J Oral Pathol Med 1990;19:271–272.

[335] Schulten EA, ten Kate RW, van der Waal I. Oral manifestations of HIV infection in 75 Dutch patients. J Oral Pathol Med 1989;18:42–46.

[336] Ramirez V, Gonzalez A, de la Rosa E, et al. Oral lesions in Mexican HIV-infected patients. J Oral Pathol Med 1990;19:482–485.

[337] Luangjamekorn L, Silverman S Jr, Gallo J,McKnight M, Migliorati C. Findings in 50 AIDS virus-infected patients with positive oral Candida cultures. J Dent Assoc Thai 1990;40:157–164.

[338] Laskaris G, Potouridou I, Laskaris M, Stratigos J. Gingival lesions of HIV infection in 178 Greek patients. Oral Surg Oral Med Oral Pathol 1992;74:168–171.

[339] Gillespie GM, Marino R. Oral manifestations of HIV infection: a pan-American perspective. J Oral Pathol Med 1993;22:2–7.

[340] Dreizen S. Oral candidiasis. Am J Med 1984;77:28–33.

[341] Braun-Falco O. International Workshop on Oral and Gastrointestinal Candidosis: From Pathology to Therapy. Introduction. Mycoses 1989;32(suppl 2): 6–8.

[342] Samson J. Oral candidiasis: epidemiology, diagnosis and treatment. Schweiz Monatsschr Zahnmed 1990; 100:548–559.

[343] Zegarelli DJ. Fungal infections of the oral cavity. Otolaryngol Clin North Am 1993;26:1069–1089.

[344] Lynch DP. Oral candidiasis: History, classification, and clinical presentation. Oral Surg Oral Med Oral Pathol 1994;78:189–193.

[345] Chandrasekar PH, Molinari JA. Oral candidiasis: forerunner of acquired immunodeficiency syndrome

[346] Scully C, Epstein JB, Porter S, Luker J. Recognition of oral lesions of HIV infection. 1. Candidosis. Br Dent J 1990;169:295–296.

[347] Stevens DA. Fungal infections in AIDS patients. Br J Clin Pract Symp Suppl 1990;71:11–22.

[348] Imam N, Carpenter CC, Mayer KH, Fisher A, Stein M, Danforth SB.Hierarchical pattern of mucosal Candida infections in HIV-seropositive women. Am J Med 1990;89:142–146.

[349] Di Silverio A, Brazzelli V, Brandozzi G, Barbarini G, Maccabruni A, Sacchi S. Prevalence of dermatophytes and yeasts (Candida spp., Malassezia furfur) in HIV patients. A study of former drug addicts. Mycopathologia 1991;114:103–107.

[350] Felix DH, Wray D. The prevalence of oral candidiasis in HIV-infected individuals and dental attenders in Edinburgh. J Oral Pathol Med 1993;22:418–420.

[351] Franker CK, Lucatorto FM, Johnson BS, Jacobson JJ. Characterization of the mycoflora from oral mucosal surfaces of some HIV-infected patients. Oral Surg Oral Med Oral Pathol 1990;69:683–687.

[352] Miyasaki SH, Hicks JB, Greenspan D, et al. The identification and tracking of Candida albicans isolates from oral lesions in HIV-seropositive individuals. J Acquir Immune Defic Syndr 1992;5:1039–1046.

[353] Powderly WG. Mucosal candidiasis caused by nonalbicans species of Candida in HIV-positive patients. AIDS 1992;6:604–605.

[354] Sullivan D, Bennett D, Henman M, et al. Oligonucleotide fingerprinting of isolates of Candida species other than *C. albicans* and of atypical Candida species from human immunodeficiency virus-positive and AIDS patients. J Clin Microbiol 1993;31:2124–2133.

[355] Coleman DC, Bennett DE, Sullivan DJ, et al. Oral Candida in HIV infection and AIDS: new perspectives/new approaches. Crit Rev Microbiol 1993; 19:61–82.

[356] Syrjanen S, Valle SL, Antonen J, et al. Oral candidal infection as a sign of HIV infection in homosexual men. Oral Surg Oral Med Oral Pathol 1988;65:36–40.

[357] Korting HC. Clinical spectrum of oral candidosis and its role in HIV-infected patients. Mycoses 1989;32 (suppl 2):23–29.

[358] Schiodt M, Bakilana PB, Hiza JF, et al. Oral candidiasis and hairy leukoplakia correlate with HIV infection in Tanzania. Oral Surg Oral Med Oral Pathol 1990;69:591–596.

[359] Dodd CL, Greenspan D, Katz MH, Westenhouse JL, Feigal DW, Greenspan JS. Oral candidiasis in HIV infection: pseudomembranous and erythematous candidiasis show similar rates of progression to AIDS. AIDS 1991;5:1339–1343.

[360] Katz MH, Greenspan D, Westenhouse J, et al. Progression of AIDS in HIV-infected homosexual and bisexual men with hairy leukoplakia and oral candidiasis. AIDS 1992;6:95–100.

[361] Greenspan D, Gange SJ, Phelan JA, et al. Incidence of oral lesions in HIV-1–infected women: reduction with HAART. J Dent Res 2004;83:145–150.

[362] Torssander J, Morfeldt-Manson L, Biberfeld G, Karlsson A, Putkonen PO, Wasserman J. Oral Candida albicans in HIV infection. Scand J Infect Dis 1987;19: 291–295.

[363] Hauman CH, Thompson IO, Theunissen F, Wolfaardt P. Oral carriage of Candida in healthy and HIV seropositive persons. Oral Surg Oral Med Oral Pathol 1993;76:570–572.

[364] Fetter A, Partisani M, Koenig H, Kremer M, Lang JM. Asymptomatic oral Candida albicans carriage in HIV infection: frequency and predisposing factors. J Oral Pathol Med 1993;22:57–59.

[365] Tylenda CA, Larsen J, Yeh CK, Lane HC, Fox PC. High levels of oral yeasts in early HIV-1 infection. J Oral Pathol Med 1989;18:520–524.

[366] Schmidt-Westhausen A, Schiller RA, Pohle HD, Reichart PA. Oral Candida and Enterobacteriaceae in HIV-1 infection: correlation with clinical candidiasis and antimycotic therapy. J Oral Pathol Med 1991;20: 467–472.

[367] McCarthy GM, Mackie ID, Koval J, Sandhu HS, Daley TD. Factors associated with increased frequency of HIV-related oral candidiasis. J Oral Pathol Med 1991; 20:332–336.

[368] McCarthy GM. Host factors associated with HIVrelated oral candidiasis. A review. Oral Surg Oral Med Oral Pathol 1992;73:181–186.

[369] Lode H, Hoffken G. Oral candidosis and its role in immunocompromised patients. Mycoses 1989; 32(suppl 2):30–33.

[370] Lynch DP, Gibson DK. The use of calcofluor white in the histopathological diagnosis of oral candidiasis. Oral Surg Oral Med Oral Pathol 1987;63:698–703.

[371] Axell T, Simonsson T, Birkhed D, Rosenborg J, Edwardsson S. Evaluation of a simplified diagnostic aid (Oricult-N) for detection of oral candidoses. Scand J Dent Res 1985;93:52–55.

[372] Hamilton JN,Thompson SH, Schiedt MJ,McQuade MJ, Van Dyke T, Plowman K. Correlation of subclinical candidal colonization of the dorsal tongue surface with the Walter Reed staging scheme for patients infected with HIV-1. Oral Surg Oral Med Oral Pathol 1992;73:47–51.

[373] Samaranayake LP, Holmstrup P. Oral candidiasis and human immunodeficiency virus infection. J Oral Pathol Med 1989;18:554–564.

[374] Greenspan D. Treatment of oral candidiasis in HIV infection. Oral Surg Oral Med Oral Pathol 1994;78: 211–215.

[375] Epstein JB. Oral and pharyngeal candidiasis. Topical agents for management and prevention. Postgrad Med 1989;85:257–269.

[376] Lewis MA, Samaranyake LP, Lamey PJ. Diagnosis and treatment of oral candidosis. J Oral Maxillofac Surg 1991;49:996–1002.

[377] Rindum JL, Holmstrup P, Pedersen M, Rassing MR, Stoltze K. Miconazole chewing gum for treatment of chronic oral candidosis. Scand J Dent Res 1993;101: 386–390.

[378] Pons V, Greenspan D, Debruin M. Therapy for oropharyngeal candidiasis in HIV-infected patients: a randomized, prospective multicenter study of oral fluconazole versus clotrimazole troches. The Multicenter Study Group. J Acquir Immune Defic Syndr 1993;6:1311–1316.

[379] Narani N, Epstein JB. Classification of oral lesions of HIV infection. J Clin Periodontol 2001;28:137–145.

[380] Shagase L, Feller L, Blignaut E. Necrotising ulcerative gingivitis/periodontitis as indicators of HIVinfection. SADJ 2004;59:105–108. (AIDS)? Oral Surg Oral Med Oral Pathol 1985;60:532–534.

[381] Dupont B, Drouhet E. Fluconazole in the management of oropharyngeal candidosis in a predominantly HIV antibody-positive group of patients. J Med Vet Mycol 1988;26:67–71.

[382] Just-Nubling G, Gentschew G, Dohle M, Bottinger C, Helm EB, Stille W. Fluconazole in the treatment of oropharyngeal candidosis in HIV-positive patients. Mycoses 1990;33:435–440.

[383] Blatchford NR. Treatment of oral candidosis with itraconazole: a review. J Am Acad Dermatol 1990;23: 565–567.

[384] Smith DE, Midgley J, Allan M, Connolly GM, Gazzard BG. Itraconazole versus ketaconazole in the treatment of oral and oesophageal candidosis in patients infected with HIV. AIDS 1991;5:1367–1371.

[385] Tschechne B, Brunkhorst U, Ruhnke M, Trautmann M, Dempe S, Deicher H. Fluconazole in therapy of candidiasis of the oropharyngeal space in patients with HIV infection.Results of an open multicenter study of assessing the effectiveness and tolerance of fluconazole. Med Klin 1991;86:508–511.

[386] Korting HC, Blecher P, Froschl M, Braun-Falco O. Quantitative assessment of the efficacy of oral ketoconazole for oral candidosis in HIV-infected patients. Mycoses 1992;35:173–176.

[387] Bruatto M, Marinuzzi G, Raiteri R, Sinicco A. Susceptibility to ketoconazole of Candida albicans strains from sequentially followed HIV-1 patients with recurrent oral candidosis.Mycoses 1992;35:53–56.

[388] Silverman S Jr, McKnight ML, Migliorati C, et al. Chemotherapeutic mouth rinses in immunocompromised patients. Am J Dent 1989;2:303–307.

[389] Budtz-Jorgensen E. Etiology, pathogenesis, therapy, and prophylaxis of oral yeast infections.Acta Odontol Scand 1990;48:61–69.

[390] Just-Nubling G, Gentschew G, Meissner K, et al. Fluconazole prophylaxis of recurrent oral candidiasis in HIV-positive patients. Eur J Clin Microbiol Infect Dis 1991;10:917–921.

[391] Reents S, Goodwin SD, Singh V.Antifungal prophylaxis in immunocompromised hosts. Ann Pharmacother 1993;27:53–60.

[392] Korting HC, Ollert M, Georgii A, Froschl M. In vitro susceptibilities and biotypes of Candida albicans isolates from the oral cavities of patients infected with human immunodeficiency virus. J Clin Microbiol 1988;26:2626–2631.

[393] Fan-Havard P, Capano D, Smith SM, Mangia A, Eng RH. Development of resistance in Candida isolates from patients receiving prolonged antifungal therapy. Antimicrob Agents Chemother 1991;35:2302–2305.

[394] Gallagher PJ, Bennett DE, Henman MC, et al. Reduced azole susceptibility of oral isolates of Candida albicans from HIV-positive patients and a derivative exhibiting colony morphology variation. J Gen Microbiol 1992; 138:1901–1911.

[395] Heinic GS, Stevens DA, Greenspan D, et al. Fluconazole-resistant Candida in AIDS patients. Report of two cases. Oral Surg Oral Med Oral Pathol 1993;76:711–715.

[396] Boken DJ, Swindells S, Rinaldi MG. Fluconazoleresistant Candida albicans. Clin Infect Dis 1993;17: 1018–1021.

[397] Ng TT, Denning DW. Fluconazole resistance in Candida in patients with AIDS—a therapeutic approach. J Infect 1993;26:1117–1125.

[398] Redding S, Smith J, Farinacci G, et al. Resistance of Candida albicans to fluconazole during treatment of oropharyngeal candidiasis in a patient with AIDS: documentation by in vitro susceptibility testing and DNA subtype analysis. Clin Infect Dis 1994;18: 240–242.

[399] Cameron ML, Schell WA, Bruch S, Bartlett JA, Waskin HA, Perfect JR. Correlation of in vitro fluconazole resistance of Candida isolates in relation to therapy and symptoms of individuals seropositive for human immunodeficiency virus type 1. Antimicrob Agents Chemother 1993;37:2449–2453.

[400] Pfaller MA, Rhine-Chalberg J, Redding SW, et al. Variations in fluconazole susceptibility and electrophoretic karyotype among oral isolates of Candida albicans from patients with AIDS and oral candidiasis. J Clin Microbiol 1994;32:59–64.

[401] Schmid J, Odds FC, Wiselka MJ, Nicholson KG, Soll DR. Genetic similarity and maintenance of Candida albicans strains from a group of AIDS patients, demonstrated by DNA fingerprinting. J Clin Microbiol 1992;30:935–941.

[402] Powderly WG, Robinson K, Keath EJ. Molecular epidemiology of recurrent oral candidiasis in human immunodeficiency virus-positive patients: evidence for two patterns of recurrence. J Infect Dis 1993;168:

463–466.

[403] Challacombe SJ. Immunologic aspects of oral candidiasis. Oral Surg Oral Med Oral Pathol 1994;78: 202–210.

[404] Coogan MM, Sweet SP, Challacombe SJ. Immunoglobulin A (IgA), IgA1, and IgA2 antibodies to Candida albicans in whole and parotid saliva in human immunodeficiency virus infection and AIDS. Infect Immun 1994;62:892–896.

[405] Plettenberg A, Reisinger E, Lenzner U, et al. Oral candidosis in HIV-infected patients. Prognostic value and correlation with immunological parameters. Mycoses 1990;33:421–425.

[406] Greenspan D, Greenspan JS, Conant M, Petersen V, Silverman S Jr, de Souza Y Oral "hairy" leucoplakia in male homosexuals: evidence of association with both papillomavirus and a herpes-group virus. Lancet 1984;2:831–834.

[407] Greenspan JS, Greenspan D, Lennette ET, et al. Replication of Epstein-Barr virus within the epithelial cells of oral "hairy" leukoplakia, an AIDS-associated lesion. N Engl J Med 1985;313:1564–1571.

[408] Greenspan D, Greenspan JS, Hearst NG, et al. Relation of oral hairy leukoplakia to infection with the human immunodeficiency virus and the risk of developing AIDS. J Infect Dis 1987;155:475–481.

[409] Reichart PA, Langford A, Gelderblom HR, Pohle HD, Becker J, Wolf H. Oral hairy leukoplakia: observations in 95 cases and review of the literature. J Oral Pathol Med 1989;18:410–415.

[410] Sciubba J, Brandsma J, Schwartz M, Barrezueta N. Hairy leukoplakia: an AIDS-associated opportunistic infection. Oral Surg Oral Med Oral Pathol 1989; 67:404–410.

[411] Itin PH. Oral hairy leukoplakia—10 years on. Dermatology 1993;187:159–163.

[412] Greenspan D, Hollander H, Friedman-Kien A, Freese UK, Greenspan JS. Oral hairy leucoplakia in two women, a haemophiliac, and a transfusion recipient. Lancet 1986;2:978–979.

[413] Rindum JL, Schiodt M, Pindborg JJ, Scheibel E. Oral hairy leukoplakia in three hemophiliacs with human immunodeficiency virus infection. Oral Surg Med Oral Pathol 1987;63:437–440.

[414] Greenspan JS, Mastrucci MT, Leggott PJ, et al. Hairy leukoplakia in a child. AIDS 1988;2:143.

[415] Kabani S, Greenspan D, de Souza Y, Greenspan JS, Cataldo E. Oral hairy leukoplakia with extensive oral mucosal involvement. Report of two cases. Oral Surg Oral Med Oral Pathol 1989;67:411–415.

[416] Syrjanen S, Laine P, Niemela M, Happonen RP. Oral hairy leukoplakia is not a specific sign of HIV infection but related to immunosuppression in general. J Oral Pathol Med 1989;18:28–31.

[417] Ramael M, Colebunders R, Colpaert C, et al. The prevalence of hairy leukoplakia in HIV seropositive and HIV seronegative immunocompromised patients. Int J STD AIDS 1992;3:251–254.

[418] Epstein JB, Priddy RW, Sherlock CH. Hairy leukoplakia-like lesions in immunosuppressed patients following bone marrow transplantation. Transplantation 1988;46:462–464.

[419] Epstein JB, Sherlock CH, Greenspan JS. Hairy leukoplakia-like lesions following bone-marrow transplantation. AIDS 1991;5:101–102.

[420] Epstein JB, Sherlock CH, Wolber RA. Hairy leukoplakia after bone marrow transplantation. Oral Surg Oral Med Oral Pathol 1993;75:690–695.

[421] Greenspan D, Greenspan JS, de Souza Y, Levy JA, Ungar AM. Oral hairy leukoplakia in an HIV-negative renal transplant recipient. J Oral Pathol Med 1989;18:32–34.

[422] Macleod RI, Logan LQ, Soames JV, Ward MK. Oral hairy leukoplakia in an HIV-negative renal transplant patient. Br Dent J 1990;169:208–209.

[423] Euvrard S, Kanitakis J, Pouteil-Nobel C, Chardonnet Y, Touraine JL, Thivolet J. Pseudo oral hairy leukoplakia in a renal allograft recipient. J Am Acad Dermatol 1994;30:300–303.

[424] Schmidt-Westhausen A, Gelderblom HR, Neuhaus P, Reichart PA. Epstein-Barr virus in lingual epithelium of liver transplant patients. J Oral Pathol Med 1993;22: 274–276.

[425] Schmidt-Westhausen A, Gelderblom HR, Reichart PA. Oral hairy leukoplakia in an HIV-seronegative heart transplant patient. J Oral Pathol Med 1990;19:192–194.

[426] Ficarra G, Miliani A, Adler-Storthz K, et al. Recurrent oral condylomata acuminata and hairy leukoplakia: an early sign of myelodysplastic syndrome in an HIV-seronegative patient. J Oral Pathol Med 1991;20: 398–402.

[427] Eisenberg E, Krutchkoff D, Yamase H. Incidental oral hairy leukoplakia in immunocompetent persons. A report of two cases. Oral Surg Oral Med Oral Pathol 1992;74:332–333.

[428] Felix DH, Watret K, Wray D, Southam JC. Hairy leukoplakia in an HIV-negative, nonimmunosuppressed patient. Oral Surg Oral Med Oral Pathol 1992;74: 563–566.

[429] Naher H, Gissmann L, von Knebel Doeberitz C, et al. Detection of Epstein-Barr virus-DNA in tongue epithelium of human immunodeficiency virusinfected patients. J Invest Dermatol 1991;97:421–424.

[430] Walling DM, Etienne W, Ray AJ, et al. Persistence and transition of Epstein-Barr virus genotypes in the pathogenesis of oral hairy leukoplakia. J Infect Dis 2004;190:387–395.

[431] Hille JJ, Webster-Cyriaque J, Palefski JM, et al. Mechanisms of expression of HHV8, EBV and HPV in selected HIV-associated lesions. Oral Dis 2002;8(suppl 2):161–168.

[432] Corso B, Eversole LR, Hutt-Fletcher L. Hairy leukoplakia: Epstein-Barr virus receptors on oral keratinocyte plasma membranes. Oral Surg Oral Med Oral Pathol 1989;67:416–421.

[433] Sugihara K, Reupke H, Schmidt-Westhausen A, Pohle HD, Gelderblom HR, Reichart PA. Negative staining EM for the detection of Epstein-Barr virus in oral hairy leukoplakia. J Oral Pathol Med 1990;19:367–370.

[434] Madinier I, Doglio A, Cagnon L, Lefebvre JC, Monteil RA. Epstein-Barr virus DNA detection in gingival tissues of patients undergoing surgical extractions. Br J Oral Maxillofac Surg 1992;30:237–243.

[435] Adler-Storthz K, Ficarra G, Woods KV, Gaglioti D, Di Pietro M, Shillitoe EJ. Prevalence of Epstein-Barr virus and human papillomavirus in oral mucosa of HIVinfected patients. J Oral Pathol Med 1992;21:164–170.

[436] Felix DH, Jalal H, Cubie HA, Southam JC, Wray D, Maitland NJ. Detection of Epstein-Barr virus and human papillomavirus type 16 DNA in hairy leukoplakia by *in situ* hybridisation and the polymerase chain reaction. J Oral Pathol Med 1993;22:277–281.

[437] Green TL, Greenspan JS, Greenspan D, de Souza YG. Oral lesions mimicking hairy leukoplakia: a diagnostic dilemma. Oral Surg Oral Med Oral Pathol 1989; 67:422–426.

[438] Schulten EA, Snijders PJ, ten Kate RW, et al. Oral hairy leukoplakia in HIV infection: a diagnostic pitfall. Oral Surg Oral Med Oral Pathol 1991;71:32–37.

[439] Fisher DA, Daniels TE, Greenspan JS. Oral hairy leukoplakia unassociated with human immunodeficiency virus: pseudo oral hairy leukoplakia. J Am Acad Dermatol 1992;27:257–258.

[440] Kanas RJ, Abrams AM, Recher L, Jensen JL, Handlers JP, Wuerker RB. Oral hairy leukoplakia: a light microscopic and immunohistochemical study. Oral Surg Oral Med Oral Pathol 1988;66:334–340.

[441] Cubie HA, Felix DH, Southam JC, Wray D. Application of molecular techniques in the rapid diagnosis of EBV-associated oral hairy leukoplakia. J Oral Pathol Med 1991;20:271–274.

[442] Greenspan JS, Rabanus JP, Petersen V, Greenspan D. Fine structure of EBV-infected keratinocytes in oral hairy leukoplakia. J Oral Pathol Med 1989;18:565–572.

[443] el-Labban N, Pindborg JJ, Rindum J, Nielsen H. Further ultrastructural findings in epithelial cells of hairy

leukoplakia. J Oral Pathol Med 1990;19:24–34.

[444] Kratochvil FJ, Riordan GP, Auclair PL, Huber MA, Kragel PJ. Diagnosis of oral hairy leukoplakia by ultrastructural examination of exfoliative cytologic specimens. Oral Surg Oral Med Oral Pathol 1990;70: 613–618.

[445] Migliorati CA, Jones AC, Baughman PA. Use of exfoliative cytology in the diagnosis of oral hairy leukoplakia. Oral Surg Oral Med Oral Pathol 1993;76: 704–710.

[446] Walling DM, Flaitz CM, Adler-Storthz K, et al. Anon-invasive technique for studying oral epithelial Epstein-Barr virus infection and disease. Oral Oncol 2003;39:436–444.

[447] Greenspan JS, Greenspan D. Oral hairy leukoplakia: diagnosis and management. Oral Surg Oral Med Oral Pathol. 1989;67:396–403.

[448] Resnick L, Herbst JS, Ablashi DV, et al. Regression of oral hairy leukoplakia after orally administered acyclovir therapy. JAMA 1988;259:384–388.

[449] Glick M, Pliskin ME. Regression of oral hairy leukoplakia after oral administration of acyclovir. Gen Dent 1990;38:374–375.

[450] Greenspan D, de Souza YG, Conant MA, et al. Efficacy of desciclovir in the treatment of Epstein-Barr virus infection in oral hairy leukoplakia. J Acquir Immune Defic Syndr 1990;3:571–578.

[451] Newman C, Polk BF. Resolution of oral hairy leukoplakia during therapy with 9–(1,3–dihydroxy-2–propoxymethyl)guanine (DHPG). Ann Intern Med 1987;107:348–350.

[452] Phelan JA, Klein RS. Resolution of oral hairy leukoplakia during treatment with azidothymidine. Oral Surg Oral Med Oral Pathol 1988;65:717–720.

[453] Kessler HA, Benson CA, Urbanski P. Regression of oral hairy leukoplakia during zidovudine therapy. Arch Intern Med 1988;148:2496–2497.

[454] Katz MH, Greenspan D, Heinic GS, et al. Resolution of hairy leukoplakia: an observational trial of zidovudine versus no treatment. J Infect Dis 1991;164: 1240–1241.

[455] Walling DM, Flaitz CM, Nichols CM. Epstein-Barr virus replication in oral hairy leukoplakia: response, persistence and resistance to treatment with valacyclovir. J Infect Dis 2003;188:883–890.

[456] Schofer H, Ochsendorf FR, Helm EB, Milbradt R.Treatment of oral "hairy" leukoplakia in AIDS patients with vitamin A acid (topically) or acyclovir (systemically). Dermatologica 1987;174:150–151.

[457] Lozada-Nur F. Podophyllin resin 25% for treatment of oral hairy leukoplakia: an old treatment for a new lesion. J Acquir Immune Defic Syndr 1991;4:543–546.

[458] Lozada-Nur F, Costa C. Retrospective findings of the clinical benefits of podophyllum resin 25% sol on hairy leukoplakia. Clinical results in nine patients. Oral Surg Oral Med Oral Pathol 1992;73:555–558.

[459] Herbst JS, Morgan J, Raab-Traub N, Resnick L. Comparison of the efficacy of surgery and acyclovir therapy in oral hairy leukoplakia. J Am Acad Dermatol 1989;21:753–756.

[460] Moniaci D, Greco D, Flecchia G, Raiteri R, Sinicco A. Epidemiology, clinical features and prognostic value of HIV-1 related oral lesions. J Oral Pathol Med 1990; 19:477–481.

[461] Greenspan D, Greenspan JS, Overby G, et al. Risk factors for rapid progression from hairy leukoplakia to AIDS: a nested case-control study. J Acquir Immune Defic Syndr 1991;4:652–658.

[462] Greenspan D, Greenspan JS. Significance of oral hairy leukoplakia. Oral Surg Oral Med Oral Pathol 1992; 73:151–154.

[463] Klein RS, Quart AM, Small CB. Periodontal disease in heterosexuals with acquired immunodeficiency syndrome. J Periodontol 1991;62:535–540.

[464] Levine RA, Glick M. Rapidly progressive periodontitis as an important clinical marker for HIV disease.

Compendium 1991;12:478–482.

[465] Riley C, London JP, Burmeister JA. Periodontal health in 200 HIV-positive patients. J Oral Pathol Med 1992; 21:124–127.

[466] Masouredis CM, Katz MH, Greenspan D, et al. Prevalence of HIV-associated periodontitis and gingivitis in HIV-infected patients attending an AIDS clinic. J Acquir Immune Defic Syndr 1992;5:479–483.

[467] Friedman RB, Gunsolley J, Gentry A, Dinius A, Kaplowitz K, Settle J. Periodontal status of HIV seropositive and AIDS patients. J Periodontol 1991; 62:623–627.

[468] Barr C, Lopez MR, Rua-Dobles A. Periodontal changes by HIV serostatus in a cohort of homosexual and bisexual men. J Clin Periodontol 1992;19:794–801.

[469] Yeung SC, Stewart GJ, Cooper DA, Sindhusake D. Progression of periodontal disease in HIV seropositive patients. J Periodontol 1993;64:651–657.

[470] Murray PA, Grassi M, Winkler JR. The microbiology of HIV-associated periodontal lesions. J Clin Periodontol 1989;16:636–642.

[471] Lucht E, Heimdahl A, Nord CE. Periodontal disease in HIV-infected patients in relation to lymphocyte subsets and specific micro-organisms. J Clin Periodontol 1991;18:252–256.

[472] Gornitsky M, Clark DC, Siboo R, et al. Clinical documentation and occurrence of putative periodontopathic bacteria in human immunodeficiency virus-associated periodontal disease. J Periodontol 1991;62:576–585.

[473] Moore LV, Moore WE, Riley C, Brooks CN, Burmeister JA, Smibert RM. Periodontal microflora of HIV positive subjects with gingivitis or adult periodontitis. J Periodontol 1993;64:48–56.

[474] Rosenstein DI, Riviere GR, Elott KS. HIV-associated periodontal disease: new oral spirochete found. J Am Dent Assoc 1993;124:76–80.

[475] Ryder MI. Periodontal considerations in the patient with HIV. Curr Opin Periodontol 1993;43–51.

[476] Winkler JR, Murray PA, Grassi M, Hammerle C. Diagnosis and management of HIV-associated periodontal lesions. J Am Dent Assoc. 1989;(suppl);25S–34S.

[477] Greenspan D, Greenspan JS. Management of the oral lesions of HIV infection. J Am Dent Assoc 1991; 122:26–32.

[478] Hammerle C, Grassi M, Winkler JR. HIV periodontopathies. The diagnosis and therapy of HIV-associated gingivitis/periodontitis. Schweiz Monatsschr Zahnmed 1992;102:940–950.

[479] Robinson PG. The significance and management of periodontal lesions in HIV infection. Oral Dis 2002;8(suppl 2):91–97.

[480] Dodd CL, Greenspan D, Greenspan JS. Oral Kaposi's sarcoma in a woman as a first indication of HIV infection. J Am Dent Assoc 1991;122:61–63.

[481] Epstein JB, Silverman S Jr. Head and neck malignancies associated with HIV infection. Oral Surg Oral Med Oral Pathol 1992;73:193–200.

[482] Regezi JA, MacPhail LA, Daniels TE, de Souza YG, Greenspan JS, Greenspan D. Human immunodeficiency virus-associated oral Kaposi's sarcoma. A heterogeneous cell population dominated by spindleshaped endothelial cells. Am J Pathol 1993;143:240–249.

[483] Kaul A, Pearson JD, Petty R, Williams DM, Dalgleish AG. Vascular endothelium: a potential role in HIV infection and the pathogenesis of Kaposi's sarcoma: observations and speculations. Mol Aspects Med 1991;12:297–312.

[484] Peterman TA, Jaffe HW, Friedman-Kien AE, Weiss RA. The aetiology of Kaposi's sarcoma. Cancer Surv 1991; 10:23–37.

[485] Henke-Gendo C, Schulz TF. Transmission and disease association of Kaposi's sarcoma-associated herpesvirus: recent developments. Curr Opin Infect Dis 2004;17:53–57.

[486] Chang Y, Cesarman E, Pessin MS, et al. Identification of herpesvirus-like DNA sequences in AIDS-associated Kaposi's sarcoma. Science 1994;266(5192):1865–1869.

[487] Moore PS, Chang Y. Detection of herpesvirus-like DNA sequences in Kaposi's sarcoma in patients with and those without HIV infection. N Engl J Med 1995;332: 1181–1185.

[488] Koelle DM, Huang ML, Chandran B,Vieira J, Piepkorn M, Corey L. Frequent detection of Kaposi's sarcomaassociated herpesvirus (human herpesvirus 8) DNA in saliva of human immunodeficiency virus-infected men: clinical and immunologic correlates. J Infect Dis 1997;176:94–102.

[489] Martin JN. Diagnosis and epidemiology of human herpesvirus 8 infection. Semin Hematol 2003;40:133–142.

[490] Pauk J, Huang ML, Brodie SJ, et al. Mucosal shedding of human herpesvirus 8 in men. N Engl J Med 2000; 343:1369–1377.

[491] Casper C, Redman M, Huang ML, et al. HIV infection and human herpesvirus-8 oral shedding among men who have sex with men. J Acquir Immune Defic Syndr 2004;35:233–238.

[492] Flaitz CM, Jin YT, Hicks MJ, Nichols CM,Wang YW, Su IJ. Kaposi's sarcoma-associated herpesvirus-like DNA sequences (KSHV/HHV-8) in oral AIDS-Kaposi's sarcoma: a PCR and clinicopathologic study. Oral Surg Oral Med Oral Pathol Oral Radiol Endod 1997;83:259–264.

[493] Di Alberti L, Ngui SL, Porter SR, et al. Presence of human herpesvirus 8 variants in the oral tissues of human immunodeficiency virus-infected individuals. J Infect Dis 1997;175:703–707.

[494] Triantos D, Horefti E, Paximadi E, et al. Presence of human herpesvirus-8 in saliva and non-lesional oral mucosa in HIV-infected and oncologic immunocompromised patients. Oral Microbiol Immunol 2004;19: 201–204.

[495] Teo CG. Viral infections in the mouth. Oral Dis 2002;8(suppl 2):88–90.

[496] Bubman D, Cesarman E. Pathogenesis of Kaposi's sarcoma. Hematol Oncol Clin North Am 2003;17:717–745.

[497] Aoki Y, Tosato G. Pathogenesis and manifestations of human herpesvirus-8–associated disorders. Semin Hematol 2003;40:143–153.

[498] De Paoli P. Human herpesvirus 8: an update.Microbes Infect 2004;6:328–335.

[499] Leao JC, Porter S, Scully C. Human herpesvirus 8 and oral health care: an update. Oral Surg Oral Med Oral Pathol Oral Radiol Endod 2000;90:694–704.

[500] Porter SP, Di Alberti L, Kumar N.Human herpes virus 8 (Kaposi's sarcoma herpesvirus). Oral Oncol 1998; 34:5–14.

[501] Goedert JJ. The epidemiology of acquired immunodeficiency syndrome malignancies. Semin Oncol 2002;27:390–401.

[502] Reichart PA. Oral manifestations in HIV infection: fungal and bacterial infections, Kaposi's sarcoma.Med Microbiol Immunol (Berl) 2003;192:165–169.

[503] Regezi JA, Jordan RC. Oral Kaposi's sarcoma: biopsy accessions as an indication of declining incidence. Oral Surg Oral Med Oral Pathol Oral Radiol Endod 2002;94:399.

[504] Langford A, Pohle HD, Reichart P. Primary intraosseous AIDS-associated Kaposi's sarcoma. Report of two cases with initial jaw involvement. Int J Oral Maxillofac Surg 1991;20:366–368.

[505] Lausten LL, Ferguson BL, Barker BF, et al. Oral Kaposi sarcoma associated with severe alveolar bone loss: case report and review of the literature. J Periodontol 2003;74:1668–1675.

[506] Epstein JB, Scully C.Neoplastic disease in the head and neck of patients with AIDS. Int J Oral Maxillofac Surg 1992;21:219–226.

[507] Regezi JA, MacPhail LA, Daniels TE, et al. Oral Kaposi's sarcoma: a 10–year retrospective histopathologic study. J Oral Pathol Med 1993;22:292–297.

[508] Newland JR, Adler-Storthz K. Cytomegalovirus in intraoral Kaposi's sarcoma. Oral Surg Oral Med Oral Pathol 1989;67:296–300.

[509] Chak LY, Gill PS, Levine AM, Meyer PR, Anselmo JA, Petrovich Z. Radiation therapy for acquired immunodeficiency syndrome-related Kaposi's sarcoma.J Clin Oncol 1988;6:863–867.

[510] Schweitzer VG,Visscher D. Photodynamic therapy for treatment of AIDS-related oral Kaposi's sarcoma. Otolaryngol Head Neck Surg 1990;102:639–649.

[511] Baumann R, Tauber MG, Opravil M, et al. Combined treatment with zidovudine and lymphoblast interferon-alpha in patients with HIV-related Kaposi's sarcoma. Klin Wochenschr 1991;69:360–367.

[512] de Wit R, Danner SA, Bakker PJ, Lange JM, Eeftinck Schattenkerk JK, Veenhof CH. Combined zidovudine and interferon-alpha treatment in patients with AIDSassociated Kaposi's sarcoma. J Intern Med 1991;229: 35–40.

[513] Epstein JB, Lozada-Nur F, McLeod WA, Spinelli J. Oral Kaposi's sarcoma in acquired immunodeficiency syndrome. Review of management and report of the efficacy of intralesional vinblastine. Cancer 1989;64: 2424–2430.

[514] Epstein JB. Treatment of oral Kaposi sarcoma with intralesional vinblastine. Cancer 1993;71:1722–1725.

[515] Lucatorto FM, Sapp JP. Treatment of oral Kaposi's sarcoma with a sclerosing agent in AIDS patients. A preliminary study. Oral Surg Oral Med Oral Pathol 1993;75:192–198.

[516] Shiboski CH, Winkler JR. Gingival Kaposi's sarcoma and periodontitis. A case report and suggested treatment approach to the combined lesions. Oral Surg Oral Med Oral Pathol 1993;76:49–53.

[517] Birnbaum W, Hodgson TA, Reichart PA. Prognostic significance of HIV-associated oral lesions with their relation to therapy. Oral Dis 2002;8(suppl 2):110–114.

[518] Greenwood I, Zakrzewska JM, Robinson PG. Changes in the prevalence of HIV-associated mucosal disease at a dedicated clinic over 7 years. Oral Dis 2002;8: 90–94.

[519] Mbopi-Keou FX, Legoff J, Piketty C, et al. Salivary production of IgA and IgG to human herpes virus 8 latent and lytic antigens by patients in whom Kaposi's sarcoma has regressed. AIDS 2004;18:338–340.

[520] Ziegler JL, Beckstead JA, Volberding PA, et al. Non- Hodgkin's lymphoma in 90 homosexual men. Relation to generalized lymphadenopathy and the acquired immunodeficiency syndrome. N Engl J Med 1984;311: 565–570.

[521] Levine AM. Non-Hodgkin's lymphomas and other malignancies in the acquired immune deficiency syndrome. Semin Oncol 1987;14(suppl 3):34–39.

[522] Leess FR, Kessler DJ, Mickel RA. Non-Hodgkin's lymphoma of the head and neck in patients with AIDS. Arch Otolaryngol Head Neck Surg 1987;113: 1104–1106.

[523] Kaplan LD. AIDS-associated lymphomas. Infect Dis Clin North Am 1988;2:525–532.

[524] Jordan RC, Chong L, Dipierdomenico S, et al. Oral lymphoma in HIV infection. Oral Dis 1997;3(suppl 1): S135–S137.

[525] Jordan RC, Chong L, Dipierdomenico S, et al. Oral lymphoma in human immunodeficiency virus infection: a report of six cases and review of the literature. Otolaryngol Head Neck Surg 1998;119:672–677.

[526] Carbone AIDS-related non-Hodgkin's lymphomas: from pathology and molecular pathogenesis to

treatment A. Hum Pathol 2002;33:392–404.

[527] Ioachim HL, Dorsett B, Cronnin W, Maya M, Wahl S. Acquired immunodeficiency syndrome-associated lymphomas: clinical, pathologic, immunologic, and viral characteristics of 111 cases. Hum Pathol 1991;22:659–673.

[528] Green TL, Eversole LR. Oral lymphomas in HIVinfected patients: association with Epstein-Barr virus DNA. Oral Surg Oral Med Oral Pathol 1989;67: 437–442.

[529] Goldschmidts WL, Bhatia K, Johnson JF, et al. Epstein-Barr virus genotypes in AIDS-associated lymphomas are similar to those in endemic Burkitt's lymphomas. Leukemia 1992;6:875–878.

[530] Palmer GD, Morgan PR, Challacombe SJ. T-cell lymphoma associated with periodontal disease and HIV infection. A case report. J Clin Periodontol 1993;20: 378–380.

[531] Groot RH, van Merkesteyn JP, Bras J. Oral manifestations of non-Hodgkin's lymphoma in HIV-infected patients. Int J Oral Maxillofac Surg 1990;19:194–196.

[532] Colmenero C, Gamallo C, Pintado V, Patron M, Sierra I, Valencia E. AIDS-related lymphoma of the oral cavity. Int J Oral Maxillofac Surg 1991;20:2–6.

[533] Langford A, Dienemann D, Schurman D, et al. Oral manifestations of AIDS-associated non-Hodgkin's lymphomas. Int J Oral Maxillofac Surg 1991;20:136–141.

[534] Rubin MM, Gatta CA, Cozzi GM. Non-Hodgkin's lymphoma of the buccal gingiva as the initial manifestation of AIDS. J Oral Maxillofac Surg 1989;47: 1311–1313.

[535] Kaugars GE, Burns JC. Non-Hodgkin's lymphoma of the oral cavity associated with AIDS. Oral Surg Oral Med Oral Pathol 1989;67:433–436.

[536] Dodd CL, Greenspan D, Schiodt M, et al. Unusual oral presentation of non-Hodgkin's lymphoma in association with HIV infection. Oral Surg Oral Med Oral Pathol 1992;73:603–608.

[537] Hicks MJ, Flaitz CM, Nichols CM, Luna MA, Gresik MV. Intraoral presentation of anaplastic large-cell Ki-1 lymphoma in association with HIV infection. Oral Surg Oral Med Oral Pathol 1993;76:73–81.

[538] Dodd CL, Greenspan D, Heinic GS, Rabanus JP, Greenspan JS. Multi-focal oral non-Hodgkin's lymphoma in a AIDS patient. Br Dent J 1993;175:373–377.

[539] De Weese TL, Hazuka MB, Hommel DJ, Kinzie JJ, Daniel WE. AIDS-related non-Hodgkin's lymphoma: the outcome and efficacy of radiation therapy. Int J Radiat Oncol Biol Phys 1991;20:803–808.

[540] Beck K. Mycobacterial disease associated with HIV infection. J Gen Intern Med 1991;6(suppl 1):S19–S23.

[541] Young LS. Mycobacterial diseases and the compromised host. Clin Infect Dis 1993;17:436–441.

[542] Joshi VV, Oleske JM, Saad S, Connor EM, Rapkin RH, Minnefor AB. Pathology of opportunistic infections in children with acquired immune deficiency syndrome. Pediatr Pathol 1986;6:145–150.

[543] Rutstein RM, Cobb P, McGowan KL, Pinto-Martin J, Starr SE.Mycobacterium avium intracellulare complex infection in HIV-infected children. AIDS 1993;7:507–512.

[544] Collins FM. Mycobacterial disease, immunosuppression, and acquired immunodeficiency syndrome. Clin Microbiol Rev 1989;2:360–367.

[545] Horsburgh CR Jr, Selik RM. The epidemiology of disseminated nontuberculous mycobacterial infection in the acquired immunodeficiency syndrome (AIDS). Am Rev Respir Dis 1990;139:4–7.

[546] Berlin OG, Zakowski P, Bruckner DA, Clancy MN, Johnson BL Jr. Mycobacterium avium: a pathogen of patients with acquired immunodeficiency syndrome. Diagn Microbiol Infect Dis 1984;2:213–218.

[547] Hawkins CC, Gold JW, Whimbey E, et al. Mycobacterium avium complex infections in patients with the acquired immunodeficiency syndrome. Ann Intern Med 1986;105:184–188.

[548] Klatt EC, Jensen DF, Meyer PR. Pathology of Mycobacterium avium-intracellulare infection in acquired immunodeficiency syndrome. Hum Pathol 1987;18: 709–714.

[549] Jacobson MA, Hopewell PC, Yajko DM, et al. Natural history of disseminated Mycobacterium avium complex infection in AIDS. J Infect Dis 1991;164: 994–998.

[550] Horsburgh CR Jr, Mason 3rd UG, Farhi DC, Iseman MD. Disseminated infection with Mycobacterium avium-intracellulare. A report of 13 cases and a review of the literature.Medicine 1985;64:36–48.

[551] Young LS, Inderlied CB, Berlin OG, Gottlieb MS. Mycobacterial infections in AIDS patients, with an emphasis on the Mycobacterium avium complex. Rev Infect Dis 1986;8:1024–1033.

[552] Tenholder MF, Moser 3rd RJ, Tellis CJ. Mycobacteria other than tuberculosis. Pulmonary involvement in patients with acquired immunodeficiency syndrome. Arch Intern Med 1988;148:953–955.

[553] Wallace JM, Hannah JB. Mycobacterium avium complex infection in patients with the acquired immunodeficiency syndrome. A clinicopathologic study. Chest 1988;93:926–932.

[554] Horsburgh CR Jr. Mycobacterium avium complex infection in the acquired immunodeficiency syndrome. N Engl J Med 1991;324:1332–1338.

[555] Masur H,Tuazon C, Gill V, et al.Effect of combined clofazimine and ansamycin therapy on Mycobacterium avium-Mycobacterium intracellulare bacteremia in patients with AIDS. J Infect Dis 1987;155:127–129.

[556] Levin RH, Bolinger AM. Treatment of nontuberculous mycobacterial infections in pediatric patients. Clin Pharm 1988;7:545–551.

[557] Guthertz LS, Damsker B, Bottone EJ, Ford EG, Midura TF, Janda JM. Mycobacterium avium and Mycobac576. Liang GS, Daikos GL, Serfling U, et al. An evaluation of oral ulcers in patients with AIDS and AIDS-related complex. J Am Acad Dermatol 1993;29:563–568.

[558] Hoy J, Mijch A, Sandland M, Grayson K, Lucas R, Dwyer B. Quadruple-drug therapy for Mycobacterium avium-intracellulare bacteremia in AIDS patients. J Infect Dis 1990;161:801–805.

[559] Benson CA, Kessler HA, Pottage JC Jr, Trenholme GM. Successful treatment of acquired immunodeficiency syndrome-related Mycobacterium avium complex disease with a multiple drug regimen including amikacin. Arch Intern Med 1991;151:582–585.

[560] Garrelts JC. Clofazimine: a review of its use in leprosy and Mycobacterium avium complex infection. Drug Intell Clin Pharm 1991;25:525–531.

[561] Kemper CA, Meng TC, Nussbaum J, et al. Treatment of Mycobacterium avium complex bacteremia in AIDS with a four-drug oral regimen. Rifampin, ethambutol, clofazimine, and ciprofloxacin. The California Collaborative Treatment Group. Ann Intern Med 1992;116: 466–472.

[562] Abrams DI, Mitchell TF, Child CC, Shiboski SC, Brosgart CL, Mass MM. Clofazimine as prophylaxis for disseminated Mycobacterium avium complex infection in AIDS. J. Infect Dis 1993;167:1459–1463.

[563] Benson CA, Ellner JJ. Mycobacterium avium complex infection and AIDS: advances in theory and practice. Clin Infect Dis 1993;17:7–20.

[564] Centers for Disease Control US. Department of Health and Human Services. Diagnosis and management of mycobacterial infection and disease in persons with human immunodeficiency virus infection. Ann Intern Med 1987;106:254–256.

[565] Goodman PC. Pulmonary tuberculosis in patients with acquired immunodeficiency syndrome. J Thorac Imaging 1990;5:38–45.

[566] Sunderam G, McDonald RJ, Maniatis T, Oleske J, Kapila R, Reichman LB. Tuberculosis as a manifestation of the acquired immunodeficiency syndrome (AIDS). JAMA 1986;256:362–366.

[567] Braun MM, Byers RH, Heyward WL, et al. Acquired immunodeficiency syndrome and extrapulmonary tuberculosis in the United States. Arch Intern Med 1990;150:1913–1916.

[568] Horsburgh CR Jr, Pozniak A. Epidemiology of tuberculosis in the era of HIV. AIDS 1993;7(suppl 1): S109–S114.

[569] Yoder KM. Tuberculosis: a reemerging hazard for oral healthcare workers. J Dent Hyg 1993;67:208–213.

[570] Pitchenik AE, Fertel D. Medical management of AIDS patients. Tuberculosis and nontuberculous mycobacterial disease. Med Clin North Am 1992;76: 121–171.

[571] Barnes PF, Le HQ, Davidson PT. Tuberculosis in patients with HIV infection. Med Clin North Am 1993;77:1369–1390.

[572] Miller B. Preventive therapy for tuberculosis.Med Clin North Am 1993;77:1263–1275.

[573] Cohn DL, Dobkin JF. Treatment and prevention of tuberculosis in HIV infection. AIDS 1993;7(suppl 1): S195–S202.

[574] Johnson MP, Chaisson RE. Tuberculosis and HIV disease. AIDS Clin Rev 1993;94;73–93.

[575] Brudney K, Dobkin J. Resurgent tuberculosis in New York City. Human immunodeficiency virus, homelessness, and the decline of tuberculosis control programs. Am Rev Respir Dis 1991;144:745–749

[576] Liang GS, Daikos GL, Serfling U, et al. An evaluation of oral ulcers in patients with AIDS and AIDS-related complex. J Am Acad Dermatol 1993;29:563–568.

[577] Langford A, Pohle HD, Gelderblom H, Zhang X, Reichart PA. Oral hyperpigmentation in HIV-infected patients. Oral Surg Oral Med Oral Pathol 1989;67:301–307.

[578] Langford AA, Gelderblom H, Kunze RO, Pohle HD, Reichart PA.Hyperpigmentation of the oral mucosa in HIV infection. Schweiz Monatsschr Zahnmed 1990; 100:1037–1041.

[579] Ficarra G, Shillitoe EJ, Adler-Storthz K, et al. Oral melanotic macules in patients infected with human immunodeficiency virus. Oral Surg Oral Med Oral Pathol 1990;70:748–755.

[580] Greenberg RG, Berger TG. Nail and mucocutaneous hyperpigmentation with azidothymidine therapy. J Am Acad Dermatol 1990;22:327–330.

[581] Tadini G, D'Orso M, Cusini M, Alessi E. Oral mucosa pigmentation: a new side effect of azidothymidine therapy in patients with acquired immunodeficiency syndrome. Arch Dermatol 1991;127:267–268.

[582] Porter SR, Glover S, Scully C. Oral hyperpigmentation and adrenocortical hypofunction in a patient with acquired immunodeficiency syndrome.Oral Surg Oral Med Oral Pathol 1990;70:59–60.

[583] Zhang X, Langford A, Gelderblom H, Reichart P. Ultrastructural findings in oral hyperpigmentation of HIV-infected patients. J Oral Pathol Med 1989;18:471–474.

[584] Langford A, Ruf B. Diagnosis and differential diagnosis of oral hyperpigmentation. Quintessenz 1990;41: 1989–2001.

[585] Winkler JR, Robertson PB. Periodontal disease associated with HIV infection. Oral Surg Oral Med Oral Pathol 1992;73:145–150.

[586] Williams CA,Winkler JR, Grassi M, Murray PA. HIVassociated periodontitis complicated by necrotizing stomatitis. Oral Surg Oral Med Oral Pathol 1990;69: 351–355.

[587] Melnick SL, Engel D, Truelove E, et al. Oral mucosal lesions: association with the presence of antibodies to the human immunodeficiency virus. Oral Surg Oral Med Oral Pathol 1989;68:37–43.

[588] Felix DH, Wray D, Smith GL, Jones GA. Oro-antral fistula: an unusual complication of HIV-associated periodontal disease. Br Dent J 1991;171:61–62.

[589] Scully C, McCarthy G. Management of oral health in persons with HIV infection. Oral Surg Oral Med Oral Pathol 1992;73:215–225.

[590] Anneroth G, Anneroth I, Lynch DP. Acquired immune deficiency syndrome (AIDS) in the United States in 1986: etiology, epidemiology, clinical manifestations, and dental implications. J Oral Maxillofac Surg 1986; 44:956–964.

[591] Schiodt M, Greenspan D, Daniels TE, et al. Parotid gland enlargement and xerostomia associated with labial sialadenitis in HIV-infected patients. J Autoimmun 1989;2:415–425.

[592] Schiodt M, Greenspan D, Levy JA, et al.Does HIV cause salivary gland disease? AIDS 1989;3:819–822.

[593] Zeitlen S, Shaha A. Parotid manifestations of HIV infection. J Surg Oncol 1991;47:230–232.

[594] Schiodt M. HIV-associated salivary gland disease: a review. Oral Surg Oral Med Oral Pathol 1992;73:164–167. terium intracellulare infections in patients with and without AIDS. J Infect Dis 1989;160:1037–1041.

[595] Fox PC, van der Ven PF, Sonies BC, Weiffenbach JM, Baum BJ. Xerostomia: evaluation of a symptom with increasing significance. J Am Dent Assoc 1985;110: 519–525.

[596] Couderc LJ, D'Agay MF, Danon F, Harzic M, Brocheriou C, Clauvel JP. Sicca complex and infection with human immunodeficiency virus. Arch Intern Med 1987;147:898–901.

[597] Kaye BR. Rheumatologic manifestations of infection with human immunodeficiency virus (HIV). Ann Intern Med 1989;111:158–167.

[598] Chapnik JS, Noyek AM, Berris B, et al. Parotid gland enlargement in HIV infection: clinical/imaging findings. J Otolaryngol 1990;19:189–194.

[599] Knox WF, McWilliam LJ, Banerjee SS. Benign lymphoepithelial lesion of salivary gland in a patient with AIDS. J Clin Pathol 1990;43:780–781.

[600] Terry JH, Loree TR, Thomas MD, Marti JR.Major salivary gland lymphoepithelial lesions and the acquired immunodeficiency syndrome. Am J Surg 1991;162: 324–329.

[601] Fox PC. Saliva and salivary gland alterations in HIV infection. J Am Dent Assoc 1991;122:46–48.

[602] Schiodt M, Dodd CL, Greenspan D, et al. Natural history of HIV-associated salivary gland disease. Oral Surg Oral Med Oral Pathol 1992;74:326–331.

[603] Rosenberg ZS, Joffe SA, Itescu S. Spectrum of salivary gland disease in HIV-infected patients: characterization with Ga-67 citrate imaging. Radiology 1992;184: 761–764.

[604] Scully C, Davies R, Porter S, Eveson J, Luker J. HIVsalivary gland disease. Salivary scintiscanning with technetium pertechnetate. Oral Surg Oral Med Oral Pathol 1993;76:120–123.

[605] Ryan JR, Ioachim HL,Marmer J,Loubeau JM.Acquired immune deficiency syndrome-related lymphadenopathies presenting in the salivary gland lymph nodes. Arch Otolaryngol 1985;111:554–556.

[606] Shaha A, Thelmo W, Jaffee BM. Is parotid lymphadenopathy a new disease or part of AIDS? Am J Surg 1988;156:297–300.

[607] Vargas PA, Mauad T, Boehm GM, et al. Parotid gland involvement in advanced AIDS. Oral Dis 2003;9:55–61.

[608] Lecatsas G, Houff S, Macher A, et al. Retrovirus-like particles in salivary glands, prostate and testes of AIDS patients. Proc Soc Exp Biol Med 1985;178:653–655.

[609] Schiodt M, Atkinson JC, Greenspan D, et al. Sialochemistry in human immunodeficiency virus associated salivary gland disease. J Rheumatol 1992;19:26–29.

[610] Fox PC. Salivary gland involvement in HIV-1 infection. Oral Surg Oral Med Oral Pathol 1992;73:168–170.

[611] Yeung SC, Kazazi F, Randle CG, et al. Patients infected with human immunodeficiency virus type 1 have low levels of virus in saliva even in the presence of periodontal disease. J Infect Dis 1993;167:803–809.

[612] Barr CE, Miller KL, Lopez MR, et al. Recovery of infectious HIV-1 from whole saliva. J Am Dent Assoc 1992; 123:36–48.

[613] Barr CE, Lopez MR, Rua-Dobles A, Miller LK, Mathur-Wagh U, Turgeon LR. HIV-associated oral lesions; immunologic, virologic and salivary parameters. J Oral Pathol Med 1992;21:295–298.

[614] Mandel ID, Barr CE, Turgeon L. Longitudinal study of parotid saliva in HIV-1 infection. J Oral Pathol Med 1992;21:209–213.

[615] Yeh CK, Fox PC, Goto Y, Austin HA, Brahim JS, Fox CH. Human immunodeficiency virus (HIV) and HIV infected cells in saliva and salivary glands of a patient with systemic lupus erythematosus. J Rheumatol 1992; 19:1810–1812.

[616] Epstein JB, Scully C, Porter SR. The risk of transmission of human immunodeficiency virus in dental practice. Oral Health 1992;82:33–38.

[617] Moore BE, Flaitz CM, Coppenhaver DH, et al. HIV recovery from saliva before and after dental treatment. Inhibitors may have a critical role in viral inactivation. J Am Dent Assoc 1993;124:67–74.

[618] Branson BM. FDA approves OraQuick for use in saliva. AIDS Clin Care 2004;16:39.

[619] Oral HIV test approved by FDA. Lancet 2004;363:1125.

[620] Pinheiro A, Marcenes W, Zakrzewska JM, et al. Dental and oral lesions in HIV infected patients: a study in Brazil. Int Dent J 2004;54:131–137.

[621] Mulligan R, Phelan JA, Brunelle J, et al. Baseline characteristics of participants in the oral health component of the Women's Interagency HIV Study. Community Dent Oral Epidemiol 2004;32:86–98.

[622] Abelson DC, Barton J, Mandel ID. The effect of chewing sorbitol-sweetened gum on salivary flow and cemental plaque pH in subjects with low salivary flow. J Clin Dent 1990;2:3–5.

[623] Fox RI, Michelson P. Approaches to the treatment of SjoÅNgren's syndrome. J Rheumatol 2000;suppl 61:15–21.

[624] Fox RI, Stern M, Michelson P. Update in SjoÅNgren syndrome. Curr Opin Rheumatol 2000;12:391–398.

[625] Karpatkin S, Nardi MA. Immunologic thrombocytopenic purpura in human immunodeficiency virus–seropositive patients with hemophilia. Comparison with patients with classic autoimmune thrombocytopenic purpura, homosexuals with thrombocytopenia, and narcotic addicts with thrombocytopenia. J Lab Clin Med 1988;111:441–448.

[626] Rarick MU, Espina B, Mocharnuk R, Trilling Y, Levine AM. Thrombotic thrombocytopenic purpura in patients with human immunodeficiency virus infection: a report of three cases and review of the literature. Am J Hematol 1992;40:103–109.

[627] Najean Y, Rain JD. The mechanism of thrombocytopenia in patients with HIV infection. J Lab Clin Med 1994;123:415–420.

[628] Ficarra G. Oral lesions of iatrogenic and undefined etiology and neurologic disorders associated with HIV infection. Oral Surg Oral Med Oral Pathol 1992;73:201–211.

[629] van der Waal I. Organ-specific manifestations of HIV infection. IV. Oral manifestations of HIV infection: comments on the present classification. AIDS 1993;7(suppl 1):S223–224.

[630] Cabrera VP, Rodu B. Differential diagnosis of oral mucosal petechial hemorrhages. Compendium 1991; 12:418–422.

[631] Speight PM, Zakrzewska J, Fletcher CD. Epithelioid angiomatosis affecting the oral cavity as a first sign of HIV infection. Br Dent J 1991;171:367–370.

[632] Nishioka GJ, Chilcoat CC, Aufdemorte TB, Clare N.The gingival biopsy in the diagnosis of thrombotic thrombocytopenic purpura. Oral Surg Oral Med Oral Pathol 1988;65:580–585.

[633] Costello C, Treacy M, Lai L. Treatment of immune thrombocytopenic purpura in homosexual men. Scand J Haematol 1986;36:507–510.

[634] Reichart PA. Oral ulceration and iatrogenic disease in HIV infection. Oral Surg Oral Med Oral Pathol 1992; 73:212–214.

[635] Silverman Jr S, Gallo J, Stites DP. Prednisone management of HIV-associated recurrent oral aphthous ulcerations. J Acquir Immune Defic Syndr 1992;5:952–953.

[636] Youle M, Clarbour J, Farthing C, et al. Treatment of resistant aphthous ulceration with thalidomide in patients positive for HIV antibody. BMJ 1989;298:432.

[637] Erlich KS, Mills J. Other virus infections in AIDS. II. Herpes simplex virus. Immunol Ser 1989;44:534–554.

[638] Corey JP, Seligman I. Otolaryngology problems in the immune compromised patient—an evolving natural history. Otolaryngol Head Neck Surg 1991;104:196–203.

[639] Eversole LR. Viral infections of the head and neck among HIV-seropositive patients. Oral Surg Oral Med Oral Pathol 1992;73:155–163.

[640] Katz MH, Mastrucci MT, Leggott PJ, Westenhouse J, Greenspan JS, Scott GB. Prognostic significance of oral lesions in children with perinatally acquired human immunodeficiency virus infection. Am J Dis Child 1993;147:45–48.

[641] Jones AC, Migliorati CA, Baughman RA. The simultaneous occurrence of oral herpes simplex virus, cytomegalovirus, and histoplasmosis in an HIVinfected patient. Oral Surg Oral Med Oral Pathol 1992;74:334–339.

[642] Heinic GS, Northfelt DW, Greenspan JS, MacPhail LA, Greenspan D. Concurrent oral cytomegalovirus and herpes simplex virus infection in association with HIV infection. A case report. Oral Surg Oral Med Oral Pathol 1993;75:488–494.

[643] Miller RG, Whittington WL, Coleman RM, Nigida Jr SM. Acquisition of concomitant oral and genital infection with herpes simplex virus type 2. Sex Transm Dis 1987;14:41–43.

[644] Cohen SG, Greenberg MS. Chronic oral herpes simplex virus infection in immunocompromised patients. Oral Surg Oral Med Oral Pathol 1985;59:465–471.

[645] Reichart PA. Oral manifestations of recently described viral infections, including AIDS. Curr Opin Dent 1991;1:377–383.

[646] Barrett AP, Buckley DJ, Greenberg ML, Earl MJ. The value of exfoliative cytology in the diagnosis of oral herpes simplex infection in immunosuppressed patients. Oral Surg Oral Med Oral Pathol 1986;62:175–178.

[647] Bagg J, Mannings A, Munro J, Walker DM. Rapid diagnosis of oral herpes simplex or zoster virus infections by immunofluorescence: comparison with Tzanck cell preparations and viral culture. Br Dent J 1989;167: 235–238.

[648] Epstein JB, Page JL, Anderson GH, Spinelli J. The role of an immunoperoxidase technique in the diagnosis of oral herpes simplex virus infection in patients with leukemia. Diagn Cytopathol 1987;3:205–209.

[649] Laga Jr EA, Toth BB, Rolston KV, Tarrand JJ. Evaluation of a rapid enzyme-linked immunoassay for the diagnosis of herpes simplex virus in cancer patients with oral lesions. Oral Surg Oral Med Oral Pathol 1993;75:168–172.

[650] Mintz GA, Rose SL. Diagnosis of oral herpes simplex virus infections: practical aspects of viral culture. Oral Surg Oral Med Oral Pathol 1984;58:486–492.

[651] Declerq E. Antivirals for the treatment of herpesvirus infections. J Antimicrob Chemother 1993;32(suppl A): 121–132.

[652] Perry CM, Wagstaff AJ. Famciclovir. A review of its pharmacological properties and therapeutic efficacy in herpesvirus infections. Drugs 1995;50:396–415.

[653] Cirelli R, Herne K, McCrary M, Lee P, Tyring SK. Famciclovir: review of clinical efficacy and safety. Antiviral Res 1995;29:141–151.

[654] Alrabiah FA, Sachs SL. New antiherpesvirus agents. Their targets and therapeutic potential. Drugs 1996; 52:17–32.

[655] Perry CM, Faulds D. Valaciclovir. A review of its antiviral activity, pharmacokinetic properties and therapeutic efficacy in herpesvirus infections. Drugs 1996;52:754–772.

[656] Stein GE. Pharmacology of new antiherpes agents: famciclovir and valacyclovir. J Am Pharm Assoc 1997;37:157–163.

[657] Acosta EP, Fletcher CV. Valacyclovir. Ann Pharmacother 1997;31:185–191.

[658] Hamuy R, Berman B. Treatment of herpes simplex virus infections with topical antiviral agents. Eur J Dermatol 1998;8:310–319.

[659] Snoeck R. Antiviral therapy of herpes simplex. Int J Antimicrob Agents 2000;16:157–169.

[660] Emmert DH. Treatment of common cutaneous herpes simplex virus infections. Am Fam Physician 2000; 61:1697–1708.

[661] Safrin S. Treatment of acyclovir-resistant herpes simplex virus infections in patients with AIDS. J Acquir Immune Defic Syndr 1992;5(suppl 1):S29–S32.

[662] Safrin S, Kemmerly S, Plotkin B, et al. Foscarnetresistant herpes simplex virus infection in patients with AIDS. J Infect Dis 1994;169:193–196.

[663] Marks GL, Nolan PE, Erlich KS, Ellis MN. Mucocutaneous dissemination of acyclovir-resistant herpes simplex virus in a patient with AIDS. Rev Infect Dis 1989;11:474–476.

[664] Butler S, Molinari JA, Plezia RA, Chandrasekar P, Venkat H. Condyloma acuminatum in the oral cavity: four cases and a review. Rev Infect Dis 1988;10:544–550.

[665] Zunt SL, Tomich CE. Oral condyloma acuminatum. J Dermatol Surg Oncol 1989;15:591–594.

[666] Syrjanen SM, Syrjanen KJ, Lamberg MA. Detection of human papillomavirus DNA in oral mucosal lesions using in situ DNA-hybridization applied on paraffin sections. Oral Surg Oral Med Oral Pathol 1986;62: 660–667.

[667] Eversole LR, Laipis PJ, Merrell P, Choi E. Demonstration of human papillomavirus DNA in oral condyloma acuminatum. J Oral Pathol 1987;16:266–272.

[668] Luomanen M. Experience with a carbon dioxide laser for removal of benign oral soft-tissue lesions. Proc Finn Dent Soc 1992;88:49–55.

[669] Vilmer C, Cavelier-Balloy B, Pinquier L, Blanc F, Dubertret L. Focal epithelial hyperplasia and multifocal human papillomavirus infection in an HIV-seropositive man. J Am Acad Dermatol 1994;30: 497–498.

[670] Syrjanen S, von Krogh G, Kellokoski J, Syrjanen K. Two different human papillomavirus (HPV) types associated with oral mucosal lesions in an HIV-seropositive man. J Oral Pathol Med 1989;18:366–370.

[671] Schulten EA, ten Kate RW, van der Waal I. Oral findings in HIV-infected patients attending a department of internal medicine: the contribution of intraoral examination towards the clinical management of HIV disease. Q J Med 1990;76:741–745.

[672] Laskaris G, Hadjivassiliou M, Stratigos J. Oral signs and symptoms in 160 Greek HIV-infected patients. J Oral Pathol Med 1992;21:120–123.

[673] de Villiers EM. Prevalence of HPV 7 papillomas in the oral mucosa and facial skin of patients with human immunodeficiency virus. Arch Dermatol 1989;125:1590.

[674] Greenspan D, de Villiers EM, Greenspan JS, de Souza YG, zur Hausen H. Unusual HPV types in oral warts in association with HIV infection. J Oral Pathol 1988;17:482–488.

[675] DeRossi SS, Laudenbach J. The management of oral human papillomavirus with topical cidofir: a case report. Cutis 2004;73:191–193.

[676] Quinnan Jr GV, Masur H, Rook AH, et al. Herpesvirus infections in the acquired immune deficiency syndrome. JAMA 1984;252:72–77.

[677] Perronne C, Lazanas M, Leport C, et al. Varicella in patients infected with the human immunodeficiency virus. Arch Dermatol 1990;126:1033–1036.

[678] Kelley R, Mancao M, Lee F, Sawyer M, Nahmias A, Nesheim S. Varicella in children with perinatally acquired human immunodeficiency virus infection. J Pediatr 1994;124:271–273.

[679] Jura E, Chadwick EG, Josephs SH, et al. Varicella-zoster virus infections in children infected with human immunodeficiency virus. Pediatr Infect Dis J 1989;8: 586–590.

[680] Patterson LE, Butler KM, Edwards MS. Clinical herpes zoster shortly following primary varicella in two HIVinfected children. Clin Pediatr 1989;28:354.

[681] Gulick RM, Heath-Chiozzi M, Crumpacker CS. Varicella-zoster virus disease in patients with human immunodeficiency virus infection. Arch Dermatol 1990;126:1086–1088.

[682] Hoppenjans WB, Bibler MR, Orme RL, Solinger AM. Prolonged cutaneous herpes zoster in acquired immunodeficiency syndrome. Arch Dermatol 1990; 126:1048–1050.

[683] Gnann JW, Whitley RJ. Natural history and treatment of varicella-zoster in high-risk populations. J Hosp Infect 1991;18(suppl A):317–329.

[684] Leibovitz E, Kaul A, Rigaud M, Bebenroth D, Krasinski K, Borkowsky W. Chronic varicella zoster in a child infected with human immunodeficiency virus: case report and review of the literature. Cutis 1992;49: 27–31.

[685] Srugo I, Israele V, Wittek AE, Courville T, Viman VM, Brunell PA. Clinical manifestations of varicella-zoster virus infections in human immunodeficiency virusinfected children. Am J Dis Child 1993;147:742–745.

[686] Wallace MR, Hooper DG, Pyne JM, Graves SJ, Malone JL. Varicella immunity and clinical disease in HIVinfected adults. South Med J 1994;87:74–76.

[687] Sindrup JH, Weismann K, Sand Petersen C, et al. Skin and oral mucosal changes in patients infected with human immunodeficiency virus. Acta Derm Venereol 1988;68:440–443.

[688] Jensen JL, Kanas RJ, De Boom GW. Multiple oral and labial ulcers in an immunocompromised patient. J Am Dent Assoc 1987;114:235–236.

[689] Van de Perre P, Bakkers E, Batungwanayo J, et al. Herpes zoster in African patients: an early manifestation of HIV infection. Scand J Infect Dis 1988;20:277–282.

[690] Moskow BS, Hernandez G. Aggressive periodontal destruction and herpes zoster in a suspected AIDS patient. J Parodontol 1991;10:359–369.

[691] Balfour Jr HH. Acyclovir and other chemotherapy for herpes group viral infections. Annu Rev Med 1984;35:279–291.

[692] Straus SE. The management of varicella and zoster infections. Infect Dis Clin North Am 1987;1:367–382.

[693] Hermans PE, Cockerill 3rd FR. Antiviral agents. Mayo Clin Proc 1987;62:1108–1115.

[694] Straus SE, Ostrove JM, Inchauspe G, et al. NIH conference. Varicella-zoster virus infections. Biology,

natural history, treatment, and prevention. Ann Intern Med 1988;108:221–237.

[695] Huff JC. Antiviral treatment in chickenpox and herpes zoster. J Am Acad Dermatol 1988;18:204–206.

[696] Balfour Jr HH. Varicella zoster virus infections in immunocompromised hosts. A review of the natural history and management. Am J Med 1988;85:68–73.

[697] Sellitti TP, Huang AJ, Schiffman J, Davis JL. Association of herpes zoster ophthalmicus with acquired immunodeficiency syndrome and acute retinal necrosis. Am J Ophthalmol 1993;116:297–301.

[698] Tricot G, De Clercq E, Boogaerts MA, Verwilghen RL. Oral bromovinyldeoxyuridine therapy for herpes simplex and varicella-zoster virus infections in severely immunosuppressed patients: a preliminary clinical trial. J Med Virol 1986;18:11–20.

[699] Safrin S, Berger TG, Gilson I, et al. Foscarnet therapy in five patients with AIDS and acyclovir-resistant varicella-zoster virus infection. Ann Intern Med 1991; 115:19–21.

[700] Cole NL, Balfour Jr HH. Varicella-zoster virus does not become more resistant to acyclovir during therapy. J Infect Dis 1986;153:605–608.

[701] Jacobson MA, Berger TG, Fikrig S, et al. Acyclovirresistant varicella zoster virus infection after chronic oral acyclovir therapy in patients with the acquired immunodeficiency syndrome (AIDS). Ann Intern Med 1990;112:187–191.

[702] Balfour Jr HH, Benson C, Braun J, et al. Management of acyclovir-resistant herpes simplex and varicellazoster virus infections. J Acquir Immune Defic Syndr 1994;7:254–260.

[703] Lyall EG, Ogilvie MM, Smith NM, Burns S. Acyclovir resistant varicella zoster and HIV infection. Arch Dis Child 1994;70:133–135.

[704] Zambon JJ, Reynolds HS, Genco RJ. Studies of the subgingival microflora in patients with acquired immunodeficiency syndrome. J Periodontol 1990;61: 699–704.

[705] Watkins KV, Richmond AS, Langstein IM. Nonhealing extraction site due to Actinomyces naeslundii in a patient with AIDS. Oral Surg Oral Med Oral Pathol 1991;71:675–677.

[706] Cockerell CJ, Le Boit PE. Bacillary angiomatosis: a newly characterized, pseudoneoplastic, infectious, cutaneous vascular disorder. J Am Acad Dermatol 1990;22:501–512.

[707] Cockerell CJ. The clinicopathologic spectrum of bacillary (epithelioid) angiomatosis. Prog AIDS Pathol 1990;2:111–226.

[708] Cotell SL, Noskin GA. Bacillary angiomatosis. Clinical and histologic features, diagnosis, and treatment. Arch Intern Med 1994;154:524–528.

[709] Koehler JE, Le Boit PE, Egbert BM, Berger TG. Cutaneous vascular lesions and disseminated catscratch disease in patients with the acquired immunodeficiency syndrome (AIDS) and AIDS-related complex. Ann Intern Med 1988;109:449–455.

[710] Le Boit PE, Berger TG, Egbert BM, et al. Epithelioid haemangioma-like vascular proliferation in AIDS: manifestation of cat scratch disease bacillus infection? Lancet 1988;1:960–963.

[711] Pilon VA, Echols RM. Cat-scratch disease in a patient with AIDS. Am J Clin Pathol 1989;92:236–240.

[712] Szaniawski WK, Don PC, Bitterman SR, Schachner JR. Epithelioid angiomatosis in patients with AIDS. Report of seven cases and review of the literature. J Am Acad Dermatol 1990;23:41–48.

[713] Schwartzman WA, Marchevsky A, Meyer RD. Epithelioid angiomatosis or cat scratch disease with splenic and hepatic abnormalities in AIDS: case report and review of the literature. Scand J Infect Dis 1990;22: 121–133.

[714] Kemper CA, Lombard CM, Deresinski SC, Tompkins LS. Visceral bacillary epithelioid angiomatosis: possible manifestations of disseminated cat scratch disease in the immunocompromised host: a report of

two cases. Am J Med 1990;89:216–122.

[715] Relman DA, Loutit JS, Schmidt TM, Falkow S, Tompkins LS. The agent of bacillary angiomatosis. An approach to the identification of uncultured pathogens. N Engl J Med 1990;323:1573–1580.

[716] Cockerell CJ, Tierno PM, Friedman-Kien AE, Kim KS. Clinical, histologic, microbiologic, and biochemical characterization of the causative agent of bacillary (epithelioid) angiomatosis: a rickettsial illness with features of bartonellosis. J Invest Dermatol 1991;97: 812–817.

[717] McDonald G. Cat-scratch disease. Postgrad Med 1992; 92:47.

[718] Birtles RJ, Harrison TG, Taylor AG. Cat scratch disease and bacillary angiomatosis: aetiological agents and the link with AIDS. Commun Dis Rep CDR Rev 1993;3:R107–110.

[719] Tappero JW, Mohle-Boetani J, Koehler JE, et al. The epidemiology of bacillary angiomatosis and bacillary peliosis. JAMA 1993;269:770–775.

[720] Marasco WA, Lester S, Parsonnet J. Unusual presentation of cat scratch disease in a patient positive for antibody to the human immunodeficiency virus. Rev Infect Dis 1989;11:793–803.

[721] Abrams J, Farhood AI. Infection-associated vascular lesions in acquired immunodeficiency syndrome patients. Hum Pathol 1989;20:1025–1026.

[722] Berger TG, Tappero JW, Kaymen A, Le Boit PE. Bacillary (epithelioid) angiomatosis and concurrent Kaposi's sarcoma in acquired immunodeficiency syndrome. Arch Dermatol 1989;125:1543–1547.

[723] Le Boit PE, Berger TG, Egbert BM, Beckstead JH, Yen TS, Stoler MH. Bacillary angiomatosis. The histopathology and differential diagnosis of a pseudoneoplastic infection in patients with human immunodeficiency virus disease. Am J Surg Pathol 1989;13: 909–920.

[724] Walford N, Van der Wouw PA, Das PK, Ten Velden JJ, Hulsebosch HJ. Epithelioid angiomatosis in the acquired immunodeficiency syndrome: morphology and differential diagnosis. Histopathology 1990;16: 83–88.

[725] Glick M, Cleveland DB. Oral mucosal bacillary epithelioid angiomatosis in a patient with AIDS associated with rapid alveolar bone loss: case report. J Oral Pathol Med 1993;22:235–239.

[726] Rudikoff D, Phelps RG, Gordon RE, Battone EJ. Acquired immunodeficiency syndrome-related bacillary vascular proliferation (epithelioid angiomatosis): rapid response to erythromycin therapy. Arch Dermatol 1989;125:706–707.

[727] van der Wouw PA, Hadderingh RJ, Reiss P, Hulsebosch HJ, Walford N, Lange JM. Disseminated cat-scratch disease in a patient with AIDS. AIDS 1989;3:751–753.

[728] Mui BS, Mulligan ME, George WL. Response of HIV associated disseminated cat scratch disease to treatment with doxycycline. Am J Med 1990;89:229–231.

[729] Holley Jr HP. Successful treatment of cat-scratch disease with ciprofloxacin. JAMA 1991;265:1563–1565.

[730] Innocenzi D, Cerio R, Barduagni O, Bosman C, Carlesimo OA. Bacillary epithelioid angiomatosis in acquired immunodeficiency syndrome (AIDS)—clinicopathological and ultrastructural study of a case with a review of the literature. Clin Exp Dermatol 1993;18:133–137.

[731] Salomon D, Saurat JH. Erythema multiforme major in a 2–month-old child with human immunodeficiency virus (HIV) infection. Br J Dermatol 1990;123:797–800.

[732] Belfort Jr R, de Smet M, Whitcup SM, et al. Ocular complications of Stevens-Johnson syndrome and toxic epidermal necrolysis in patients with AIDS. Cornea 1991;10:536–538.

[733] Lewis DA, Brook MG. Erythema multiforme as a presentation of human immunodeficiency virus seroconversion illness. Int J STD AIDS 1992;3:56–57.

[734] Schuval SJ, Bonagura VR, Ilowite NT. Rheumatologic manifestations of pediatric human

immunodeficiency virus infection. J Rheumatol 1993;20:1578–1582.

[735] Porteous DM, Berger TG. Severe cutaneous drug reactions (Stevens-Johnson syndrome and toxic epidermal necrolysis) in human immunodeficiency virus infection. Arch Dermatol 1991;127:740–741.

[736] Saiag P, Caumes E, Chosidow O, Revuz J, Roujeau JC. Drug-induced toxic epidermal necrolysis (Lyell syndrome) in patients infected with the human immunodeficiency virus. J Am Acad Dermatol 1992; 26:567–574.

[737] Azon-Masoliver A, Vilaplana J. Fluconazole-induced toxic epidermal necrolysis in a patient with human immunodeficiency virus infection. Dermatology 1993;187:268–269.

[738] Schlienger RG, Haefeli WE, Bircher A, Leib SL, Luscher TF. Drug-induced Stevens-Johnson syndrome in a patient with AIDS. Schweiz Rundsch Med Prax 1993;82:888–892.

[739] Krippaehne JA, Montgomery MT. Erythema multiforme: a literature review and case report. Spec Care Dentist 1992;12:125–130.

[740] Williams DM. Non-infectious diseases of the oral soft tissue: a new approach.Adv Dent Res 1993;7:213–219.

[741] Corticosteroids for erythema multiforme? Pediatr Dermatol 1989;6:229–250.

[742] Lozada-Nur F, Gorsky M, Silverman Jr S. Oral erythema multiforme: clinical observations and treatment of 95 patients. Oral Surg Oral Med Oral Pathol 1989;67:36–40.

[743] Lozada-Nur F, Cram D, Gorsky M. Clinical response to levamisole in thirty-nine patients with erythema multiforme. An open prospective study. Oral Surg Oral Med Oral Pathol 1992;74:294–298.

[744] Schofield JK, Tatnall FM, Leigh IM. Recurrent erythema multiforme: clinical features and treatment in a large series of patients. Br J Dermatol 1993;128: 542–545.

[745] Stein DK, Sugar AM. Fungal infections in the immunocompromised host. Diagn Microbiol Infect Dis 1989; 12(suppl 4):221S–228S.

[746] de Almeida OP, Scully C. Oral lesions in the systemic mycoses. Curr Opin Dent 1991;1:423–428.

[747] Samaranayake LP. Oral mycoses in HIV infection. Oral Surg Oral Med Oral Pathol 1992;73:171–180.

[748] Grant IH, Armstrong D. Fungal infections in AIDS. Cryptococcosis. Infect Dis Clin North Am 1988;2: 457–464.

[749] Sugar AM. Overview: cryptococcosis in the patient with AIDS.Mycopathologia 1991;114:153–157.

[750] Stern JJ, Hartman BJ, Sharkey P, et al. Oral fluconazole therapy for patients with acquired immunodeficiency syndrome and cryptococcosis: experience with 22 patients. Am J Med 1988;85:477–480.

[751] Hostetler JS, Denning DW, Stevens DA. US experience with itraconazole in aspergillus, cryptococcus and histoplasma infections in the immunocompromised host. Chemotherapy 1992;8(suppl 1):12–22.

[752] Laroche R, Dupond B, Touze JE, et al. Cryptococcal meningitis associated with acquired immunodeficiency syndrome (AIDS) in African patients: treatment with fluconazole. J Med Vet Mycol 1992;30: 71–78.

[753] Dismukes WE. Management of cryptococcosis. Clin Infect Dis 1993;17(suppl 2):S507–512.

[754] Como JA, Dismukes WE. Oral azole drugs as systemic antifungal therapy. N Engl J Med 1994;330:263–272.

[755] Lynch DP, Naftolin LZ. Oral Cryptococcus neoformans infection in AIDS. Oral Surg Oral Med Oral Pathol 1987;64:449–453.

[756] Glick M,Cohen SG, Cheney RT,Crooks GW,Greenberg MS. Oral manifestations of disseminated Cryptococcus neoformans in a patient with acquired immunodeficiency syndrome. Oral Surg Oral Med

Oral Pathol 1987;64:454–459.

[757] Heimdahl A, Nord CE. Oral yeast infections in immunocompromised and seriously diseased patients. Acta Odontol Scand 1990;48:77–84.

[758] Tzerbos F, Kabani S, Booth D. Cryptococcosis as an exclusive oral presentation. J Oral Maxillofac Surg 1992;50:759–760.

[759] Heinic GS, Greenspan D, MacPhail LA, Greenspan JS. Oral Geotrichum candidum infection associated with HIV infection. A case report. Oral Surg Oral Med Oral Pathol 1992;73:726–728.

[760] Hay RJ. Histoplasmosis. Semin Dermatol 1993;12:310–314.

[761] Cobb CM, Shultz RE, Brewer JH, Dunlap CL. Chronic pulmonary histoplasmosis with an oral lesion. Oral Surg Oral Med Oral Pathol 1989;67:73–76.

[762] Cohen PR, Bank DE, Silvers DN, Grossman ME. Cutaneous lesions of disseminated histoplasmosis in human immunodeficiency virus-infected patients. J Am Acad Dermatol 1990;23:422–428.

[763] Oda D, MacDougall L, Fritsche T, Worthington P, Mac-Dougall L. Oral histoplasmosis as a presenting disease in acquired immunodeficiency syndrome. Oral Surg Oral Med Oral Pathol 1990;70:631–636.

[764] Eisig S, Boguslaw B, Cooperband B, Phelan J. Oral manifestations of disseminated histoplasmosis in acquired immunodeficiency syndrome: report of two cases and review of the literature. J Oral Maxillofac Surg 1991;49:310–313.

[765] Heinic GS, Greenspan D, MacPhail LA, et al. Oral Histoplasma capsulatum infection in association with HIV infection: a case report. J Oral Pathol Med 1992; 21:85–89.

[766] Swindells S, Durham T, Johansson SL, Kaufman L. Oral histoplasmosis in a patient infected with HIV. A case report. Oral Surg Oral Med Oral Pathol 1994;77: 126–130.

[767] Mandell W, Goldberg DM, Neu HC. Histoplasmosis in patients with the acquired immune deficiency syndrome. Am J Med 1986;81:974–978.

[768] Dobleman TJ, Scher N, Goldman M, Doot S. Invasive histoplasmosis of the mandible. Head Neck 1989;11: 81–84.

[769] Scully C, de Almeida OP. Orofacial manifestations of the systemic mycoses. J Oral Pathol Med 1992;21:289–294.

[770] Stein DK, Sugar AM. Fungal infections in the immunocompromised host. Diagn Microbiol Infect Dis 1989; 12(suppl 4):221S–228S.

[771] Wheat LJ. Diagnosis and management of histoplasmosis. Eur J Clin Microbiol Infect Dis 1989;8:480–490.

[772] Saag MS, Dismukes WE. Treatment of histoplasmosis and blastomycosis. Chest 1988;93:848–851.

[773] Quinones CA, Reuben AG, Hamill RJ, Musher DM, Gorin AB, Sarosi GA. Chronic cavitary histoplasmosis. Failure of oral treatment with ketoconazole. Chest 1989;95:914–916.

[774] Hay RJ. Antifungal therapy and the new azole compounds. J Antimicrob Chemother 1991;28(suppl A): 35–46.

[775] Negroni R, Taborda A, Robies AM, Archevala A. Itraconazole in the treatment of histoplasmosis associated with AIDS. Mycoses 1992;35:281–287.

[776] Berger TG. Treatment of bacterial, fungal, and parasitic infections in the HIV-infected host. Semin Dermatol 1993;12:296–300.

[777] Rinaldi MG. Zygomycosis. Infect Dis Clin North Am 1989;3:19–41.

[778] Ng KH, Chin CS, Jalleh RD, Siar CH, Ngui CH, Singaram SP. Nasofacial zygomycosis. Oral Surg Oral Med Oral Pathol 1991;72:685–688.

[779] Jones AC, Bentsen TY, Freedman PD. Mucormycosis of the oral cavity. Oral Surg Oral Med Oral Pathol 1993;75:455–460.

[780] Clark R, Greer DL, Carlisle T, Carroll B. Cutaneous zygomycosis in a diabetic HTLV-I-seropositive man. J Am Acad Dermatol 1990;22:956–959.

[781] Hopwood V, Hicks DA, Thomas S, Evans EG. Primary cutaneous zygomycosis due to Absidia corymbifera in a patient with AIDS. J Med Vet Mycol 1992;30:399–402.

[782] Graybill JR. Treatment of systemic mycoses in patients with AIDS. Arch Med Res 1993;24:403–412.

[783] Klapholz A, Salomon N, Perlman DC, Talavera W. Aspergillosis in the acquired immunodeficiency syndrome. Chest 1991;100:1614–1618.

[784] Denning DW, Follansbee SE, Scolaro M, Norris S, Edelstein H, Stevens DA. Pulmonary aspergillosis in the acquired immunodeficiency syndrome. N Engl J Med 1991;324:654–662.

[785] Morace G, Tamburrini E, Manzara S, Antinori A, Maiuro G, Dettori G. Epidemiological and clinical aspects of mycoses in patients with AIDS-related pathologies. Eur J Epidemiol 1990;6:398–403.

[786] Shannon MT, Sclaroff A, Colm SJ. Invasive aspergillosis of the maxilla in an immunocompromised patient. Oral Surg Oral Med Oral Pathol 1990;70:425–427.

[787] Hostetler JS, Stevens DA. The treatment of aspergillosis, cryptococcosis and histoplasmosis in immunocompromised patients. Report of experience in the United States.Med Klin 1991;86(suppl 1):8–10.

[788] Brown MM, Thompson A, Goh, Forster GE, Swash M. Bell's palsy and HIV infection. J Neurol Neurosurg Psychiatry 1988;51:425–426.

[789] Belec L, Gherardi R, Georges AJ, et al. Peripheral facial paralysis and HIV infection: report of four African cases and review of the literature. J Neurol 1989; 236:411–414.

[790] Murr AH, Benecke Jr JE. Association of facial paralysis with HIV positivity. Am J Otol 1991;12:450–451.

[791] Belec L, Georges AJ, Bouree P, et al. Peripheral facial nerve palsy related to HIV infection: relationship with the immunological status and the HIV staging in Central Africa. Cent Afr J Med 1991;37:88–93.

[792] Linstrom CJ, Pincus RL, Leavitt EB, Urbina MC. Otologic neurotologic manifestations of HIV-related disease. Otolaryngol Head Neck Surg 1993;108:680–687.

[793] Uldry PA, Regli F. Isolated and recurrent peripheral facial paralysis in human infection with human immunodeficiency virus (HIV). Schweiz Med Wochenschr 1988;118:1029–1031.

[794] Hutton KP, Rogers 3rd RS. Recurrent aphthous stomatitis. Dermatol Clin 1987;5:761–768.

[795] Scully C, Porter S. Recurrent aphthous stomatitis: current concepts of etiology, pathogenesis and management. J Oral Pathol Med 1989;18:21–27.

[796] MacPhail LA, Greenspan D, Feigal DW, Lennette ET, Greenspan JS. Recurrent aphthous ulcers in association with HIV infection. Description of ulcer types and analysis of T-lymphocyte subsets. Oral Surg Oral Med Oral Pathol 1991;71:678–683.

[797] MacPhail LA, Greenspan D, Greenspan JS. Recurrent aphthous ulcers in association with HIV infection. Diagnosis and treatment. Oral Surg Oral Med Oral Pathol 1992;73:283–288.

[798] Siegel RD, Granich R. Recurrent aphthous ulcers in association with HIV infection. Oral Surg Oral Med Oral Pathol 1993;76:406–407.

[799] Phelan JA, Eisig S, Freedman PD, Newsome N, Klein RS. Major aphthous-like ulcers in patients with AIDS. Oral Surg Oral Med Oral Pathol 1991;71:68–72.

[800] Reyes-Teran G, Ramirez-Amador V, De la Rosa E, Gonzalez-Guevara M, Ponce de Leon S. Major recurrent oral ulcers in AIDS: report of three cases. J Oral Pathol Med 1992;21:409–411.

[801] Muzyka BC, Glick M. Major aphthous ulcers in patients with HIV disease. Oral Surg Oral Med Oral

Pathol 1994;77:116–120.

[802] Thompson AC, Nolan A, Lamey PJ. Minor aphthous oral ulceration: a double-blind cross-over study of beclomethasone dipropionate aerosol spray. Scott Med J 1989;34:531–532.

[803] Vincent SC, Lilly GE. Clinical, historic, and therapeutic features of aphthous stomatitis. Literature review and open clinical trial employing steroids. Oral Surg Oral Med Oral Pathol 1992;74:79–86.

[804] Chadwick B, Addy M, Walker DM. Hexetidine mouthrinse in the management of minor aphthous ulceration and as an adjunct to oral hygiene. Br Dent J 1991;171:83–87.

[805] Grinspan D. Significant response of oral aphthosis to thalidomide treatment. J Am Acad Dermatol 1985;12: 85–90.

[806] Strazzi S, Lebbe C, Geoffray C, et al. Aphthous ulcers in HIV-infected patients: treatment with thalidomide. Genitourin Med 1992;68:424–425.

[807] Ghigliotti G, Repetto T, Farris A, Roy MT, De Marchi R. Thalidomide: treatment of choice for aphthous ulcers in patients seropositive for human immunodeficiency virus. J Am Acad Dermatol 1993;28:271–272.

[808] Ruah CB, Stram JR, Chasin WD. Treatment of severe recurrent aphthous stomatitis with colchicine. Arch Otolaryngol Head Neck Surg 1988;114:671–675.

[809] Hutchinson VA, Angenend JL, Mok WL, Cummins JM, Richards AB. Chronic recurrent aphthous stomatitis: oral treatment with low-dose interferon alpha. Mol Biother 1990;2:160–164.

[810] Marder MZ, Barr CE, Mandel ID. Cytomegalovirus presence and salivary composition in acquired immunodeficiency syndrome. Oral Surg Oral Med Oral Pathol 1985;60:372–376.

[811] Lucht E, Albert J, Linde A, et al. Human immunodeficiency virus type 1 and cytomegalovirus in saliva. J Med Virol 1993;39:156–162.

[812] Schubert MM. Oral manifestations of viral infections in immunocompromised patients. Curr Opin Dent 1991;1:384–397.

[813] Epstein J, Scully C. Cytomegalovirus: a virus of increasing relevance to oral medicine and pathology. J Oral Pathol Med 1993;22:348–353.

[814] Glick M, Cleveland DB, Salkin LM, Alfaro-Miranda M, Fielding AF. Intraoral cytomegalovirus lesion and HIV-associated periodontitis in a patient with acquired immunodeficiency syndrome. Oral Surg Oral Med Oral Pathol 1991;72:716–720.

[815] Kanas RJ, Jensen JL, Abrams AM, Wuerker RB. Oral mucosal cytomegalovirus as a manifestation of the acquired immune deficiency syndrome. Oral Surg Oral Med Oral Pathol 1987;64:183–189.

[816] Langford A, Kunze R, Timm H, Ruf B, Reichart P. Cytomegalovirus associated oral ulcerations in HIV-infected patients. J Oral Pathol Med 1990;19:71–76.

[817] Jones AC, Freedman PD, Phelan JA, Baughman RA, Kerpel SM. Cytomegalovirus infections of the oral cavity. A report of six cases and review of the literature. Oral Surg Oral Med Oral Pathol 1993;75:76–85.

[818] Heinic GS, Greenspan D, Greenspan JS. Oral CMV lesions and the HIV infected. Early recognition can help prevent morbidity. J Am Dent Assoc 1993;124: 99–105.

[819] Epstein JB, Sherlock CH, Wolber RA. Oral manifestations of cytomegalovirus infection. Oral Surg Oral Med Oral Pathol 1993;75:443–451.

[820] Schubert MM, Epstein JB, Lloid ME, Cooney E. Oral infections due to cytomegalovirus in immunocompromised patients. J Oral Pathol Med 1993;22:268–273.

[821] Pedersen A, Hornsleth A. Recurrent aphthous ulceration: a possible clinical manifestation of reactivation of varicella zoster or cytomegalovirus infection. J Oral Pathol Med 1993;22:64–68.

[822] Syrjanen S, Leimola-Virtanen R, Schmidt-Westerhausen A, et al. Oral ulcers in AIDS patients frequently associated with cytomegalovirus (CMV) and Epstein-Barr virus (EBV) infection. J Oral Pathol Med 1999;28:204–209.

[823] Dodd CL, Winkler JR, Heinic GS, Daniels TE, Yee K, Greenspan D. Cytomegalovirus infection presenting as acute periodontal infection in a patient infected with the human immunodeficiency virus. J Clin Periodontol 1993;20:282–285.

[824] Flaitz CM, Hicks MJ, Nichols CM. Cytomegaloviral infection of the mandible in acquired immunodeficiency syndrome. J Oral Maxillofac Surg 1994;52: 305–308.

[825] Langford A, Kunze R, Schmelzer S, Wolf H, Pohle HD, Reichart P. Immunocytochemical detection of herpes viruses in oral smears of HIV-infected patients. J Oral Pathol Med 1992;21:49–57.

[826] Meyers JD. Treatment of herpesvirus infections in the immunocompromised host. Scand J Infect Dis Suppl 1985;47:128–236.

[827] Meyers JD. Chemoprophylaxis of viral infection in immunocompromised patients. Eur J Cancer Clin Oncol 1989;25:1369–1374.

[828] Balfour Jr HH, Fletcher CV, Dunn D. Cytomegalovirus infections in the immunocompromised transplant patient. Prevention of cytomegalovirus disease with oral acyclovir. Transplant Proc 1991;23(suppl 1): 17–19.

[829] De Armond B. Future directions in the management of cytomegalovirus infections. J Acquir Immune Defic Syndr 1991;4(suppl 1):S53–56.

[830] Griffiths PD. Current management of cytomegalovirus disease. J Med Virol 1993;suppl 1;106–111.

[831] Nelson MR, Erskine D, Hawkins DA, Gazzard BG. Treatment with corticosteroids—a risk factor for the development of clinical cytomegalovirus disease in AIDS. AIDS 1993;7:375–378.

[832] Gellis SE. Warts and molluscum contagiosum in children. Pediatr Ann 1987;16:69–76.

[833] Epstein WL. Molluscum contagiosum. Semin Dermatol. 1992;11:184–189.

[834] Porter CD, Blake NW, Cream JJ, Archard LC. Molluscum contagiosum virus. Mol Cell Biol Hum Dis Ser 1992;1:233–257.

[835] Katzman M, Elmets CA, Lederman MM. Molluscum contagiosum and the acquired immunodeficiency syndrome. Ann Intern Med 1985;102:413–414.

[836] Sarma DP, Weilbaecher TG. Molluscum contagiosum in the acquired immunodeficiency syndrome. J Am Acad Dermatol 1985;13:682–683.

[837] Delescluse J, Goens J. Molluscum contagiosum disclosing HTLV III infection. Dermatologica 1986;172: 283–285.

[838] Katzman M, Carey JT, Elmets CA, Jacobs GH, Lederman MM. Molluscum contagiosum and the acquired immunodeficiency syndrome: clinical and immunological details of two cases. Br J Dermatol 1987;116:131–138.

[839] Cotton DW, Cooper C, Barrett DF, Leppard BJ. Severe atypical molluscum contagiosum infection in an immunocompromised host. Br J Dermatol 1987;116: 871–876.

[840] Prose NS, Mendez H, Menikoff H, Miller HJ. Pediatric human immunodeficiency virus infection and its cutaneous manifestations. Pediatr Dermatol 1987; 4:67–74.

[841] Matis WL, Triana A, Shapiro R, Eldred L, Polk BF, Hood AF. Dermatologic findings associated with human immunodeficiency virus infection. J Am Acad Dermatol 1987;17:746–751.

[842] Petersen CS, Gerstoft J. Molluscum contagiosum in HIV-infected patients. Dermatology 1992;184:19–21.

[843] Schwartz JJ, Myskowski PL. Molluscum contagiosum in patients with human immunodeficiency virus

[844] Barsh LI. Molluscum contagiosum of the oral mucosa. Report of a case. Oral Surg Oral Med Oral Pathol 1966;22:42–46.
[845] Phelan JA, Saltzman BR, Friedland GH, Klein RS. Oral findings in patients with acquired immunodeficiency syndrome. Oral Surg Oral Med Oral Pathol 1987;64:50–56.
[846] Ficarra G, Gaglioti D. Facial molluscum contagiosum in HIV-infected patients. Int J Oral Maxillofac Surg 1989;18:200–201.
[847] Sugihara K, Reichart PA, Gelderblom HR. Molluscum contagiosum associated with AIDS: a case report with ultrastructural study. J Oral Pathol Med 1990;19:235–239.
[848] Laskaris G, Sklavounou A. Molluscum contagiosum of the oral mucosa. Oral Surg Oral Med Oral Pathol 1984;58:688–691.
[849] Svirsky JA, Sawyer DR, Page DG. Molluscum contagiosum of the lower lip. Int J Dermatol 1985;24:668–669.
[850] Whitaker SB, Wiegand SE, Budnick SD. Intraoral molluscum contagiosum. Oral Surg Oral Med Oral Pathol 1991;72:334–336.
[851] Betlloch I, Pinazo I, Mestre F, Altes J, Villalonga C. Molluscum contagiosum in human immunodeficiency virus infection: response to zidovudine. Int J Dermatol 1989;28:351–352.
[852] Garrett SJ, Robinson JK, Roenigk Jr HH. Trichloroacetic acid peel of molluscum contagiosum in immunocompromised patients. J Dermatol Surg Oncol 1992;18:855–858.

第6章
常见呼吸道病毒及肺部黏膜免疫
David B. Huang

肺脏在对人体细胞供氧及代谢废物排出的过程中发挥着至关重要的作用。肺脏每天吸入的气体达上万升,因此它持续暴露于各种气体、颗粒和空气传播的病原体中。尽管如此,宿主肺黏膜表面强有力的防御系统仍然能够使下呼吸道内保持无菌状态。肺黏膜表面含有上皮细胞及诸如T细胞和树突状细胞(dendritric cell,DC)等其他细胞,这些细胞通过激活体液免疫应答及细胞介导的免疫应答,分泌炎性介质(如细胞因子、趋化因子和抗微生物肽)对暴露的微生物作出反应。若宿主肺脏免疫系统遭受破坏,尤其是当肺脏暴露于强毒性或大量病原体时,则可导致呼吸道感染。肺部感染通常是上呼吸道常驻菌群的吸入、气溶胶的吸入及传染性病原体在肺脏的系统性转移造成的。本章主要介绍导致呼吸道感染的常见病毒,以及针对这些病毒感染的肺脏黏膜免疫应答。

导致呼吸道感染的常见病毒

许多病毒可导致呼吸道感染。呼吸道病毒感染的靶位点是上皮纤毛细胞。大多数情况下,病毒感染仅限于上呼吸道,然而下呼吸道感染在感染人群中也占了相当大的比重。在世界范围内,大约90%的"普通感冒"是由病毒引起的,且大部分发生于冬季。这些病毒可在人群中传播,主要传播方式为手-手接触。本章重点从病原学、流行病学、临床症状、致病机理及诊断和治疗等方面介绍导致呼吸道感染的常见病毒,如腺病毒、冠状病毒包括严重急性呼吸综合征冠状病毒(severe acute respiratory syndrome-associated coronavirus,SARS-CoV)、流感病毒、鼻病毒和呼吸道合胞病毒(respiratory syncytial virus,RSV)(表6.1)。

表6.1 引起呼吸道感染的常见病毒

病毒	流行病学	临床症状	致病机理	诊断	治疗
腺病毒	原发性感染发生于幼年,具有季节性,多发于冬春夏三季	细支气管炎、肺炎、咽结膜热、出血性膀胱炎、腹泻、中枢神经系统疾病	裂解性、潜伏或慢性感染,致癌性转化	病毒分离、抗原检测、PCR或血清学诊断技术	自限性

续表

病毒	流行病学	临床症状	致病机理	诊断	治疗
冠状病毒，包括SARS-CoV	具有季节性，多发于冬春季。SARS-CoV于2002年11月首次在中国广东省发现，导致8000余人感染，800余人死亡	上呼吸道和下呼吸道疾病、发热、头痛、寒战、黏液脓性鼻涕、咽痛、咳嗽、腹泻、神经症状，SARS-CoV的症状与之相似。SARS-CoV的总体病死率为7%~17%，但是在医疗卫生条件较差或年龄超过65岁的患者中病死率高达50%	SARS-CoV可导致肺透明质膜形成、间质浸润和肺泡细胞脱落	病毒分离、抗原检测、RT-PCR或血清学诊断技术	自限性；类固醇可能对SARS-CoV感染患者具有一定疗效
流感病毒	平均感染率为10%~20%，在低龄和老龄人群中可能高达50%。共暴发过31次大流行。1918-1919年的大流行在世界范围内致2100万人死亡	发热、寒战、头痛、干咳、咽痛、鼻塞、声音嘶哑、肌痛、不适、厌食和眼部症状、肌炎、心脏并发症、中毒性休克综合征和中枢神经系统并发症。可伴发继发性细菌感染	红细胞凝集素和神经氨酸酶是病毒表面抗原。M1和M2组成膜蛋白。潜伏期为18~72h。上呼吸道和下呼吸道黏膜发生弥漫性炎症反应	病毒分离、鸡胚培养、抗原检测、PCR（科研用）或血清学诊断技术	在症状出现后的48h内，使用M2抑制剂（金刚烷胺、金刚乙胺）和神经氨酸酶抑制剂（扎那米韦、奥塞米韦）
鼻病毒	原发性感染发生于幼年。具有季节性，好发于秋春夏季	累及鼻、咽或下呼吸道，症状持续时间平均为7天，25%的感染者可持续达2周	潜伏期为8~10h。对黏膜上皮只产生轻微的损伤	细胞培养进行病毒分离（细胞系有WI-38、MRC-5和M-HeLa）、PCR和血清学诊断技术	自限性
呼吸道合胞病毒	原发性感染发生于幼年。具有季节性，好发于冬春季。危险因素包括低龄、男性、社会经济地位较低	细支气管炎、假膜性喉炎、气管支气管炎和肺炎；不常见的表现有中枢神经和心血管症状及出疹	膜蛋白（F、G）参与致病过程。感染的表现包括支气管周围淋巴细胞浸润和支气管上皮水肿	病毒分离、EIA（灵敏度60%~70%，特异性90%~95%）、RT-PCT（科研用）或血清学诊断技术	支持疗法；对于重症婴幼儿患者，病毒唑、支气管扩张剂、糖皮质激素、RSV-IVIG或帕利珠单抗具有一定疗效

EIA：酶免疫测定；RT-PCR：逆转录聚合酶链反应；SARS：严重急性呼吸综合征

腺病毒

1953年，在儿童摘除的腺样增殖体和扁桃体中分离到一种病原体，在培养数周后发现是一种可引起细胞病变的传染性病原体，即腺病毒[1]。病毒感染后2~5天，连续传代的上皮细胞变大变圆，且细胞间以丝状物相连。从患有呼吸道症状的新兵的腺样组织和肺脏分泌物及患有结膜炎的船厂工人的眼中也分离到腺病毒。大约5%的5岁以下幼儿的上呼吸道感染和大约10%的儿童肺炎是由腺病毒引起的。

腺病毒具有一种独特的特性，即高度的潜在致癌性。它是第一种被证明对啮齿类动物具有潜在致癌性的人类病毒。经过改造后的腺病毒可以作为载体，从而将遗传物质导入不同类型的细胞，进行基因治疗和病原体免疫。根据红细胞凝集类型、对啮齿类动物的致癌能力和基因组DNA中G+C含量的差异，至少可将腺病毒分为51个血清型[2]。但是仅有不到一半的血清型可使人类致病。所有的血清型都具有相似的形态和核酸组成，并且可以产生特征性的致细胞病变效应。

腺病毒颗粒为中等大小、无包膜的二十面体结构，表面有纤维状突起，基因组为双链DNA，分子质量约为$23×10^6$Da。位于病毒壳粒上的纤维状突起呈节杆状，具有头节，主要起吸附作用（图6.1）。腺病毒与细胞受体 CAR（柯萨奇－腺病毒受体）结合，并在核内体中发生内化，病毒在此完成最初的脱衣壳过程。病毒的外层蛋白称为衣壳，由252个称为壳粒的亚单位组成，壳粒以20条边和12个顶角构成的六邻体形式排列。纤维突起和六邻体上的主要型特异性中和表位可与中和抗体结合。

腺病毒合成多种病毒蛋白，包括 E1A 和 E1B 区编码的转化蛋白家族，E2A 和 E2B 区编码负责病毒基因组复制的三种蛋白质，E3 区编码调节宿主免疫及细胞因子反应的蛋白质，E4 区编码促进病毒 mRNA 转录的蛋白质。

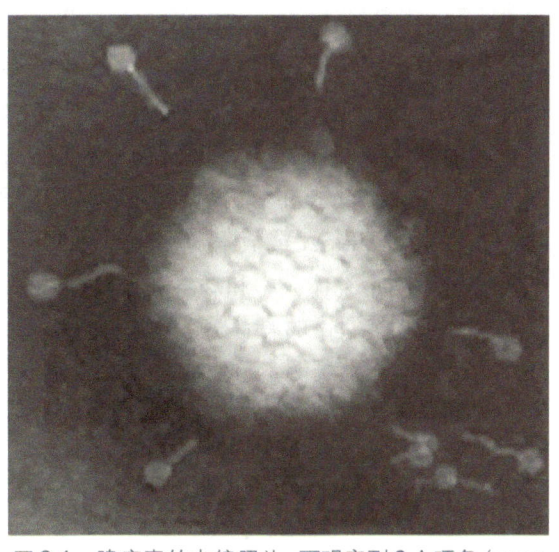

图6.1 腺病毒的电镜照片，可观察到6个顶角（www.clinical-virology.org/gallery/images/em/adenovirus2.gif）。

大部分人在幼年都发生过腺病毒的原发性感染[3]。感染后有些无症状，有些表现为呼吸道疾病，如肺炎、假膜性喉炎或支气管炎[1]。第二次世界大战期间，也有腺病毒感染引发急性呼吸系统疾病的报道，主要是士兵的居住条件拥挤和精神压力过大造成的[4]。腺病毒感染具有季节性，多发于冬末、春季和夏初。腺病毒也可引起非呼吸系统的感染，如胃肠炎、结膜炎、膀胱炎和皮疹。腺病毒感染的潜伏期为 4~5 天，最常见的症状为咳嗽、发热、咽痛和流涕，通常持续 3~5 天。腺病毒的血清学分类具有重要的临床意义，因为病毒血清型、患者年龄和临床疾病谱之间有一定的关系。在婴幼儿中，腺病毒 7 型导致暴发性细支气管炎和肺炎；在儿童中，腺病毒 1 型、2 型和 4~6 型与上呼吸道疾病有关；在青少年，尤其是入伍军人中，腺病毒 3 型、4 型和 7 型与急性呼吸道疾病、气管支气管炎和肺炎有关；在免疫缺陷患者中，腺病毒 5 型、31 型、34 型、35 型和 39 型与肺炎及其播散相关。腺病毒的传播途径有直接接触传播、粪－口传播及偶发的水源传播。由于腺病毒在多种物理和化学因素及不利的 pH 条件下仍然能保持稳定，因此它可在体外长时间存活。

腺病毒与上皮细胞相互作用可引起裂解性感染[5]、隐性或慢性感染[1]，或致癌性转化[6]。裂解性感染通过抑制宿主的大分子合成及 mRNA 向胞浆转运而导致细胞死亡，在此过程中每个细胞可释放多达 10^6 个病毒颗粒。自然杀伤细胞和淋巴细胞识别被感染的细胞，从而激发细胞因子反应，诱导细胞毒性 T 细胞（cytotoxic T cell，CTL）及中和（或）非中和抗体来对抗病毒感染。隐性或慢性感染累及淋巴细胞。即使人体能够产生中和抗体反应，仍然能够在淋巴细胞和扁桃体中检测到腺病毒序列，并且这些部位可长期释放少量病毒。当腺病毒基因组整合入宿主细胞基因组 DNA，并随着宿主基因组的复制而复制时，就会发生致癌性转化，但是不会产生病毒颗粒。三种类型的感染都会产生病毒特异性蛋白（T 抗原），提示有腺病毒存在。

腺病毒感染的确诊方法包括抗原检测、聚合酶链反应（polymerase chain reaction，

PCR）、病毒分离和血清学检测[7]。因为腺病毒可长时间分泌，所以即使分离出腺病毒也并不意味着患病。血凝抑制试验或用型特异性抗血清进行中和试验可对腺病毒分型。患者的痰液、鼻咽拭子、粪便、尿液或结膜刮片都可以作为病毒培养的来源，在人单层上皮细胞中进行培养。培养 2~5 天可以观察到典型的细胞病变。免疫荧光或酶联免疫吸附试验（enzyme-linked immunosorbent assay，ELISA）可用来检测样本中的腺病毒抗原。血清学诊断需要通过 ELISA 或放射免疫法（radioimmunoassay，RIA）检测到抗体 4 倍升高，这些抗体可以固定补体、中和病毒或阻止血凝。

在免疫功能正常的患者中，大部分腺病毒感染都是自限性的，只需进行对症治疗。对于免疫力低下的严重病例，单独或联合使用西多福韦、病毒唑、阿糖腺苷或人免疫球蛋白也有不同程度的治疗效果[8~10]。但是，这些治疗药物的整体疗效还不确定，还有待于深入研究。

包括 SARS-CoV 在内的冠状病毒

1937 年，冠状病毒首次从鸡中分离得到。1965 年，Tyrrell 和 Bynoe[11] 从普通感冒患者的鼻腔冲洗液中分离出冠状病毒，并在人胚气管纤维细胞和鼻上皮细胞中进行了连续传代。这些病毒培养物可使志愿者产生呼吸道症状。与此同时，Hamre 和 Procknow[12,13] 报道了冠状病毒 229E 株的致细胞病变效应，此病毒株是从患有急性呼吸道疾病的医学生中分离到的。在此之后，又报道了大量的引起疾病的动物冠状病毒。

SARS-CoV 于 2002 年 11 月发现[14]。该病毒最初在中国广东省发现，随后迅速传播至香港及东南亚、欧洲和北美各国，最终扩散至全世界。截至 2003 年 6 月，全球感染病例超过 8000 例，死亡 800 多例。科学家们迅速测定了 SARS-CoV 基因组序列，发现它与已知的人和动物冠状病毒具有相关性[14]。

在电镜下，冠状病毒颗粒为中等大小（80~150nm）。由于病毒外膜覆盖有冠状表面蛋白，因此命名为冠状病毒（图 6.2 和图 6.3）。冠状病毒科有 2 个属，即冠状病毒属（*Coronavirus*）

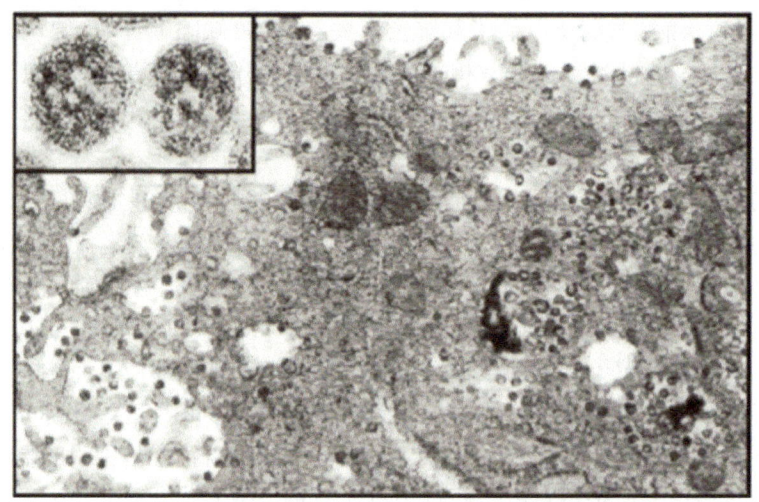

图 6.2　冠状病毒感染的 Vero E6 细胞的电镜照片，病毒位于与浆膜相连的液泡里，并且聚集在浆膜表面呈线状。左上角为更高放大倍数下的冠状病毒（www.cdc.gov/mmwr/preview/mmwrhtml/mm5212a1.html）。

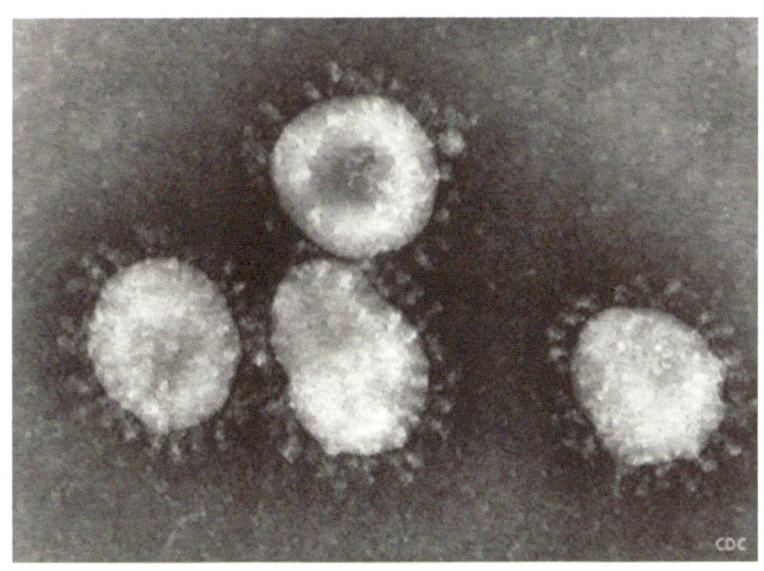

图 6.3 冠状病毒电镜照片（www.fda.gov/fdac/features/2003/403_sars.html）。

和环状病毒属（*Torovirus*）。冠状病毒属的基因组为不分节段的单股正链 RNA，5′ N 端有甲基化帽子结构，3′ 端有 polyA 尾。基因组 RNA 编码一个大的多聚蛋白，后者经由病毒编码的蛋白酶消化后形成多种结构和非结构蛋白。结构蛋白包括血凝素酯酶（HE）表面蛋白、位于病毒包膜上的介导受体结合和细胞融合的表面刺突糖蛋白（S 蛋白，一种小包膜蛋白）、介导病毒出芽和包膜形成的膜糖蛋白（M）及与基因组 RNA 结合的核衣壳蛋白。S 蛋白介导病毒与宿主细胞膜上的唾液酸受体结合。S 蛋白抗体可中和病毒感染。目前，有两株冠状病毒可进行细胞培养：229E 和 OC43。当两株冠状病毒共同感染同一个细胞时可发生基因重组。冠状病毒的正链基因组可翻译出病毒聚合酶，后者催化负链基因组的合成。负链基因组是合成 mRNA 的模板，该 mRNA 是一组嵌套式且 3′ 端含有 polyA 尾的转录产物。病毒颗粒的装配是在内质网膜胞质小泡中出芽时完成的，然后病毒颗粒转移至细胞表面，并在细胞死亡时释放[15]。

目前研究最多的两株冠状病毒是 OC43 和 229E，超过 85% 的成人中都有这两株病毒的抗体。呼吸道冠状病毒可在人群中传播，多发于温带地区的冬春季。该病毒感染大约占成人上呼吸道感染的 15%。在病毒活跃高峰期间，由冠状病毒造成的呼吸道疾病占比高达 35%。在美国，OC43 和 229E 是造成大规模流行的主要毒株[16,17]。大约有一半的呼吸道冠状病毒感染者会发病，这些患者体内抗体滴度升高。若感染后抗体水平迅速下降，则可能会发生再次感染。

SARS-CoV 可导致严重急性非典型肺炎，这些患者都有明确的与 SARS 患者的接触史或疫区的旅居史（如中国大陆、中国香港、河内、中国台湾或新加坡）。流行病学调查发现大量的病例都来自医院，大多为医务工作者、探视者、其他疾病患者及与 SARS-CoV 感染者直接接触的家庭成员。2003 年 6 月，SARS-CoV 进入流行末期，总体病死率为 7%~17%。在高龄患者（> 65 岁）及医疗卫生条件较差的患者中，病死率则高达 50%。

冠状病毒感染者可发展为上呼吸道疾病，出现感冒症状，如发热、头痛、不适、咳嗽、咽痛、黏液脓性鼻涕和寒战等[11,18]。另外，冠状病毒感染也会累及肠道、神经系统和下呼吸道（如肺炎和胸腔积液）。这些症状可持续2~18天，平均为7天。病毒抗原多样性特征及免疫应答的血清型特异性决定了冠状病毒可发生再次感染。相对于青少年而言，老年人更易患严重呼吸系统感染。SARS-CoV感染者最常见的症状为发热、头痛、不适、肌痛、干咳、呼吸困难和腹泻，偶尔也有鼻塞和咽痛的症状。在25%的患者中，尤其是年龄大于50岁的老年患者或医疗条件较差的患者，肺部疾病可发展成为急性呼吸窘迫综合征（acute respiratory distress syndrome，ARDS）[19]，后者的病死率约为10%。SARS-CoV感染患者的实验室检测指标经常出现异常，如淋巴细胞减少及肌酸激酶、乳酸脱氢酶和谷草转氨酶水平升高。

呼吸道冠状病毒包括SARS-CoV，可感染多种哺乳动物和鸟类。由于大多数冠状病毒不能培养，因此病毒血清型的数量还无法确定。呼吸道分泌物的气溶胶使冠状病毒与鼻咽部上皮细胞的病毒受体相结合，随后病毒在上皮细胞中复制，导致纤毛上皮细胞出现细胞溶解效应，并释放细胞因子和趋化因子，如CXCL10/IFN-γ-诱导蛋白-10和CCL2/单核细胞趋化蛋白-1[20]。这些炎症介质是感染后多种呼吸道症状的病因。冠状病毒的潜伏期和排毒期为3~5天[18]。SARS-CoV的潜伏期为4~7天，在一些病例中其排毒期为数周[21]。SARS-CoV感染的肺部组织学表现为透明质膜形成、间质淋巴细胞和单核细胞浸润、肺间隔肺泡细胞脱落[22]。

呼吸道冠状病毒分离自气管和鼻咽部上皮的临床样本。通过细胞免疫荧光法、分泌物酶联免疫试验或RT-PCR可对病毒进行快速抗原检测[23,24]。有些毒株，如229E和OC43，可以在人类二倍体成纤维细胞系中培养繁殖。SARS-CoV可从上呼吸道、下呼吸道、血液、粪便和尿液样本中通过RT-PCR进行鉴别分离，并可在Vero E6细胞和恒河猴胚胎肾细胞中培养。单份血清样本SARS-CoV抗体阳转或恢复期抗体滴度比急性期4倍或4倍以上升高可作为SARS-CoV感染的检测依据[25]。在感染早期的很短时间内可检出IgM，感染一周后可检出IgG。因为冠状病毒感染始于鼻咽部，所以IgA可能是抵御病毒感染的主要抗体成分。

冠状病毒感染多为自限性，其治疗主要采用支持疗法。有个别研究报道称，类固醇对于SARS-CoV的治疗可能有效[26]。在体外试验中，干扰素（interferon，IFN）对SARS-CoV有抑制作用，而病毒唑没有。目前，人们正在从各种各样的抗病毒药物中筛选SARS-CoV的有效治疗方法。

流感病毒

1679年，Sydenham首次对流感病毒暴发进行了报道，然而直到1933年才确定了此次暴发是由流感病毒引起的[27]。流感的感染率高达40%。每1~3年流感病毒引起的发热性呼吸道疾病就会流行一次，而每10~20年就会在世界范围内造成一次大流行[28]。流感多发于冬季，并有一定的流行特点，儿童最早发病，然后是成人出现流感样症状，最后因肺炎、慢性阻塞性肺疾病恶化和充血性心衰而入院治疗的患者大量增多。流感流行时平均感染率为10%~20%，但是在某些特殊人群中，感染率则可高达50%。儿童的感染率是最高的，而在老年人（≥65岁）和医疗条件比较差的患者中重症和死亡病例是最多的。在美国，每年大约有3.6万人死于流感。到目前为止，流感的大流行共发生过31次，其中最大的一次发生于1918~1919年，全球共有2000万~4000万人因此死亡[29]。

流感病毒属于正黏病毒科，根据其抗原性、结构、基因特征及流行病学等方面的差异可分为甲、乙、丙三个型别。甲型流感病毒研究最多，又可根据两种表面抗原——血细胞凝集素（hemagglutinin，HA）和神经氨酸苷酶（neuraminidase，NA），进一步分为不同的亚型。流感病毒毒株的命名包括病毒型别、最初分离地、毒株编号和分离年份。流感病毒含有8个节段，每个节段均为线性的单股负链RNA，核糖核蛋白核心排列成螺旋状的核衣壳，表面覆盖着脂质包膜和大约500个表面突起，后者具有HA或NA活性（图6.4）。HA突出于脂质包膜，呈球杆状，参与病毒与细胞膜表面含神经氨酸的黏多糖受体的结合。甲型流感病毒至少含有15个HA亚型和9个NA亚型。NA呈蘑菇状，具有酶活性，在病毒侵入细胞的早期催化糖蛋白清除末端的唾液酸。病毒编码的其他膜蛋白还包括位于病毒包膜上的M2蛋白和位于病毒基质内的M1蛋白。病毒包膜内的8个独立的核衣壳片段与核蛋白、三种聚合酶蛋白成分（PB1、PB2、PB3）相结合，构成交叉反应性和病毒特异性CTL反应的重要靶位点。

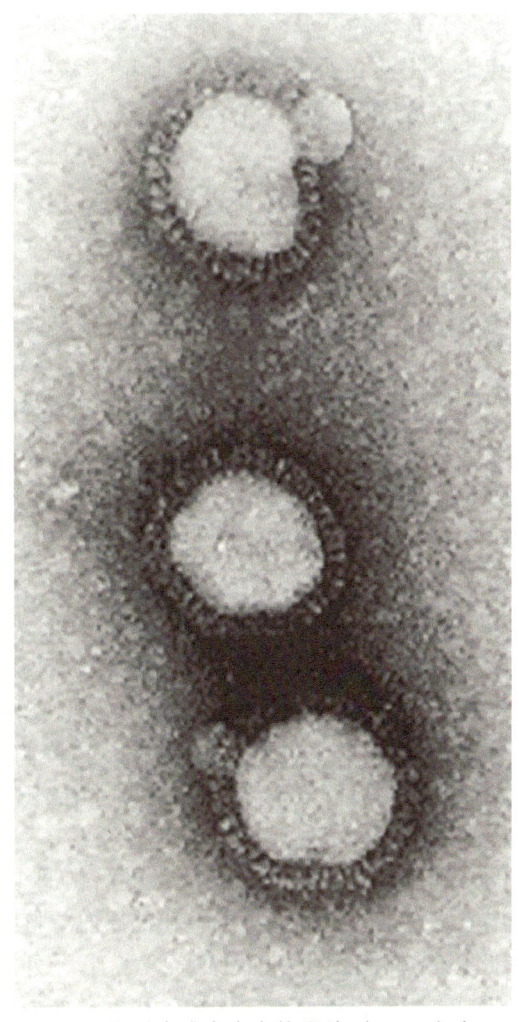

图6.4　甲型流感病毒电镜照片（www.virology.net/Big_Virology/BVRNAortho.html）。

流感病毒引起呼吸道相关疾病，其流行趋势呈U形曲线，并且在抗体水平较低的儿童和老人中感染率最高[30]。学龄儿童容易感染流感病毒，因为教室内拥挤的空间有利于气溶胶的传播。在北半球，流感的流行多发生于10月至次年4月，南半球则多发生于5月至9月。流感大流行的毒株变异非常大，且大流行通常是在新的毒株突然出现并感染几乎没有免疫力的人群时发生。基础性疾病是重症流感的危险因素，如心血管和肺部疾病、糖尿病、肾功能障碍、血红蛋白病和免疫缺陷等[31]。

流感病毒之所以能够持续流行和大流行，原因之一就是它具有改变抗原结构的独特能力，即两种表面糖蛋白HA和NA的抗原变异。甲型流感病毒的HA和NA编码基因相对不稳定，在经历连续的突变之后就会发生抗原结构改变。流感病毒较小的变异称之为抗原漂移，较大的变异称之为抗原转换。在病毒复制过程中，在 HA 或 NA 分子的主要抗原位点上发生的相对较小的变异或者点突变的积累可造成抗原漂移[32]。甲型流感病毒的抗原漂移速度比乙型快。抗原转换可产生人群没有抵抗力的新毒株。较大的抗原转换则会引发流感大流行。

吸入含有病毒的小颗粒气溶胶（＜10μm）可感染流感病毒。喷嚏、咳嗽和说话都可以产生气溶胶。在实验条件下，含有 137~300 倍半数组织培养感染剂量（the median tissue-culture infective dose，$TCID_{50}$）病毒的滴鼻液具有感染性；而通过气溶胶感染时，含有 0.6~3.0 倍 $TCID_{50}$ 病毒的气溶胶则具有感染性[33,34]。尽管在感染后 24h 内即可检测到流感病毒的增殖，但是流感的潜伏期一般为 1~4 天。对于大多数感染者而言，感染 5~10 天后，人体就不再通过呼吸道分泌物排毒，但是在严重免疫缺陷个体中，排毒期可持续数月。虽然相对低的湿度和温度有利于流感病毒的存活，但是在不同的温度和湿度条件下，流感病毒也能保持相对稳定[35]。患者的组织病理学表现为典型的、简单的急性炎症，其特点为咽喉、气管和支气管黏膜的弥漫性炎症（充血和水肿）、柱状上皮细胞空泡形成和纤毛柱状上皮基底层细胞脱落。单个细胞表现为萎缩、核固缩和纤毛丢失。在上皮细胞中可检测到病毒抗原，但是在基底层细胞中则检测不到。在上皮炎症损伤区有淋巴细胞和组织细胞存在。

在重症病例中，病变在组织学上表现为弥漫性坏死性气管支气管炎，伴发支气管黏膜溃疡和脱落、弥漫性出血、透明质膜形成和中性粒细胞浸润减少。病毒在宿主细胞内复制，并通过减少宿主细胞的蛋白质合成、降解和阻碍细胞 mRNA 的转录、降解共表达蛋白及诱导细胞凋亡等方式导致宿主细胞死亡[36,37]。凋亡引起的细胞死亡与病毒复制过程中双链 RNA 诱导 Fas 抗原有关，或者病毒 *PB1* 基因的第二个可读框编码的 PB1-F2 蛋白对线粒体的毒性作用有关[38]。流感病毒的潜伏期为 18~72h，它可在细胞死亡前的几个小时内释放出来，感染邻近的上皮细胞和外周血单核细胞。上皮细胞及外周血单核细胞感染后可刺激细胞因子的分泌，进而出现全身症状。外周血单核细胞，如中性粒细胞、淋巴细胞和单核细胞，感染病毒后会导致趋化和吞噬能力的缺失，以及增殖和协同刺激能力的降低[39,40]。外周血单核细胞的功能缺失与病毒复制和特定病毒蛋白，如 HA、NA 和核蛋白的直接毒性作用有关。

流感病毒感染后可激发人体产生体液和细胞免疫应答，这对于疾病恢复和再感染防御都是至关重要的[41]。在病毒亚型内可发生不同程度的交叉免疫保护，但在亚型之间则不能产生交叉免疫保护。IFN 和 CTL 在急性流感的恢复中起到最重要的作用。血清和呼吸道分泌物中的抗体可抵御病毒的再感染，并能降低疾病的严重程度。流感病毒的全身性抗体反应包括针对 NA、HA、膜基质蛋白及核蛋白的 IgM、IgG 和 IgA 抗体[42]。血清 IgG 中和抗体是抵御流感病毒感染的最重要抗体。但是针对某一型流感病毒的抗体对另一型别的保护能力十分有限，甚至完全没有。在感染后 4~7 周，抗体水平达到高峰。抗 NA 抗体与血凝抑制抗体（hemagglutinin-inhibiting antibody，HAI）平行产生[43]，并可作为检测流感病毒血凝素之间抗原相关性的重要方法。研究表明，血清 HAI 抗体效价＞1：40 或血清中和滴度＞1：8 时都可以抵御流感病毒的感染。NA 抗体检测方法为 NA 抑制试验或 ELISA。NA 抗体可通过降低感染细胞中病毒的释放效率来抵御病毒感染，从而降低疾病的严重程度[44,45]。针对病毒内部蛋白（膜基质蛋白和核蛋白）的抗体具有交叉保护作用，但是不能完全避免病毒感染。鼻腔分泌物中含有 IgG 和 IgA。其中，HA IgG 为 IgG1 亚型，与血清中 IgG 亚型一致，提示鼻腔分泌物中的 IgG1 来源于血清中 IgG1 的扩散[46]。鼻腔 HA 特异性 IgA 为多聚体，属于 IgA1 亚型。IgA1 亚型在鼻腔局部产生，由黏膜记忆细胞诱导的外周淋巴组织分泌。

细胞免疫应答对于疾病恢复和再感染预防非常重要。CD4 T 细胞和 CD8 T 细胞都能有效地清除甲型流感病毒。病毒特异性 CD8 CTL 识别人类白细胞抗原（human leukocyte antigen，HLA）-I 类分子，并且通过裂解感染细胞和表达抗病毒细胞因子来介导免疫应答的产生。CD4 T 细胞能识别 HA、膜基质蛋白和核衣壳蛋白上的表位，并刺激 B 细胞产生针对 HA、NA 的抗体并表达抗病毒细胞因子[47,48]。动物和人体研究表明，流感病毒可激发 1 型和 2 型辅助性 T 细胞（Th1 和 Th2）应答。抗体（通过补体和抗体依赖的细胞毒作用）或 CTL 可以裂解被感染的上皮细胞[49]。感染 14 天时，CTL 数量达到高峰。HLA-I 类限制性 CTL 可降低甲型流感病毒在上皮细胞中的复制水平及持续时间[50]。

流感病毒感染后可发生不同的并发症，最早的症状和体征为突然发热（37.7℃）和干咳。流感病毒普通感染的症状为发热、寒战、头痛、干咳、咽痛、鼻塞、声音嘶哑、肌痛、不适、食欲不振和眼部症状。儿童流感的症状通常为中耳炎、恶心和呕吐。对于大多数个体而言，疾病和症状持续数天后可自行缓解消失。咳嗽和不适可持续两周或更长时间。流感病毒感染可能引起的肺部并发症为原发性流感病毒肺炎和继发性细菌感染。在怀疑患有心血管和肺部基础性疾病的感染者中可并发原发性流感病毒肺炎。流感症状一般持续三天，而这些患者在三天后病情迅速恶化，体检发现双侧肺脏均有病变，但痰液中正常菌群没有发生改变。65 岁以上并且患有心、肺、代谢及其他基础性疾病的老年人容易发生继发性细菌性肺炎，虽然在随后的 1~2 周内症状得以缓解，但是发热和细菌性肺炎的症状和体征在短暂的间隔期后会复发。支气管上皮的物理性损伤和纤毛活性障碍造成肺部细菌不能及时清除，有可能引发继发性细菌感染。革兰氏染色及痰液培养通常会检测到金黄色葡萄球菌（*Staphylococcus aureus*）、肺炎链球菌（*Streptococcus pneumoniae*）和流感嗜血杆菌（*Haemophilus influenzae*）。肺外并发症也有报道，包括肌炎、心脏并发症（心肌炎和心包炎）、中毒性休克综合征、中枢神经系统并发症（格林-巴利综合征、横贯性脊髓炎和脑病）和 Reye 氏综合征。

与病毒培养相比，流感和流感样疾病的临床诊断的灵敏度和特异性分别为 63%~78% 和 55%~71%。在呼吸道分泌物、鼻拭子、咽拭子、鼻腔冲洗液或鼻咽拭子样本中分离到病毒或检测到病毒抗原就可以确诊流感病毒感染。将流感病毒在恒河猴肾细胞、猕猴肾细胞或 Madin-Darby 犬肾细胞系中培养可发生典型的致细胞病变效应。流感病毒也可在鸡胚中培养，3~7 天内可检测到病毒[51]。利用酶联免疫和直接免疫荧光法可快速检测呼吸道分泌物中的病毒抗原。常用的直接免疫荧光法检测试剂盒有 Directigen Flu A+B（Becton-Dickenson，Cockeysville，MO）、Flu OIA（Biostar，Boulder，CO）、QuickVue Influenza A+B test（Quide Corp，San Diego，CA）和 ZstaFlu（ZymeTX，Oklahoma City，OK）。与病毒培养相比，这些试剂盒的灵敏度为 40%~80%，特异性为 85%~100%[52~55]。这些检测方法在复杂性及操作和结果解释的技术难度及费时上各有不同。与咽拭子和含漱液相比，鼻咽拭子和吸入物样本中的病毒检测灵敏度更高。核酸杂交和 PCR 扩增通常在研究中使用，其灵敏度更高，但工作量大，技术要求高。血清学检测用于流感的回顾性诊断，如补体结合和血凝素抑制试验（包括急性期和恢复期的双份血清样本）。

流感病毒的治疗药物包括 M2 抑制剂（金刚烷胺、金刚乙胺）和 NA 抑制剂（扎那米韦、奥塞米韦）。美国 CDC 建议对于患有可能危及生命的流感相关疾病或具有严重流感并发症高危因素且在发病后两天内的患者应该进行抗病毒药物治疗[56]。研究表明，M2 抑制剂（金刚烷胺、金刚乙胺）对于实验室诱导的和自然感染的甲型流感病毒感染都有一定的治疗效果。只有不足 1% 的未暴露人群具有耐药性[57~59]。M2 抑制剂可以抑制病毒的 M2 离子通道活性，后者可以酸化病毒的内环境，阻断膜基质蛋白和核蛋白的相互作用，并将核糖核蛋白转运至细胞核内以完成宿主细胞的复制[60]。金刚烷胺最常见的副作用为中枢神经系统症状，包括失眠、头晕、注意力不集中等。NA 抑制剂在人体攻击试验模型和临床试验中证明是有效的。只在 1% 的成人和 6% 的儿童中分离到对奥塞米韦治疗敏感性降低的流感病毒。NA 可裂解糖蛋白上充当流感病毒吸附宿主受体的末端唾液酸，并增强病毒在呼吸道中的通过性[61,62]。NA 抑制剂通常具有良好的耐受性，最常见的副反应是胃肠道症状。

鼻病毒

1914 年，Kruse 最早发现了感冒的传染特性。他将感冒患者的鼻腔分泌物过滤除菌后滴入健康志愿者的鼻腔内，结果这些受试者产生了感冒样的症状[63]。但是，直到 20 世纪 40 年代才有学者从感冒患者的鼻腔分泌物中分离到鼻病毒（rhinovirus）[64]。鼻病毒来源于希腊词根"*rhin*"，意为鼻。从 20 世纪 50 年代起，在对鼻病毒的分离和特征研究、高敏感人胚肺细胞系的培育研究[65]、已知鼻病毒和免疫类型的分型研究[66]和流行病学研究中发现鼻病毒是引发普通感冒的一个病因[67]。据估计，高达 35% 的成人感冒是由鼻病毒引起的，并且多发于春季、夏季和秋初。

鼻病毒为单股正链RNA病毒，属于小核糖核酸病毒科，含有4种结构蛋白（VP1~VP4），结构蛋白外有突起，可与中和抗体相互作用。这些结构蛋白位于呈二十面体对称的无包膜衣壳上。鼻病毒的非结构蛋白包括两种含有特异性病毒切割位点的蛋白酶，一种是 RNA 依赖的 RNA 聚合酶，另一种是可共价结合于病毒 RNA 5′ 端的 VPg 蛋白。每个核衣壳由 12 个壳粒组成。病毒表面有一个较深的保守性的疏水性裂隙，其作用是保持病毒衣壳的完整性并辅助病毒脱衣壳时的构象变化。基因组的 5′ 端有基因组链接蛋白，3′ 端有 PolyA 尾。鼻病毒与肠道病毒基因组的同源性为 40%~60%。鼻病毒至少可分为 110 多个型别，反映了每种血清型的原型毒株的分离年代[66]。

鼻病毒在酸性环境（pH < 5）中容易失活，在氯化铯梯度中具有较高的密度，可区分于肠道病毒。鼻病毒对有机溶剂如醚、氯仿及其他化学试剂如三氯氟甲烷、乙醇和苯酚较为耐受。鼻病毒最适宜生长温度为人类鼻腔和主气道内的 33~35℃[68]。根据受体特异性，鼻病毒可分为不同的血清型，最大的一组鼻病毒（约80%）以白细胞黏附蛋白为受体，即细胞间黏附分子 -1（ICAM-1，CD54），属于免疫球蛋白超家族成员[69]。这类受体存在于大多数人类细胞表面，包括 HeLa 细胞、成纤维细胞和呼吸道上皮细胞。只有少数的鼻病

毒与低密度脂蛋白受体结合。

在世界范围内，鼻病毒感染发生于幼年时期，并持续终生。儿童和青少年时期可快速产生鼻病毒抗体；在青年时期达到高峰，随后开始下降，最后在整个成年时期都维持不变[70,71]。由于入伍军人长期居住在拥挤的军营里，密切接触的机会增加，近距离暴露有利于传染性分泌物的传播，因此鼻病毒经常会引起入伍军人的呼吸道疾病[72]。志愿者研究表明，鼻病毒的有效传染方式包括传染性鼻腔分泌物通过手–手接触传播，以及鼻腔和结膜黏膜接触污染物而发生的自体接种传播。气溶胶可能也是鼻病毒的传播途径之一，但是有研究显示，以气溶胶形式存在的鼻病毒在 70°F 室温和 40% 的相对湿度环境中会很快失活[73]。鼻病毒感染具有季节性，在秋季达到高峰，3、4、5 月份为次高峰[70,71]。这种季节性特点部分是由于生活条件的变化，因为病毒在较高的相对湿度条件下更易存活。有研究显示，利用细胞培养可以在约 25% 的感冒患者中检测出病毒，若联合使用细胞培养和 PCR，则检出率高达 50%[74]。在 1 岁以上儿童中，鼻病毒的感染率为 1.2 次 /（人·年），在成人中为 0.7 次 /（人·年）[12,13]。病毒传播多发于家庭、学校及学龄儿童日托中心。鼻病毒二代传播多发于年轻的兄弟姐妹和母亲之间，感染率为 25%~70%[75]。另外一些可能导致病毒感染性增加的因素有疲劳、精神压力、营养不良、吸烟或居住工作条件拥挤等。

鼻病毒感染的临床表现在广义上可归类为鼻、咽或下呼吸道受累，症状包括流泪、不适、厌食、鼻溢、鼻塞、咽痛、咳嗽、喷嚏和声音嘶哑，但发热并不常见。病毒在鼻咽部定殖后，潜伏期为 24~72h。症状持续时间平均为 7 天，约 25% 的感染者可持续 2 周。通常排毒期为 7~10 天，但也有资料显示某些病例排毒期可延长至数周。

鼻病毒攻击健康志愿者后，感染率可达 95%。研究还发现，鼻病毒在受试对象的鼻腔内复制，最早可于感染后 8~10h 在鼻腔分泌物中检测到病毒，并于第 2~3 天达到排毒高峰[76]。病毒在纤毛上皮细胞中复制，细胞死亡后会有大量蛋白质（包括纤维蛋白原）从鼻黏膜中释放出来。组织学检查发现鼻黏膜上皮仅有轻微的损伤，后者可诱导炎性介质的释放，如白细胞介素 1（interleukin-1，IL-1）、IL-6、IL-8、IL-16，以及其他介质，如缓激肽、赖氨酰缓激肽、前列腺素、组胺和调节活化正常 T 细胞表达分泌因子（regulated on activation, normal T-cell expressed and secreted, RANTES)[77]。组胺促进血液向感染细胞流动，导致水肿、充血和黏液分泌增加。鼻病毒感染后，在鼻腔中可生成血清中和抗体 IgM、IgA 和 IgG[78,79]。这些抗体只对同种血清型的病毒再感染具有保护作用。IgA 是抵御鼻病毒感染的最为重要的抗体。

鼻病毒的临床诊断通常依靠临床经验。鼻病毒可从鼻腔分泌物中分离得到，可以通过直接收集分泌物或用生理盐水冲洗鼻腔黏膜表面来提高病毒收集量。鼻病毒感染的确诊需要通过细胞培养进行病毒鉴定，可用于病毒培养的细胞系有人胚肺细胞系（WI-38 和 MRC-5）、Hep-2 细胞和 M-HeLA 细胞，培养温度为 33~34℃。致细胞病变效应通常发生在病毒感染后 2~6 天。利用核酸探针的 PCR 技术越来越广泛地用于鼻病毒的鉴定[80]。中和试验可对鼻病毒感染进行血清学诊断；但是由于鼻病毒型别的多样性，此方法并不适宜用于常规诊断。

鼻病毒感染的治疗主要为支持疗法，并联合使用第一代抗组胺药物和非固醇类抗炎药物[81]。支持疗法包括休息、补水、解充血药、盐水含漱和止咳,可以缓解打喷嚏、流鼻涕、眼睛发痒和充血症状。但目前对于鼻病毒感染尚无有效的抗病毒药物。

呼吸道合胞病毒

1956年,Morris 及同事首次报道了呼吸道合胞病毒(respiratory syncytial virus,RSV)[82]。他们从感冒的黑猩猩体内鉴定出了黑猩猩鼻炎病毒（chimpanzee coryza agent, CCA）。后来,从呼吸道疾病的患者体内分离出了一株未知病毒株,并且发现患者体内针对 CCA 的特异性中和抗体增多。流行病学调查显示,95% 的 2 岁儿童体内有 CCA 抗体。随后,基于其临床和实验室表现,CCA 病毒被重新命名为呼吸道合胞病毒[83]。RSV 是婴幼儿下呼吸道感染的最常见病因。在年龄略大的儿童和成人中,RSV 是上呼吸道感染的常见病因。血清学研究显示,大部分人在幼年时期均有 RSV 感染史。小于 1 岁的儿童中,RSV 下呼吸道疾病的年感染率约为 23%[84]。

呼吸道合胞病毒属于副黏病毒科。该病毒没有血凝素和神经氨酸苷酶活性。RSV 分为 A、B 两大群[85]。两群之间的抗原相关性为 25%。两群之间的主要差异为 G、F、SH 和 NS1 蛋白的变异。在病毒暴发时,A、B 两群可同时流行。RSV 是有包膜、不分段的单股负链 RNA 病毒。RSV 基因组 RNA 编码多种蛋白质,其中 3 种蛋白质组成核衣壳,5 种蛋白质组成病毒包膜,3 种蛋白质（F、G 和 SH）组成糖基化的跨膜表面蛋白,M 和 M2 组成非糖基化膜基质蛋白,两种糖基化表面蛋白 F 和 G 在 RSV 的致病性和感染性中起主要作用。F 蛋白通过介导病毒包膜和细胞膜融合而促进病毒入侵,G 蛋白介导病毒与宿主细胞的黏附。RSV 包膜由宿主细胞膜及含有多种刺突糖蛋白的跨膜表面蛋白构成。RSV 在自然界环境不稳定,对温度和 pH 的变化非常敏感[86]。RSV 在非渗透表面可存活 3~30h,在渗透表面存活时间不超过 1h,最适宜的 pH 为 7.5。RSV 对肥皂、水和消毒剂都很敏感,很容易灭活。

RSV 存在于所有地域和气候条件下[87]。在美国,RSV 多在冬季或春季暴发。在北半球的热带地区,RSV 感染与降水量增加和温度降低有关。而在南半球的热带地区,RSV 感染与降水量减少和温度降低有关。儿童感染 RSV 可致细支气管炎、假膜性喉炎、气管-支气管炎和肺炎。在没有呼吸道疾病的儿童中仅有极少数携带 RSV（0.3%）[88]。RSV 通过近距离接触感染者的呼吸道分泌物或感染性物质传播。感染性物质与眼睛、口腔或鼻腔黏膜的接触或可能发生的感染性飞沫的吸入都会引发感染。RSV 疾病的危险因素包括年龄（重症病例多见于婴幼儿）、性别（男性比女性易感）和社会经济因素,如拥挤的居住条件、低收入、日托看护、多子女家庭及 RSV 感染 6 个月内被动吸烟[89]。RSV 感染后所产生的免疫力是不完全、易变且不持久的。日托机构的研究表明,RSV 首次暴露可使 98% 的儿童感染[88],两次暴露后感染或再感染率为 74%,三次暴露后感染或再感染率为 65%。RSV 通过鼻和眼的传播效率高于通过口腔传播。RSV 潜伏期为 2~8 天[90-92]。RSV 感染主要局限于呼吸道内,疾病早期累及上呼吸道,疾病晚期累及下呼吸道。

RSV 感染的致病机理包括病毒的体内传播、呼吸道纤毛上皮细胞的破坏（图 6.5）、支气管周围淋巴细胞浸润伴随细胞壁和周围组织水肿,从而引发支气管上皮的增生和坏死[93]。肺上皮细胞受到损伤后,会分泌调理素、胶原凝集素、多种趋化因子和细胞因子，如 IL-1β、IL-6、IL-8、IL-10、IL-11、RANTES 和巨噬细胞炎症蛋白 -1α（macrophage inflammatory protein-1α，MIP-1α）[94]。趋化因子和细胞因子又可募集一些效应分子、中性粒细胞、巨噬细胞、NK 细胞和嗜酸性细胞。炎症、坏死的上皮和分泌的黏液可造成支气管腔的堵塞。支气管腔狭窄伴随呼气的正压力，会使肺脏过度膨胀。气道完全堵塞并且残留气体被吸收后，可以导致肺不张。肺体积增加和呼气受阻时，会导致支气管炎[95]。单核细胞的肺间质浸润及伴随而来的水肿和坏死可导致肺泡充盈，从而引发肺炎[93]。

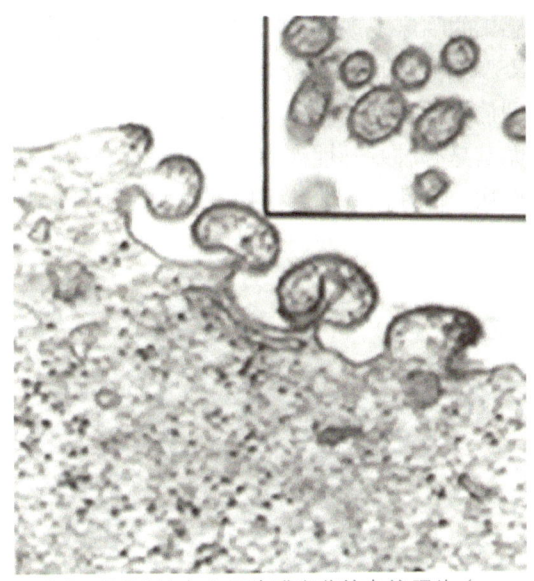

图 6.5　RSV 从宿主细胞膜出芽的电镜照片（www.epidemic.org/theFACTS/viruses/viralReplication.html）。

尽管 RSV 抗体不能阻止病毒在鼻腔内的复制，但是 RSV 特定蛋白的血清抗体能保护机体免受 RSV 感染，这为超免疫球蛋白和单克隆抗体用于重症 RSV 感染者的治疗提供了理论依据[94]。虽然针对 F 蛋白和 G 蛋白的定性及定量抗体应答并不明确，但是这些抗体应答似乎可以抵御病毒的再感染，而且受预存抗体和宿主年龄的影响[95,96]。从 RSV 感染者的鼻腔分泌物中可检测到 IgM、IgG、IgA 和 IgE[97]。IgM 出现在感染的早期，鼻咽分泌物中 IgE 和组胺反应与疾病急性期和支气管痉挛发作时的哮鸣有关，IgA 则似乎与病毒滴度降低有关。

细胞免疫对于 RSV 的清除和宿主的疾病恢复都非常重要。细胞免疫缺陷的免疫抑制个体感染 RSV 后疾病更为严重，排毒期也会延长[98]。患者的 T 细胞亚群的功能降低，IL-2 水平降低，IL-8 水平则升高[99]。RSV 感染者的 CTL 反应比较复杂。一些研究表明，CTL 和 Th 应答与临床反应和病毒清除有关。RSV 感染的细胞免疫应答可能是 Th1 和 Th2 共同作用的结果[100]。T 细胞的数量、持续时间、特异性和类型决定了 RSV 感染的免疫学和临床转归。

RSV 感染的临床表现与患者的年龄和自身患有的基础性疾病有关。RSV 感染最主要的临床表现为支气管炎、肺炎、假膜性喉炎、中耳炎、呼吸骤停和婴儿猝死综合征。在婴儿和小于 1 岁的儿童中，RSV 感染是下呼吸道感染和上呼吸道疾病的最常见病因[101,102]。约有 2% 的低龄儿童在首次感染 RSV 后需要住院治疗，而且大部分不足 6 个月[102]。临床症状包括哮鸣、干啰音、湿啰音、鼻溢、鼻塞、咳嗽、低热、呼吸困难和低氧血症[103]。低氧血症的发生预示着感染累及下呼吸道并且病毒弥漫性扩散至肺部软组织[104]。住院婴幼儿的平均动脉血氧饱和度为 87%。中耳炎是年龄较小的儿童 RSV 感染的常见并发症。RSV 感染可以引起特殊人群发病率和病死率的升高，这些特殊人群包括早产儿、低出生体重婴儿（< 2500g）、患有基础性疾病的儿童，如慢性肺部疾病、先天性心脏病、免疫抑制疾病（骨髓和器官移植，HIV）或其他慢性疾病。在年龄稍大的儿童及成人中，RSV

感染的临床表现取决于宿主的免疫状态，这类人群的 RSV 感染多为再感染。在健康个体中，RSV 再感染的危害较轻，有的无症状，有的出现上呼吸道疾病症状，如鼻塞、咳嗽、声嘶、咽痛、低热和结膜炎。临床症状平均持续 9.5 天，排毒期为 1~6 天。对于患有其他疾病，尤其是心肺基础性疾病的患者来说，RSV 感染后可能会引起重症疾病[105]。RSV 是心血管疾病和慢性阻塞性肺疾病发作的病因，尤其是经常发作的患者。

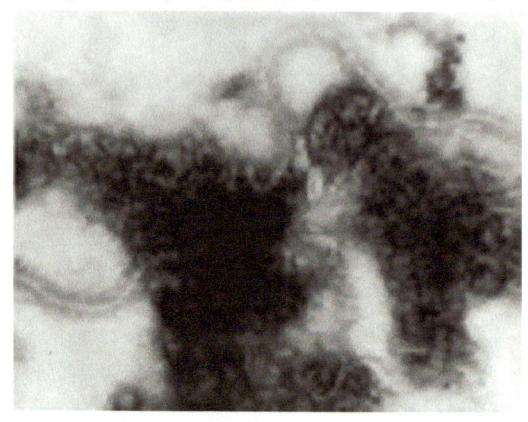

图 6.6　RSV 电镜照片（www.cdc.gov/ncidod/aip/images/rsv_germ.jpg）。

RSV 诊断依赖于临床经验，可通过病毒分离（图 6.6）、病毒抗原或核酸检测或血清学诊断技术确诊。病毒分离既费时又昂贵。RSV 分离需要的样本来自鼻咽冲洗液、气管分泌物或鼻拭子，培养 3~7 天内通常可观察到特异性的细胞病变。Shell vial 技术的应用可加速病毒鉴定[106]。由于病毒抗原检测既经济又快速，目前为大多数的临床实验室所采用。可用的抗原检测技术包括直接或间接免疫荧光法和酶联免疫法（EIA）（灵敏度为 60%~70%，特异性为 90%~95%）[107]。与其他诊断技术相比，RT-PCR 具有更高的灵敏度和特异性，但是目前主要作为科研用[107,108]。RSV 的血清学诊断通常利用酶联免疫实验和中和试验，用于大规模流行病学调查，但对于患者管理并不适用，因为恢复期血清要在一段时间后才能采集。另外，RSV 抗体滴度也不都是明显升高的，尤其是在婴儿和患有基础性疾病的患者中。

大多数轻症患者采取支持疗法，包括大量饮水、对乙酰氨基酚降温和休息。住院婴儿可能需要吸氧治疗，有时还需要机械通风，雾化吸入病毒唑、支气管扩张药物和皮质类固醇[109]。对于患有下呼吸道疾病的住院婴儿，雾化吸入病毒唑是一种被认可的抗病毒治疗方法。研究表明，这种广谱的抗病毒药物可减少长期肺脏后遗症和哮鸣的复发，并可快速改善临床症状和氧合作用[110,111]。支气管扩张药物和皮质类固醇对于婴儿支气管炎有一定的疗效。RSV 中和抗体 [RSV 静脉注射用免疫球蛋白（intravenous immunoglobulin，IVIG）多抗] 或肌注单克隆抗体（帕利珠单抗 - 人源化鼠 IgG 单抗，可结合 RSV 的 F 蛋白）的使用可将有或无慢性肺病的高危早产儿的入院风险降低 41%~50%。RSV-IVIG 对于免疫缺陷患者也有一定的治疗效果[112]。

肺部黏膜免疫

肺部防御系统包括呼吸道的解剖和机械屏障及黏膜免疫。这些屏障形成了抵御经黏膜传播的病原体的第一道防线。呼吸的气体中的大部分颗粒可通过口鼻过滤清除，而较小的颗粒（直径 < 4μm）能够到达下呼吸道。机械屏障和反射机制（咳嗽和喷嚏）可阻止和减少吸入到呼吸道内的病原体数量。黏膜防御系统包括天然屏障和宿主适应性免疫，前者包括黏液、上皮细胞和固有免疫机制（吞噬细胞）；后者包括体液免疫和细胞免疫，如分泌

型 IgA（sIgA）、CD4 T 细胞和抗原特异性 CTL[113]。

传导性气道由气管和支气管组成，内衬柱状纤毛上皮细胞，此类细胞可分泌抗微生物因子、清除黏液、通过分泌炎性趋化因子和细胞因子来募集炎性细胞和吞噬细胞进入肺组织。肺部上皮细胞有三种类型：I 型、II 型和 Clara 细胞。I 型为肺泡上皮细胞，其主要功能为气体交换。II 型上皮细胞可在气道表面分泌一种含有溶菌酶、乳铁蛋白、分泌型白细胞蛋白酶抑制剂、抗菌肽、β- 防御素、一氧化氮和细胞外超氧化物歧化酶的液体，所有这些物质都有抗微生物活性[114,115]。Clara 细胞分布于细支气管，参与肺的重建。β- 防御素参与宿主肺脏的非特异性免疫，并与记忆性 T 细胞和树突状细胞（dendritic cell，DC）相互作用。下呼吸道的体液免疫和细胞介导的宿主防御系统在肺部黏膜免疫中发挥着重要作用。正如传导性气道一样，肺泡表面也覆盖一层衬液，这些衬液中含有可杀灭微生物的物质，如表面活性剂、纤连蛋白、免疫球蛋白、补体因子、自由脂肪酸和离子结合蛋白。从免疫学角度来看，由多个组分构成的表面活性剂可以增强巨噬细胞杀伤病原体的能力，影响自由基的生成和淋巴细胞的活性并结合各种微生物，包括病毒[113]。表面活性剂与微生物结合后，可以减弱微生物的毒力，或增强中性粒细胞和肺泡巨噬细胞的吞噬能力[116]。

呼吸道中含有多种吞噬细胞，包括肺泡巨噬细胞、肺间质巨噬细胞、DC 和血管内巨噬细胞[117]。肺泡巨噬细胞分布于肺泡上皮衬液中，可抵御吸入的外源物质侵袭下呼吸道[118]。当上皮细胞和常驻巨噬细胞释放趋化因子时，如巨噬细胞炎性蛋白 -1/2（MIP-1/2）和单核细胞趋化蛋白 -1（MCP-1），肺泡巨噬细胞就会迁移到肺部。肺泡巨噬细胞通过吞噬和消灭微生物来发挥作用，并通过分泌细胞因子和趋化因子募集中性粒细胞来介导炎症反应[119]。肺间质巨噬细胞分布于肺部结缔组织，它既是吞噬细胞又是 MHC II 类抗原提呈细胞（antigen presenting cell，APC）。与肺泡巨噬细胞相比，肺间质巨噬细胞的吞噬作用依赖 Fc 受体，并且也不能产生细胞因子或氧自由基。DC 分布于气管、传导性气管、末端气道、肺泡隔、肺血管和肺胸膜上皮内，也可作为吞噬细胞和 MHC II 类 APC。这些吞噬细胞都来源于单核细胞，可迁移至淋巴组织，刺激 T 细胞免疫应答。DC 也可分泌多种趋化因子和细胞因子来刺激 T 细胞和 B 细胞免疫应答[119]。血管内巨噬细胞分布于毛细血管内皮，起到吞噬细胞的作用，清除通过血流进入肺脏的外源物质或受损物质。

在肺脏炎性反应中，趋化因子和细胞因子介导的中性粒细胞募集起着关键作用。补体因子，尤其是补体 V 因子、白三烯 B_4 和细菌细胞壁多肽也可以作为炎性介质募集中性粒细胞进入炎症区域。这些介质不仅可以募集中性粒细胞，并使其停留在肺损伤的部位，而且可以调节炎症反应的进程。这个过程中的关键的趋化因子和细胞因子包括 IL-1、TNF-α、IFN-γ、IL-8、IL-10、IL-12 和 α- 趋化因子[120]。

肺上皮通过体液免疫产生的抗体可以防止细菌黏附或生长。呼吸道体液免疫包括 sIgA、IgG 和 IgM。sIgA 是呼吸道体液免疫的主要免疫球蛋白，是防止呼吸道病毒向深层组织入侵的第一道重要的防线。sIgA 可以阻止或减少病毒的吸附，从而阻止宿主细胞内化。多聚 IgA（polymeric IgA，pIgA）也可在细胞内中和病毒，并且可以穿过上皮细胞，有效清除黏膜部位的免疫复合物及上皮细胞内的病毒。许多种病毒的减毒活疫苗都优化了 sIgA 的产生，使其对呼吸道病毒形成黏膜免疫保护。sIgA 约占鼻腔分泌物中总蛋白含量的10%，并具有抗菌和抗病毒活性[121]。其他免疫球蛋白IgG和IgM也有抗菌和抗病毒活性，并在宿主对细菌的调理作用、补体激活、凝集反应和中和活性等方面发挥辅助作用。这些抗体通过渗出的方式从血液循环中进入上呼吸道和下呼吸道。IgG2或IgG4的缺失与支气管扩张相关，主要是由于炎性反应使支气管和细支气管发生进行性扩张。

由于病毒和细胞内寄生虫在肺巨噬细胞中仍可存活，所以由$CD4^+$ Th1细胞和$CD8^+$ CTL介导的呼吸道细胞免疫对防御这些病毒和细胞内寄生虫感染至关重要。CD4/CD8比值约为2:1。据估计，人类肺上皮表面含有约4×10^8个淋巴细胞，其中95%以上为T细胞。肺脏中T细胞与B细胞的数量比为10:1。肺脏的淋巴组织沿着支气管树分布于支气管相关淋巴组织（bronchus-associated lymphoid tissue，BALT）和鼻相关淋巴组织（nasal-associated lymphoid tissue, NALT）的淋巴滤泡内，而BALT和NALT通常分布于上呼吸道、扁桃体和扁桃腺，未定型细胞在这些部位中完成向记忆性T细胞和B细胞的分化[122]。肺黏膜免疫系统可产生特异性免疫因子，可促进消除或消灭任何进入呼吸道黏膜的病毒，而不损伤黏膜表面，也不影响气体交换。与肠道内肠相关淋巴组织（gut-associated lymphoid tissue，GALT）相似，BALT是肺脏黏膜的重要组成部分，也是在抗原克隆扩增前APC向T细胞进行抗原提呈的部位。吸入的抗原穿过呼吸道上皮表面进入BALT，BALT里的APC将抗原提呈给T细胞和B细胞，从而激活它们分化为记忆细胞和效应细胞。记忆性T细胞数量的增加导致BALT里此类细胞的局部增殖或迁移。记忆性淋巴细胞位于黏膜下层和固有层。淋巴细胞主要由T细胞组成，其中40%为CD4细胞（辅助细胞），32%为CD8细胞（抑制细胞）[123]。肺脏淋巴细胞在淋巴组织和肺实质组织之间来回迁移。效应细胞位于肺上皮细胞和肺间质之间。CTL位于肺黏膜之中。

吸入的抗原到达肺泡后，被APC识别，可激活肺泡淋巴细胞。激活的肺泡淋巴细胞刺激记忆性淋巴细胞迁移至炎症区域，从而产生抗原特异性T细胞和B细胞在炎症区域的聚集。炎症反应过程的关键步骤是T细胞与内皮细胞的结合，两者的结合是通过淋巴细胞表面的白细胞功能相关抗原-1整合素与内皮细胞上的配体（如ICAM-1、ICAM-2和血管细胞黏附分子-1）的相互作用完成的。炎性因子IL-1、IFN-γ和TNF-α表达的上调可以促进内皮细胞上配体的表达。活化的淋巴细胞具有分泌抗体、杀伤细胞活性或分泌炎性因子的功能。肺内的杀伤性细胞，包括NK细胞、抗体依赖性杀伤性细胞和抗原限制性杀伤性细胞，与病原体相互作用时可分泌细胞因子。未受抗原刺激的T细胞可分泌IL-2，记忆性T细胞可分泌Th1和Th2型细胞因子。Th1型免疫应答包括细胞介导的炎性反应及细胞因子的分泌，如INF-γ、IL-2、IL-6和IL-10。Th2型免疫应答为体液免疫，可分泌细胞因子，如IL-4、IL-5、IL-10及抗体。其他一些细胞因子在Th1和Th2型免疫应答中都有分泌，如TNF-α、IL-3和粒细胞-巨噬细胞集落刺激因子（GM-CSF）。活化的肺泡上皮细胞可表达多种整合素，如ICAM-1，可使淋巴细胞、白细胞和单核细胞在炎症部位浸润和停留。

总结

呼吸道病毒是肺内、外部临床症状的常见病因，如腺病毒、SARS-CoV、流感病毒、鼻病毒和RSV。在全球范围内，这些病毒是引起发病和造成死亡的重要原因。肺部防御系统任务艰巨，既要破坏或清除持续不断的侵犯黏膜组织的外来抗原，又不能造成过度的炎症损害，要保持两者之间的平衡。肺部黏膜免疫包括固有免疫和适应性免疫，两者在预防呼吸道疾病中都是必不可少的。体液免疫（B细胞和免疫球蛋白）及细胞免疫（APC和T细胞）对于呼吸道病毒的防御尤为重要。尽管人们不停地吸入病原体和颗粒物质，但正是上述这些保护性机制阻止了病毒对肺黏膜的入侵和增殖，从而使大多数人保持健康状态。

参 考 文 献

[1] Rowe WP, Huebner RJ, Gilmore LK, Parrott RH, Ward TG. Isolation of a cytopathogenic agent from human adenoids undergoing spontaneous degeneration in tissue culture. Proc Soc Exp Biol Med 1953;84(3):570–573.

[2] De Jong JC, Wermenbol AG, Verweij-Uijterwaal MW, et al. Adenoviruses from human immunodeficiency virus-infected individuals, including two strains that represent new candidate serotypes Ad50 and Ad51 of species B1 and D, respectively. J Clin Microbiol 1999;37(12):3940–3945.

[3] Jennings LC, Anderson TP, Werno AM, Beynon KA and Murdoch DR. Viral etiology of acute respiratory tract infections in children presenting to hospital: role of polymerase chain reaction and demonstration of multiple infections. Pediatr Infect Dis J 2004;23(11):1003–1007.

[4] Hilleman MR, Werner JH. Recovery of new agent from patients with acute respiratory illness. Proc Soc Exp Biol Med 1954;85(1):183–188.

[5] Shenk T. Adenoviridae: The viruses and their replication. In: Fields BN, Knipe DM, Howley PM, eds. Virology, 3rd ed. Philadelphia: Lippincott-Raven, 1996:2111–2148.

[6] Huebner RJ, Rowe WP, Lane WT. Oncogenic effects in hamsters of human adenovirus types 12 and 18. Proc Natl Acad Sci USA 1962;48:2051–2058.

[7] Krafft AE, Russell KL, Hawksworth AW, et al. Evaluation of PCR testing of ethanol-fixed nasal swab specimens as an augmented surveillance strategy for influenza virus and adenovirus identification. J Clin Microbiol 2005;43(4):1768–1775.

[8] Schievning M, Buxbavm-Conradi H, Jager G, Kolb HJ. Intravenous ribavirin for eradication of respiratory syncytial virus (RSV) and adenovirus isolates from respiratory and/or gastrointestinal tract in recipients of allogeneic hematopoietic stem cell transplants. Hematol J. 2004;5(2):135–144.

[9] Dagan R, Schwartz RH, Insel RA, Menegus MA. Severe diffuse adenovirus 7a pneumonia in a child with combined immunodeficiency: possible therapeutic effect of human immune serum globulin containing specific neutralizing antibody. Pediatr Infect Dis 1984;3(3):246–251.

[10] Legrand F, Berrebi D, Houhou N, et al. Early diagnosis of adenovirus infection and treatment with cidofovir after bone marrow transplantation in children. Bone Marrow Transplant 2001;27(6):621–626.

[11] Tyrrell DA, Bynoe ML. Cultivation of a novel type of common-cold virus in organ cultures. Br Med J 1965;5448:1467–1470.

[12] Hamre D, Connelly AP Jr, Procknow JJ. Virologic studies of acute respiratory disease in young adults. IV. Virus isolations during four years of surveillance. Am J Epidemiol 1966;83(2):238–249.

[13] Hamre D, Procknow JJ. A new virus isolated from the human respiratory tract. Proc Soc Exp Biol Med 1966;121(1):190–193.

[14] Ksiazek TG, Erdman D, Goldsmith CS, et al. A novel coronavirus associated with severe acute respiratory syndrome. N Engl J Med 2003;348(20):1953–1966.

[15] Heath RB. The pathogenesis of respiratory viral infection. Postgrad Med J 1979;55(640):122–127.

[16] Sakai K, Kawaguchi Y, Kishino Y, Kido H. Electron immunohistochemical localization in rat bronchiolar epithelial cells of tryptase Clara, which determines the pneumotropism and pathogenicity of Sendai virus and influenza virus. J Histochem Cytochem 1993;41(1):89–93.

[17] Sakai K, Kohri T, Tashiro M, Kishino Y, Kido H. Sendai virus infection changes the subcellular localization of tryptase Clara in rat bronchiolar epithelial cells. Eur Respir J 1994;7(4):686–692.

[18] Bradburne AF, Bynoe ML, Tyrrell DA. Effects of a "new" human respiratory virus in volunteers. Br Med J 1967;3(568):767–769.

[19] Lew TW, Kwek TK, Tai D, et al. Acute respiratory distress syndrome in critically ill patients with severe acute respiratory syndrome. JAMA 2003;290(3):374–380.

[20] Cheung CY, Poon LL, Ng IH, et al. Cytokine responses in severe acute respiratory syndrome coronavirusinfected macrophages in vitro: possible relevance to pathogenesis. J Virol 2005;79(12):7819–7826.

[21] Donnelly CA, Ghani AC, Leung GM, et al. Epidemiological determinants of spread of causal agent of severe acute respiratory syndrome in Hong Kong. Lancet 2003;361(9371):1761–1766.

[22] Lee N, Hui D, Wu A, et al. A major outbreak of severe acute respiratory syndrome in Hong Kong. N Engl J Med 2003;348(20):1986–1994.

[23] Myint S, Johnston S, Sanderson G, Simpson H. Evaluation of nested polymerase chain methods for the detection of human coronaviruses 229E and OC43.Mol Cell Probes 1994;8(5):357–364.

[24] Lina B, Valette M, Foray S, et al. Surveillance of community-acquired viral infections due to respiratory viruses in Rhone-Alpes (France) during winter 1994 to 1995. J Clin Microbiol 1996;34(12):3007–3011.

[25] Peiris JS, Chu CM, Cheng VC, et al. Clinical progression and viral load in a community outbreak of coronavirus-associated SARS pneumonia: a prospective study. Lancet 2003;361(9371):1767–1772.

[26] Zhao Z, Zhang F, Xu M, et al. Description and clinical treatment of an early outbreak of severe acute respiratory syndrome (SARS) in Guangzhou, PR China. J Med Microbiol 2003;52(pt 8):715–720.

[27] Sydenham T. Classical Descriptions of Disease. London: R.Wellington, 1955.

[28] Thomson D, Thomson R. Influenza. New York: Ann Pickett-Thomas Research Labs, 1933.

[29] Crosby AW. Epidemic and Peace, 1918. Part IV.Westport, CT: Greenwood Press, 1976.

[30] Glezen WP, Keitel WA, Taber LH, Piedra PA, Clover RD, Couch RB. Age distribution of patients with medically-attended illnesses caused by sequential variants of influenza A/H1N1: comparison to agespecific infection rates, 1978–1989. Am J Epidemiol 1991;133(3):296–304.

[31] Barker WH, Mullooly JP. Impact of epidemic type A influenza in a defined adult population. Am J Epidemiol 1980;112(6):798–811.

[32] Wilson IA, Cox NJ. Structural basis of immune recognition of influenza virus hemagglutinin. Annu Rev Immunol 1990;8:737–771.

[33] Alford RH, Kasel JA, Gerone PJ, Knight V. Human influenza resulting from aerosol inhalation. Proc Soc Exp Biol Med 1966;122(3):800–804.

[34] Little JW, Douglas RG Jr, Hall WJ, Roth FK. Attenuated influenza produced by experimental intranasal inoculation. J Med Virol 1979;3(3):177–188.

[35] Hemmes JH, Winkler KC, Kool SM.Virus survival as a seasonal factor in influenza and poliomyelitis. Nature 1960;188:430–431.

[36] Katze MG, Krug RM. Metabolism and expression of RNA polymerase II transcripts in influenza virus-infected cells. Mol Cell Biol 1984;4(10):2198–2206.

[37] Katze MG, DeCorato D, Krug RM. Cellular mRNA translation is blocked at both initiation and elongation after infection by influenza virus or adenovirus.J Virol 1986;60(3):1027–1039.

[38] Sanz-Ezquerro JJ, de la Luna S, Ortin J, Nieto A. Individual expression of influenza virus PA protein induces degradation of coexpressed proteins. J Virol 1995;69(4):2420–2426.

[39] Larson HE, Parry RP, Tyrrell DA. Impaired polymorphonuclear leucocyte chemotaxis after influenza virus infection. Br J Dis Chest 1980;74(1):56–62.

[40] Roberts NJ Jr, Steigbigel RT. Effect of in vitro virus infection on response of human monocytes and lymphocytes to mitogen stimulation. J Immunol 1978;121(3):1052–1058.

[41] Mozdzanowska K, Furchner M, Zharikova D, Feng J, Gerhard W. Roles of CD4+ T-cell-independent and -dependent antibody responses in the control of influenza virus infection: evidence for noncognate CD4+ T-cell activities that enhance the therapeutic activity of antiviral antibodies. J Virol 2005;79(10):5943–5951.

[42] Murphy BR,Nelson DL,Wright PF, Tierney EL, Phelan MA, Chanock RM. Secretory and systemic immunological response in children infected with live attenuated influenza A virus vaccines. Infect Immun 1982;36(3):1102–1108.

[43] Murphy BR, Kasel JA, Chanock RM. Association of serum anti-neuraminidase antibody with resistance to influenza in man. N Engl J Med 1972;286(25):1329–1332.

[44] Schulman JL, Khakpour M, Kilbourne ED. Protective effects of specific immunity to viral neuraminidase on influenza virus infection of mice. J Virol 1968;2(8):778–786.

[45] Kilbourne ED, Laver WG, Schulman JL, Webster RG. Antiviral activity of antiserum specific for an influenza virus neuraminidase. J Virol 1968;2(4):281–288.

[46] Wagner DK, Clements ML, Reimer CB, Snyder M, Nelson DL, Murphy BR. Analysis of immunoglobulin G antibody responses after administration of live and inactivated influenza A vaccine indicates that nasal wash immunoglobulin G is a transudate from serum. J Clin Microbiol 1987;25(3):559–562.

[47] Lamb JR, Eckels DD, Lake P, Woody JN, Green N. Human T-cell clones recognize chemically synthe sized peptides of influenza haemagglutinin. Nature 1982;300(5887):66–69.

[48] Lamb JR, Woody JN, Hartzman RJ, Eckels DD. In vitro influenza virus-specific antibody production in man:antigen-specific and HLA-restricted induction of helper activity mediated by cloned human T lymphocytes.J Immunol 1982;129(4):1465–1470.

[49] Hashimoto G, Wright PF, Karzon DT. Antibodydependent cell-mediated cytotoxicity against influenza virus-infected cells. J Infect Dis 1983;148(5):785–794.

[50] McMichael AJ, Gotch FM, Noble GR, Beare PA. Cytotoxic T-cell immunity to influenza. N Engl J Med 1983;309(1):13–17.

[51] Newton DW, Mellen CF, Baxter BD, Atmar RL, Menegus MA. Practical and sensitive screening strategy for detection of influenza virus. J Clin Microbiol 2002;40(11):4353–4356.

[52] Covalciuc KA,Webb KH, Carlson CA. Comparison of four clinical specimen types for detection of influenza A and B viruses by optical immunoassay (FLU OIA test) and cell culture methods. J Clin Microbiol 1999;37(12):3971–3974.

[53] Noyola DE, Clark B, O'Donnell FT, Atmar RL, Greer J, Demmler GJ. Comparison of a new neuraminidase detection assay with an enzyme immunoassay, immunofluorescence, and culture for rapid detection of influenza A and B viruses in nasal wash specimens. J Clin Microbiol 2000;38(3):1161–1165.

[54] Habib-Bein NF, Beckwith WH 3rd, Mayo D, Landry ML. Comparison of SmartCycler real-time reverse transcription-PCR assay in a public health laboratory with direct immunofluorescence and cell culture

assays in a medical center for detection of influenza A virus. J Clin Microbiol 2003;41(8):3597–3601.

[55] Landry ML, Ferguson D. Suboptimal detection of influenza virus in adults by the Directigen Flu A+B enzyme immunoassay and correlation of results with the number of antigen-positive cells detected by cytospin immunofluorescence. J Clin Microbiol 2003;41(7):3407–3409.

[56] Centers for Disease Control and Prevention. Prevention and control of influenza. Part I: antiviral agents. MMWR 1994;43:1.

[57] Hayden FG, Belshe RB, Clover RD, Hay AJ, Oakes MG, Soo W. Emergence and apparent transmission of rimantadine-resistant influenza A virus in families. N Engl J Med 1989;321(25):1696–1702.

[58] Belshe RB, Burk B, Newman F, Cerruti RL, Sim IS. Resistance of influenza A virus to amantadine and rimantadine: results of one decade of surveillance. J Infect Dis 1989;159(3):430–435.

[59] Ziegler T, Hemphill ML, Ziegler ML, et al. Low incidence of rimantadine resistance in field isolates of influenza A viruses. J Infect Dis 1999;180(4):935–939.

[60] Bui M, Whittaker G, Helenius A. Effect of M1 protein and low pH on nuclear transport of influenza virus ribonucleoproteins. J Virol 1996;70(12):8391–8401.

[61] Air GM, Ritchie LR, Laver WG, Colman PM. Gene and protein sequence of an influenza neuraminidase with hemagglutinin activity. Virology 1985;145(1):117–122.

[62] Colman PM, Ward CW. Structure and diversity of influenza virus neuraminidase. Curr Top Microbiol Immunol 1985;114:177–255.

[63] Kruse W. Die Erreger con Husten and Schupfen. Munchen Med Wochenschr 1914;61:1547.

[64] Andrewes C. The Common Cold. New York: W.W. Norton, 1965.

[65] Hayflick L, Moorhead PS. The serial cultivation of human diploid cell strains. Exp Cell Res 1961;25:585–621.

[66] Hamparian VV, Colonno RJ, Cooney MK, et al. A collaborative report: rhinoviruses—extension of the numbering system from 89 to 100. Virology 1987;159(1):191–192.

[67] Gwaltney JM Jr, Hendley JO, Simon G, Jordan WS Jr. Rhinovirus infections in an industrial population. I. The occurrence of illness. N Engl J Med 1966;275(23):1261–1268.

[68] Halperin SA, Eggleston PA, Hendley JO, Suratt PM, Groschel DH, Gwaltney JM Jr. Pathogenesis of lower respiratory tract symptoms in experimental rhinovirus infection. Am Rev Respir Dis 1983;128(5):806–810.

[69] Winther B, Greve JM, Gwaltney JM Jr, et al. Surface expression of intercellular adhesion molecule 1 on epithelial cells in the human adenoid. J Infect Dis 1997;176(2):523–525.

[70] Monto AS. A community study of respiratory infections in the tropics. 3. Introduction and transmission of infections within families. Am J Epidemiol 1968;88(1):69–79.

[71] Monto AS, Johnson KM. A community study of respiratory infections in the tropics. II. The spread of six rhinovirus isolates within the community. Am J Epidemiol 1968;88(1):55–68.

[72] Forsyth BR, Bloom HH, Johnson KM, Chanock RM. Patterns of illness in rhinovirus infections of military personnel. N Engl J Med 1963;269:602–606.

[73] Karim YG, Ijaz MK, Sattar SA, Johnson-Lussenburg CM. Effect of relative humidity on the airborne survival of rhinovirus-14. Can J Microbiol 1985;31(11):1058–1061.

[74] Makela MJ, Puhakka T, Ruuskanen O, et al. Viruses and bacteria in the etiology of the common cold. J Clin Microbiol 1998;36(2):539–542.

[75] Pereira MS, Andrews BE, Gardner SD. A study on the virus aetiology of mild respiratory infections in the primary school child. J Hyg (Lond) 1967;65(4):475–483.

[76] Douglas RG Jr, Cate TR, Gerone PJ, Couch RB. Quantitative rhinovirus shedding patterns in volunteers. Am Rev Respir Dis 1966;94(2):159–167.

[77] Doyle WJ, Boehm S, Skoner DP. Physiologic responses to intranasal dose-response challenges with histamine, methacholine, bradykinin, and prostaglandin in adult volunteers with and without nasal allergy. J Allergy Clin Immunol 1990;86:924–935.

[78] Rossen RD, Douglas G Jr, Cate TR, Couch RB, Butler WT. The sedimentation behavior of rhinovirus neutralizing activity in nasal secretion and serum following the rhinovirus common cold. J Immunol 1966;97(4):532–538.

[79] Cate TR, Rossen RD, Douglas RG Jr, Butler WT, Couch RB. The role of nasal secretion and serum antibody in the rhinovirus common cold. Am J Epidemiol 1966;84(2):352–363.

[80] Johnston SL, Sanderson G, Pattemore PK, et al. Use of polymerase chain reaction for diagnosis of picornavirus infection in subjects with and without respiratory symptoms. J Clin Microbiol 1993;31(1):111–117.

[81] Turner RB. New considerations in the treatment and prevention of rhinovirus infections. Pediatr Ann 2005;34(1):53–57.

[82] Blount RE Jr, Morris JA, Savage RE. Recovery of cytopathogenic agent from chimpanzees with coryza. Proc Soc Exp Biol Med 1956;92(3):544–549.

[83] Hall CB, Douglas RG Jr. Clinically useful method for the isolation of respiratory syncytial virus. J Infect Dis 1975;131(1):1–5.

[84] Foy HM, Cooney MK, Maletzky AJ, Grayston JT. Incidence and etiology of pneumonia, croup and bronchiolitis in preschool children belonging to a prepaid medical care group over a four-year period. Am J Epidemiol 1973;97(2):80–92.

[85] Peret TC, Hall CB, Hammond GW, et al. Circulation patterns of group A and B human respiratory syncytial virus genotypes in 5 communities in North America. J Infect Dis 2000;181(6):1891–1896.

[86] Hambling MH. Survival of the respiratory syncytial virus during storage under various conditions. Br J Exp Pathol 1964;45:647–655.

[87] Shek LP, Lee BW. Epidemiology and seasonality of respiratory tract virus infections in the tropics. Paediatr Respir Rev 2003;4(2):105–111.

[88] Henderson FW, Collier AM, Clyde WA Jr, Denny FW. Respiratory-syncytial-virus infections, reinfections and immunity. A prospective, longitudinal study in young children. N Engl J Med 1979;300(10):530–534.

[89] Holberg CJ, Wright AL, Martinez FD, Ray CG, Taussig LM, Lebowitz MD. Risk factors for respiratory syncytial virus-associated lower respiratory illnesses in the first year of life. Am J Epidemiol 1991;133(11):1135–1151.

[90] Knight V, Kapikian AZ, Kravetz HM, et al. Ecology of a newly recognized common respiratory agent RS virus. Combined clinical staff conference at the National Institutes of Health. Ann Intern Med 1961;55:507–524.

[91] Johnson KM, Chanock RM, Rifkind D, Kravetz HM, Knight V. Respiratory syncytial virus. IV. Correlation of virus shedding, serologic response, and illness in adult volunteers. JAMA 1961;176:663–667.

[92] Kravetz HM, Knight V, Chanock RM, et al. Respiratory syncytial virus. III. Production of illness and clinical observations in adult volunteers. JAMA 1961;176:657–663.

[93] Aherne W, Bird T, Court SD, Gardner PS, McQuillin J. Pathological changes in virus infections of the lower respiratory tract in children. J Clin Pathol 1970;23(1):7–18.

[94] Graham BS, Johnson TR, Peebles RS. Immunemediated disease pathogenesis in respiratory syncytial virus infection. Immunopharmacology 2000;48(3):237–247.

[95] Wohl ME, Stigol LC, Mead J.Resistance of the total respiratory system in healthy infants and infants with bronchiolitis. Pediatrics 1969;43(4):495–509.

[96] Crowe JE Jr. Immune responses of infants to infection with respiratory viruses and live attenuated respiratory virus candidate vaccines. Vaccine 1998;16:1423–1432.

[97] Munoz JL, McCarthy CA, Clark ME, Hall CB. Respiratory syncytial virus infection in C57BL/6 mice: clear-ance of virus from the lungs with virus-specific cytotoxic T cells. J Virol 1991;65(8):4494–4497.

[98] Hall CB, Walsh EE, Long CE, Schnabel KC. Immunity to and frequency of reinfection with respiratory syncytial virus. J Infect Dis 1991;163(4):693–698.

[99] Welliver RC. Immunology of respiratory syncytial virus infection: eosinophils, cytokines, chemokines and asthma. Pediatr Infect Dis J 2000;19(8):780–783.

[100] Hall CB, Powell KR, MacDonald NE, et al. Respiratory syncytial viral infection in children with compromised immune function. N Engl J Med 1986;315(2):77–81.

[101] Abu-Harb M, Bell F, Finn A, et al. IL-8 and neutrophil elastase levels in the respiratory tract of infants with RSV bronchiolitis. Eur Respir J 1999;14(1):139–143.

[102] Fleming DM, Pannell RS, Elliot AJ, Cross KW. Respiratory illness associated with influenza and respiratory syncytial virus infection. Arch Dis Child 2005;90(7):741–746.

[103] Kotaniemi-Syrjanen A, Laatikainen A, Waris M, Reijonen TM, Vainionpaa R, Korppi M. Respiratory syncytial virus infection in children hospitalized for wheezing: virus-specific studies from infancy to preschool years. Acta Paediatr 2005;94(2):159–165.

[104] Isaacs D, Bangham CR, McMichael AJ. Cell-mediated cytotoxic response to respiratory syncytial virus in infants with bronchiolitis. Lancet 1987;2(8562):769–771.

[105] Shay DK, Holman RC, Newman RD, Liu LL, Stout JW, Anderson LJ.Bronchiolitis-associated hospitalizations among US children, 1980–1996. JAMA 1999;282(15):1440–1446.

[106] Engler HD, Preuss J. Laboratory diagnosis of respiratory virus infections in 24 hours by utilizing shell vial cultures. J Clin Microbiol 1997;35(8):2165–2167.

[107] Abels S, Nadal D, Stroehle A, Bossart W.Reliable detection of respiratory syncytial virus infection in children for adequate hospital infection control management.J Clin Microbiol 2001;39(9):3135–3139.

[108] Falsey AR, Formica MA,Walsh EE. Diagnosis of respiratory syncytial virus infection: comparison of reverse transcription-PCR to viral culture and serology in adults with respiratory illness. J Clin Microbiol 2002;40(3):817–820.

[109] Kimpen JL, Schaad UB. Treatment of respiratory syncytial virus bronchiolitis: 1995 poll of members of the European Society for Paediatric Infectious Diseases.Pediatr Infect Dis J 1997;16(5):479–481.

[110] Edell D, Khoshoo V, Ross G, Salter K. Early ribavirin treatment of bronchiolitis: effect on long-term respiratory morbidity. Chest 2002;122(3):935–939.

[111] Khoshoo V, Ross G, Edell D. Effect of interventions during acute respiratory syncytial virus bronchiolitis on subsequent long term respiratory morbidity. Pediatr Infect Dis J 2002;21(5):468–472.

[112] American Academy of Pediatrics Committee on Infectious Diseases and Committee of Fetus and Newborn. Prevention of respiratory syncytial virus infections: indications for use of palivizumab and update on the use of RSV-IVIG. Pediatrics 1998;1:1211–1216.

[113] Reynolds HY. Defense mechanisms against infections. Curr Opin Pulmon Med 1999;5(3):136–142.

[114] Coonrod JD. Human alveolar lining material and antibacterial defenses.Am Rev Respir Dis 1986;134(6):

1337.

[115] Coonrod JD. The role of extracellular bactericidal factors in pulmonary host defense. Semin Respir Infect 1986;1(2):118–129.

[116] Wright JR. Immunomodulatory functions of surfactant. Physiol Rev 1997;77(4):931–962.

[117] Lohmann-Matthes ML, Steinmuller C, Franke-Ullmann G. Pulmonary macrophages. Eur Respir J 1994;7(9):1678–1689.

[118] Sibille Y, Reynolds HY. Macrophages and polymorphonuclear neutrophils in lung defense and injury. Am Rev Respir Dis 1990;141(2):471–501.

[119] MacNee W, Selby C. Neutrophil kinetics in the lungs. Clin Sci 1990;79(2):97–107.

[120] Luster AD. Chemokines—chemotactic cytokines that mediate inflammation. N Engl J Med 1998;338(7):436–445.

[121] Reynolds H. Normal and defective respiratory host defense mechanisms. In: Pennington JE, ed. Respiratory Infections: Diagnosis and Management, 2nd ed. New York: Raven, 1988:1–33.

[122] Agostini C, Chilosi M, Zambello R, Trentin L, Semenzato G. Pulmonary immune cells in health and disease: lymphocytes. Eur Respir J 1993;6(9):1378–1401.

[123] Fishman AP, Reynolds HY, Elias JA, et al. Pulmonary defense mechanisms against infection. In: Fishman AP, ed. Fishman's Pulmonary Diseases and Disorders, 3rd ed. New York: McGraw-Hill, 1998:265–274.

第 7 章
病毒性疾病的眼部表现
Steven Yeh and Mitchell P.Weikert

病毒性疾病的眼部表现是多样和复杂的，从良性到甚至危及视力的情况都可能发生。有些病毒如腺病毒，在宿主细胞感染之后直接有眼部表现，其他的需要与另一个病毒共感染才能产生眼部症状，如巨细胞病毒（cytomegalovirus，CMV）与人类免疫缺陷病毒（human immunodeficiency virus，HIV）共感染患者[1]。本章总结了常见病毒引起的眼部临床表现，当然这些病毒引起的皮肤黏膜表现已经在前面章节进行了阐述（表 7.1）。表 7.2 概括了引起眼部表现的病毒及相关的疾病表现。

表 7.1 所列章节可以获得下列病毒的更多信息

病毒性疾病	章　节*
人类疱疹病毒（human herpes virus，HHV）	8
巨细胞病毒（cytomegalovirus，CMV）	7
EB（Epstein-Barr，EB）	6
人乳头瘤病毒（human papillomavirus，HPV）	11
传染性软疣（molluscum contagiosum）	3
腺病毒（adenovirus）	
人类免疫缺陷病毒（human immunodeficiency virus，HIV）	13
麻疹（measle）	15
腮腺炎（mump）	
风疹（rubella）	21
小核糖核酸病毒（picarnovirus）	18

*译者核查原文章节有误，请读者查看相关章节

表 7.2 眼科病毒的概况

病毒科	病毒	遗传物质	眼部疾病
疱疹病毒科	HSV-1	dsDNA	角膜结膜炎、睑缘炎、角膜炎、葡萄膜炎
	HSV-2	dsDNA	角膜结膜炎、睑缘炎、角膜炎、葡萄膜炎
	VZV	dsDNA	角膜炎、葡萄膜炎、脉络视网膜炎、视神经炎、睑缘炎、结膜炎、泪小管炎、泪腺炎、浅层巩膜炎、巩膜炎、青光眼、眼外肌瘫痪、眼前段缺血、结节性脉管炎

续表

病毒科	病毒	遗传物质	眼部疾病
疱疹病毒科	EBV	dsDNA	滤泡性结膜炎、角膜炎、眼腺综合征、视乳头水肿、视神经炎、多灶性脉络膜炎、结节性巩膜表层炎、虹膜角膜内皮综合征、干燥综合征
	CMV	dsDNA	角膜结膜炎、睑缘炎、角膜炎、葡萄膜炎
	人HSV-8	dsDNA	眼睑卡波西肉瘤、结膜卡波西肉瘤
痘病毒科	传染性软疣	dsDNA	眼睑和结膜损伤、角膜结膜炎、滤泡性结膜炎
乳头瘤病毒科	乳头瘤病毒	dsDNA	结膜、眼睑和泪腺囊的良性和恶性肿瘤
腺病毒科	腺病毒	dsDNA	咽结膜热、流行性角结膜炎、非特异性滤泡性结膜炎
逆转录病毒科	HIV	dsRNA	棉絮状白斑、视网膜出血
副黏病毒科	麻疹	ssRNA	结膜炎、角膜炎、脉络视网膜炎、视网膜病变
	腮腺炎	ssRNA	结膜炎、角膜炎、脉络视网膜炎、视网膜病变、泪腺炎、浅层巩膜炎、巩膜炎、视神经炎、葡萄膜炎、眼外肌瘫痪
披膜病毒科	风疹	ssRNA	白内障、青光眼、虹膜萎缩、斜视、小眼球综合征、小角膜、眼球震颤、色素性视网膜病变
小核糖核酸病毒科	柯萨奇A24 肠道病毒70	ssRNA	急性出血性结膜炎、角膜炎、视神经炎

单纯疱疹病毒 1 型和 2 型

在美国大约有 40 万人患有单纯眼疱疹，通常与单纯疱疹 1 型有关[2]。单纯疱疹病毒 1 型（herpes simplex virus-1，HSV-1）通过接触疾病活动期患者的病损皮肤或唾液传播，也可以通过排毒携带者或污染物传播[3]。HSV-2 相关的眼部疾病是通过眼睛与感染者生殖器接触传播的[4]，占新生儿疱疹感染者中的 80%，这些新生儿在经过产道时被感染。感染 HSV-2 的新生儿中大约 20% 有眼部表现[5]。

与其他类型的疱疹病毒一样，HSV 可以潜伏在感觉神经节和自主神经节，典型潜伏是在三叉神经节和角膜细胞[6]。病毒和机体的免疫应答决定了发病程度[7]。感染可以是原发性也可以是复发性的[8]。原发性感染常见于三叉神经上颌分支支配的面部区域，然而在原发性感染或再活化期间潜伏病毒通过三叉神经眼分支的三叉神经节传播，所以被称为"后门"路径。这可能也是原发性和复发性感染经常出现在不同部位的原因。即使没有眼分支过去的皮肤黏膜受累甚至也可能发生眼部感染[9]。

有三种理论可以解释病毒如何再活化。第一种理论认为被感染神经节受到刺激时释放病毒，从而引起眼部或皮肤的疾病；第二种理论认为病毒从神经节持续少量释放；第三种理论假设 HSV 潜伏在外周组织，但是当神经节被刺激后病毒被活化。精神或生理应激、或受损的免疫系统经常会促使病毒再活化[10]。

原发性眼部疾病

眼部疱疹可以是原发性传染性疾病，也可以是复发性的，当复发时可能和免疫力减弱有关[11]。未免疫宿主首次感染 HSV 被认为是原发性感染。原发性感染通常是自限性的，很少侵袭眼睛。原发性感染累及眼睛的概率少于 1%[12]，大多数呈现亚临床表现。

接触传染携带者 2~12 天后，患者可出现疼痛、异物感、流泪和畏光症状，往往伴有不适和发热。HSV 的眼部表现包括严重的眼睑炎、滤泡性和假膜性结膜炎及耳前腺病。眼周的皮肤损伤在恢复后一般不留疤痕。50% 的患者在结膜炎发作 1~2 周后发展成角膜炎。角膜病变开始表现为粗糙点状上皮性角膜炎，继而发展成微小树枝状角膜炎，然后合并变成大的树枝状角膜炎和地图样溃疡。病毒以线性方式细胞接着细胞地扩散，从而使角膜炎呈现特征性树枝状[13]。荧光染色显示，树枝状角膜溃疡的基底部上皮细胞发生了丢失（图 7.1）。孟加拉玫瑰红染料可将树枝状角膜溃疡边缘的感染后肿胀的上皮细胞染色。在原发性眼部疱疹疾病中很少观察到牵涉基质。角膜损伤会在 2~3 周后痊愈，不留或仅留下很小的疤痕。原发性眼部 HSV 可能会使角膜丧失感觉[14,15]。原发性眼部 HSV 感染的诊断依据为特有的临床特征和两周内是否有暴露史。新生儿原发性眼部感染主要表现为结膜炎和角膜炎，并伴有水泡样皮肤损伤。新生儿和免疫受损个体发生原发性感染后症状比较严重，并具有致死的可能性[16,17]。原发性 HSV 感染可导致危及生命的脑膜炎或脑炎，对这些患者推荐使用全身抗病毒治疗[18]。

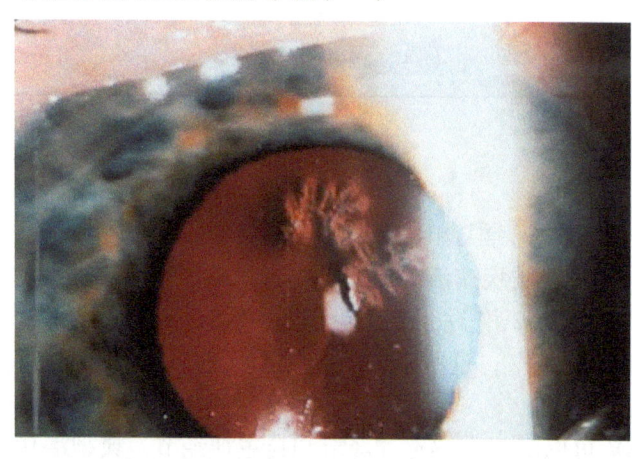

图 7.1 通过裂隙灯和后部反光照相法显示的发生在角膜上皮细胞的单纯疱疹性树枝状角膜炎。线性分支模式和"终端球状"可用来确诊疱疹性树枝状角膜炎。荧光染色显示树枝状基底部上皮细胞缺失。病毒在树枝状边缘的上皮细胞内复制。

复发性眼部疾病

25% 的单纯疱疹性角膜炎患者在初次感染两年内会复发，发作次数越多，则复发时间间隔越短[19]。HSV 引起的视觉病态主要与病毒复发感染有关，包括上皮性角膜炎、基质性角膜炎和前眼葡萄膜炎。复发性眼部疱疹与发热和不适无关，其严重程度取决于宿主的免疫应答和病毒株。这类疾病的诊断依靠临床症状和已知的原发性疱疹感染史。

在复发性眼病 HSV 中，上皮性角膜炎表现为点状或斑片样的星状格式。角膜上皮树枝状溃疡出现在角膜中心或近中心位置。虽然这种损伤通常两周以上的时间能够痊愈，但是仍有少数病例发展为大面积的地图样溃疡，尤其是经过局部皮质类固醇治疗之后。然后，这些溃疡进一步发展成以堆叠的、带有卷曲边缘的灰白色上皮细胞为特征的营养不良性溃疡。角膜炎反复发作之后可以导致上皮细胞的结构性损伤。营养不良性溃疡可持续几个月，并有基质溶解和继发穿孔。单纯疱疹病毒可以从树枝状和地图样溃疡分离培养。

基质性角膜炎被认为是一种与免疫相关的现象，但病毒和宿主免疫应答之间的相关性并不完全清楚[20]。基质性角膜炎、免疫韦斯利环和角膜缘血管炎是抗原-抗体-补体介导的反应。边界清楚呈盘形的盘状角膜炎属于基质性角膜炎的特异性亚类，是由迟发型超敏反应引起的[21]。角膜炎的两种机制可同时存在。视神经轴的炎症、血管新生和基质疤痕可导致视觉丧失。另外，其他疾病也可导致角膜炎的发生，角膜移植后也会复发。

复发性眼部 HSV 感染也可导致虹膜睫状体炎。葡萄膜炎可单独发生或者与角膜炎同时发生，与基质性角膜炎一样，可能与免疫相关[22]。单纯疱疹病毒可以在患者眼房水中被分离到。疱疹性葡萄膜炎患者可能突然出现疼痛、畏光和结膜充血的症状，眼部检查可发现严重的继发性青光眼[23]。

眼部 HSV 疾病通过临床来诊断且需要实验室研究的支持。发病后 1 周，血清抗体滴度开始升高，并可持续数周[24]。但是在复发间隔期血清抗体却没有升高。在疾病初期，可以从皮肤、角膜和结膜损伤处分离到病毒。病毒也可在树枝状溃疡早期分离到，而地图样溃疡和基质性角膜炎中分离不到。角膜削刮碎屑的吉姆萨（Giemsa）染色可发现多核上皮细胞。通过巴氏法检测细胞核内的嗜酸性包涵体也可以进行单纯疱疹病毒的确证。此外，利用荧光抗体进行角膜削刮碎屑染色可以进行 HSV 抗原的确证。酶联免疫法和 PCR 法也可用于 HSV 角膜炎的快速诊断[25,26]。

治疗

上皮性角膜炎的治疗包括局部抗病毒药物（表 7.3）。推荐如下三种疗法，疗程均为 2~3 周：

曲氟尿苷（trifluridine）（TFT，F3T，Viroptic） 1% 滴剂，8 次/天
疱疹净（idoxuridine）（IDU，Stoxil，Herplex） 0.5% 软膏，5 次/天
阿糖腺苷（vidarabine）（Ara-A，Vira-A） 5% 软膏，5 次/天

其中，曲氟尿苷的病毒耐药性及其对上皮细胞的毒性最小[27]。虽然外用阿昔洛韦眼膏在美国没有商品化，但是英国的研究表明其对上皮性角膜炎也有疗效[28]。利用 Meta 分析模型对多个疱疹性角膜炎的抗病毒治疗报告进行回顾，提出在治疗疱疹性树枝状和地图样上皮性角膜炎中，曲氟尿苷、阿昔洛韦和阿糖腺苷比疱疹净更加有效。口服阿昔洛韦和外用抗病毒治疗的效果相当，但是两者同时使用并不能加速愈合[29]。

表 7.3 HSV 的诊断

眼科疾病	治 疗
原发性眼病	
上皮性角膜炎（伴有发烧和不适）	外用曲氟尿苷和睫状肌麻痹剂
复发性眼病	
上皮性角膜炎	外用曲氟尿苷和睫状肌麻痹剂
基质性角膜炎	外用类固醇 + 外用曲氟尿苷或阿昔洛韦 + 睫状肌麻痹剂
虹膜睫状体炎	口服阿昔洛韦 400mg 5×QD 10 周 + 外用类固醇 + 外用曲氟尿苷和睫状肌麻痹剂

辅助治疗包括上皮清创术，它可以减少病毒和抗原对基质的影响。不能使用皮质激素，因为它可能促进病毒增殖、延长康复时间、增加上皮损伤范围并累及基质[30,31]。对儿童、老人或伤残患者来说，口服阿昔洛韦相比外用抗病毒治疗而言是一个更早的选择。但是，对于单独口服阿昔洛韦或者与外用阿昔洛韦联合使用治疗 HSV 角膜葡萄膜炎的有效性一直存在争议[32-34]。依据疱疹性眼病研究（herpetic eye disease study，HEDS），在发病一周

内外用曲氟尿苷治疗 HSV 上皮性角膜炎的患者，口服阿昔洛韦预防疱疹性基质性角膜炎或虹膜炎在随后的一年并没有带来额外的益处[35]。

外用泼尼松龙可用于疱疹性基质性角膜炎的治疗，能缩短基质炎症的顽固性、进程和持续时间[36]。推迟启用皮质类固醇治疗基质性角膜炎，会延迟其消退，但 HEDS 数据显示，经过 6 个月随访后，并未导致视力的恶化。外用皮质激素和曲氟尿苷联合使用可以控制基质性角膜炎的持续时间和进程[37]。外用抗病毒药物通常与类固醇药物联用，因为皮质类固醇有可能增强病毒的复制能力。活动期的基质炎症消退之后，外用皮质类固醇应该慢慢减量，从而将炎症反弹或类固醇导致的眼部副反应发生的可能性降到最低。

在 6 个月随访中，同时用曲氟尿苷和外用泼尼松龙治疗的患者，口服阿昔洛韦不能明显改变治疗失败的时间、治疗失败患者的比例或视力[38]。然而，口服阿昔洛韦（400mg，5 次 / 天）10 周治疗可以降低接受外用泼尼松龙和曲氟尿苷治疗的 HSV 虹膜睫状体炎患者的发病率。这种趋势是由 HEDS 的数据得来的，但样本量尚未达到统计学意义[39]。先前患有 HSV 眼病的患者可以从抑制性抗病毒治疗中受益，这些患者每天口服 2 次 400mg 阿昔洛韦可降低 HSV 上皮性角膜炎和基质性角膜炎的复发率。这种效果对以前患过 HSV 基质性角膜炎的患者最好[40,41]。

基质性角膜炎发展成的角膜穿孔，用氰基丙烯酸酯胶水和角膜移植处理，并在术后同时使用外用类固醇和抗病毒药物。在角膜移植后两年内，复发性疱疹性眼病的发生率为 15%~32%。术后口服阿昔洛韦可降低角膜炎的复发和移植失败风险[42]。必要时，建议外用睫状肌麻痹药物减轻角膜炎和虹膜睫状体炎引起的睫状肌痉挛所带来的不适。审慎地使用外用抗生素来治疗病毒性角膜炎的角膜溃疡以预防继发性细菌感染。

在感染后神经麻痹性角膜炎中，眼部润滑剂、修补术和隐形眼镜型绷带可用于修复角膜上皮的完整性。角膜炎复发后的治疗可能是漫长的。

在免疫受损患者中，HSV 角膜炎通常是双向的、严重的、非典型的累及角膜外周，对药物治疗有耐药性，并且经常复发。这类患者可使用全身性阿昔洛韦治疗[43]。

水痘 - 带状疱疹病毒

水痘 - 带状疱疹病毒（varicella-zoster virus，VZV）是已知的仅感染人类的疱疹病毒，大多数人在 60 岁以前呈现血清阳性。VZV 通过呼吸道分泌物经空气或者直接接触损伤的皮肤进行传播，初次感染通常导致常说的水痘。初次感染后，VZV 潜伏于三叉神经或脊髓神经节中，在成人中再次出现时就引发带状疱疹[44]。儿童的水痘很少引起眼部疾病，然而，带状疱疹性眼病（herpes zoster ophthalmicus，HZO）会引起严重的疼痛和眼部并发症[45]。

眼部水痘

眼部水痘可以表现为原发性水痘感染，以典型的水痘样皮肤损伤为主，或者在婴幼儿中表现为先天性水痘综合征。宿主暴露病毒后，病毒潜伏两周的时间，并在不同的愈合阶段表现出以水泡样损伤为主的皮疹，伴有发热和不适。皮疹可在一周内消退，这也是患者传染期结束和病毒潜伏期开始的信号。尽管大多数儿童几乎很少或不发生严重的疾病，但是婴儿或免疫缺陷的成人仍面临着潜在危及视力甚至生命的感染。

眼部水痘可表现为眼球角膜缘外周水泡状损伤，即所谓的"痘疮"，通常比较轻微并持续1~2周，这种损伤可在感染期或者甚至数月后出现。痘疮的病理生理学尚不清楚，但怀疑是免疫反应或活病毒所为。

水痘也可以导致点状或树枝状上皮性角膜炎。在感染过程中发作几次树枝状溃疡并不罕见。有一些特征可以区分单纯疱疹性树枝状溃疡和带状疱疹性树枝状溃疡，后者有时也被命名为"伪树枝状溃疡"。与单纯疱疹性树枝状溃疡不同的是，水痘性树枝状溃疡在刮擦的时候不留下溃疡基底。带状疱疹性树枝状溃疡呈典型的隆起、宽阔和多形性，与单纯疱疹性树枝状溃疡相比，清晰的分支模式和终端球形物更少。单纯疱疹性树枝状溃疡也可以通过溃疡基底的荧光染色和边缘的玫瑰红染色显示出来。

单纯疱疹和带状疱疹都可以降低角膜的感知度，所以不能通过角膜感觉缺失对两者进行鉴别。

病毒感染数周或数月后，免疫原性反应可导致盘状基质性角膜炎。外用皮质类固醇可加速症状消退，睫状肌麻痹滴剂可用来缓解睫状肌痉挛引起的不适。虹膜炎、脉络视网膜炎或视神经炎也时有发生，但是更不常见。如果不是在感染早期出现，这些病症可能是与免疫相关的，可以用皮质类固醇进行治疗[46]。

5%~16%的育龄妇女缺乏对水痘的免疫[47]。与儿童期水痘相比，先天性水痘综合征是一种更严重的全身性和眼部疾病。婴儿眼部感染后可发生脉络视网膜炎、小眼、视神经萎缩或者发育不全、先天性白内障和霍纳氏综合征[48,49]。先天性水痘目前缺乏有效的治疗方法。1995年，美国食品药品管理局（FDA）批准了一种水痘疫苗，该疫苗可降低先天性水痘综合征的发病率。

眼部的VZV感染可通过相关的全身性和皮肤症状及在感染的最初两周内血清抗体的升高来诊断。

带状疱疹性眼病

带状疱疹相对来说比较常见，20%的成人会发生[50]。与水痘相比，它更容易发生眼部感染。

尽管带状疱疹能感染三叉神经中的任何一个分支，但眼分支的易感性是其他分支的20倍。三叉神经眼分支又可分为三个小分支：额神经、泪腺神经和鼻睫神经。不管有没有眼内感染，带状疱疹感染三叉神经眼分支称之为带状疱疹性眼病（herpes zoster ophthalmicus，HZO）（图7.2）。患者首先出现皮区的疼痛和感觉过敏，在接下来的几天内出现水泡样皮肤损伤，同时或者随后出现眼部并发症。无疹性带状疱疹非常罕见，虽然表现出HZO眼病的症状，但是没有

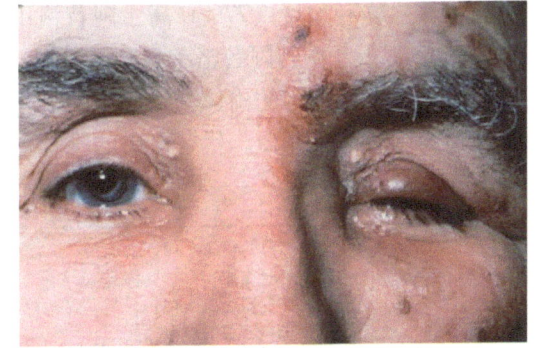

图7.2 病毒侵犯三叉神经眼分支后发生的带状疱疹性眼病。单侧眼皮可见水疱、脓疱和结痂性皮损，眼睑由损伤发展为水肿。

经典的皮肤损伤[51]。鼻尖上出现哈欣森症或带状疱疹损伤表明感染已经累及初级感觉神经——三叉神经眼分支的鼻睫神经。50%~80% 的哈欣森症患者会出现眼部炎症[52]。然而，没有出现哈欣森症的患者中仍有 61% 发生眼部感染[53]。

可能与 HZO 相关的眼部并发症包括睑缘炎、结膜炎、泪小管炎、泪腺炎、角膜炎、角膜葡萄膜炎、虹膜睫状体炎、继发性白内障、浅层巩膜炎、巩膜炎、青光眼、玻璃体炎、视网膜炎、急性视网膜坏死、视网膜脉管炎、脉络膜炎、视神经炎、眼外肌麻痹和眼前段缺血。这些并发症是由病毒增殖、免疫应答、炎症改变或者闭塞性脉管炎所致。另外，还可能包括一些眼表现，如白发症、睫毛脱落、倒睫、瘢痕性睑外翻或睑内翻、瘢痕性泪溢。任何眼部组织都会受到影响，在急性期或发病数月后都可能会出现并发症。

结膜炎的表现是多样的，包括乳突状、假膜性、膜性或滤泡性。不同形式的角膜感染包括急性上皮性角膜炎、慢性上皮性角膜炎、钱币状基质性角膜炎、基质性角膜炎、盘状角膜炎和神经麻痹性角膜炎。终端球状物和溃疡的缺失有助于急性上皮性角膜炎的树枝状溃疡与单纯疱疹相区别。从树枝状溃疡中可分离出病毒。急性上皮性角膜炎或带状疱疹皮肤损伤之后会出现慢性上皮性角膜炎或钱币状基质性角膜炎，这是自限性的，推测与免疫有关。基质性角膜炎和盘状角膜炎也与免疫有关。盘状角膜炎属于细胞介导的迟发型超敏反应，而基质性角膜炎与抗原 - 抗体 - 补体相关[54]。明显的角膜损伤后会出现神经麻痹性角膜炎，并可能导致角膜变薄和穿孔。慢性和复发性血管闭塞性脉管炎可导致带状疱疹性眼虹膜炎，点状或扇形虹膜萎缩可以将带状疱疹性眼虹膜炎与引起非缺血性弥散性虹膜萎缩的单纯疱疹性虹膜炎区分开来。广泛的角膜缘脉管炎会引起眼前端缺血。HZO 和水痘的实验室研究结果相似。

预防性外用抗生素结合良好的卫生条件可以预防 HZO 皮肤和眼睑损伤的继发性细菌感染（表7.4）。外用抗病毒制剂，如疱疹净、阿糖腺苷和曲氟尿苷，对眼部损伤的疗效甚微。尽管每天口服 5 次阿昔洛韦，每次 800mg，治疗 10 天后可减轻急性疼痛、缩短排毒持续时间并减少皮肤新囊泡的形成，但对眼部并发症是否有效并不清楚[55-57]。有些研究发现口服阿昔洛韦治疗 HZO 眼部并发症可降低发病率和严重程度[58,59]，然而其他一些研究结果并没有发现这种疗效[60]。据报道，泛西洛韦这种抗病毒药物可以迅速消除带状疱疹后神经痛，其生物利用度（77%）高于阿昔洛韦（18%）。在治疗带状疱疹性眼病时，泛西洛韦 500mg 每天 3 次与阿昔洛韦 800mg 每天 5 次具有相同的疗效，没有增加眼部并发症[61]。伐昔洛韦是阿昔洛韦的前体药物，生物利用度为 54%[62]，且在治疗免疫正常成人带状疱疹患者时与阿昔洛韦相似。伐昔洛韦的推荐剂量是 1g，每天 3 次[63]。

表 7.4 带状疱疹性眼病的诊断和治疗

眼部症状	治疗方法
鼻尖侧面的水疱样损伤（哈欣森症），三叉神经眼分支支配的皮肤区疼痛和感觉过敏（发病后三天内进行抗病毒治疗，以降低疱疹后神经痛和眼部并发症的发病率）	口服阿昔洛韦 800mg，5 次 / 天，10 天；泛昔洛韦 500mg，3 次 / 天，7 天；或泛昔洛韦 1g，3 次 / 天，7 天；配合或不配合使用抗生素软膏预防继发性细菌感染
基质角膜炎，虹膜睫状体炎	外用皮质类固醇和睫状肌麻痹剂
神经麻痹性角膜炎	积极的外用润滑剂治疗
视网膜炎，颅神经受损	静注阿昔洛韦

对于点状或树枝状上皮性角膜炎,用棉棒轻轻清创来减少角膜中病毒和抗原的数量[64]。抗病毒药物在上皮性角膜炎中的疗效尚未证实,如果诊断不明确,可以考虑使用抗病毒药物(如 HSV 上皮性角膜炎)。

外用皮质类固醇可用于免疫相关的眼部并发症的治疗,包括虹膜睫状体炎、盘状角膜炎、巩膜角膜炎和角膜葡萄膜炎。但是必须谨慎使用,并慢慢地减少使用量,将炎症复发的可能性降到最低。外用皮质类固醇不应用于治疗上皮性角膜炎。

神经麻痹性角膜炎的治疗方案包括软性隐形眼镜、润滑剂、修补术和睑缘缝合术,以促进上皮愈合。视网膜和视神经疾病的治疗方法包括静注阿昔洛韦和全身使用类固醇。

在年轻的高危患者中,带状疱疹性眼病是 AIDS 的早期临床指标[65,66]。AIDS 患者 HZO 的特征包括多处皮疹、无疱疹性眼病、进行性外层视网膜坏死(progressive outer retinal necrosis,PORN)综合征、慢性传染性假树枝状溃疡和严重的神经疾病[67]。

因为 HZO 在免疫抑制的个体中更严重和病程更长,所以应该使用静脉注射阿昔洛韦治疗[68](图 7.3)。进行性外层视网膜坏死与带状疱疹病毒感染有关,它是发生在严重免疫受损者中的一种坏死性视网膜疾病。在一项针对 38 位 PORN 患者的回顾性研究中,67% 有皮肤带状疱疹病史,41% 有 HZO 病史[69]。PORN 的早期表现为多病灶深度视网膜混浊,并迅速发展成全视网膜坏死,伴有视网膜脱落和视力预后不佳[70]。联合静脉注射治疗药物(如膦甲酸和更昔洛韦,膦甲酸钠和阿昔洛韦)或静脉注射抗病毒药物与玻璃体腔注射更昔洛韦可以阻止视网膜炎的进展并维持缓解状态[71,72]。

虽然最早被认为与 HSV 有关,但是急性视网膜坏死(acute retinal necrosis,ARN)已经归因于带状疱疹[73,74]。在免疫受损或健康患者中表现为严重的外周视网膜炎,并伴随显著的玻璃体炎症和闭塞性视网膜脉管炎,可导致视网膜脱落,也可见视神经盘炎。ARN 区别于 PORN 的特点是玻璃体炎,因为其他方面正常的患者在感染后能够产生强烈的免疫反应。此外,ARN 的预后视力往往比 PORN 更好(图 7.4)。带状疱疹、单纯疱疹和巨细胞病毒(cytomegalovirus,CMV)都与 ARN 和 PORN 有关[75-77]。坏死性疱疹性视网膜疾病代表了疱疹病毒科任一成员引起的一个疾病谱系,临床表现取决于宿主的免疫状态[78]。

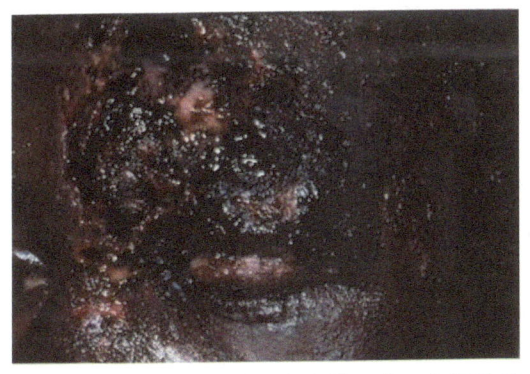

图 7.3 AIDS 患者的带状疱疹性眼病。有严重并漫长的病程,对免疫受损者推荐静脉注射抗病毒治疗。

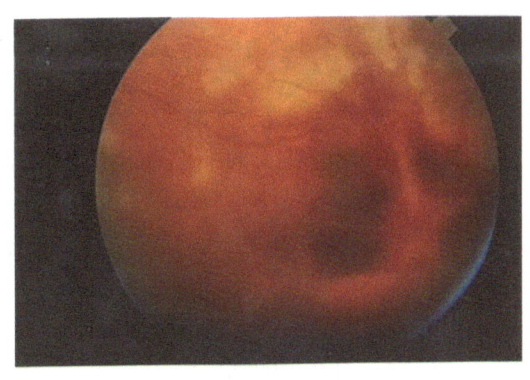

图 7.4 带状疱疹病毒感染继发的急性视网膜坏死患者的视力下降。玻璃体炎和出血使视网膜视野变模糊,并影响到视网膜血管。

静脉注射阿昔洛韦可阻止急性视网膜坏死的进程，然而它不能预防视网膜脱落[79]。曾报道泛西洛韦也有同样疗效[80]。有人报道，静脉注射阿昔洛韦或者静脉注射两种抗病毒药物，然后玻璃体腔注射更昔洛韦作为辅助治疗手段，能成功治疗疱疹性视网膜炎[81,82]。炎症发作时出现的孔源性视网膜脱离需要外科手术修复。

EB 病毒

EBV（Epstein-Barr virus，EBV）是 1964 年 Epstein 和 Barr 在电镜下观察伯基特淋巴瘤细胞时发现的。他们发现病毒颗粒与疱疹病毒科的其他成员类似[83]。在体内，EBV 通常感染 B 细胞和上皮细胞[84]，并形成 MALT 的潜伏感染[85]。EBV 与传染性单核细胞增多症（infectious mononucleosis，IM）[86,87]、地方性伯基特淋巴瘤[88]、鼻咽癌[89]和胸腺癌[90]有关。它也是干燥综合征的致病因子[91,92]。已发现在虹膜角膜内皮（iridocorneal endothelial，ICE）综合征患者中 EBV 衣壳蛋白抗体升高[93]。

在 20 世纪 70 年代，研究显示 26%~82% 的美国大学生和军官学校学生中存在 EBV 特异性抗体。也有报道称，社会经济状况低下的儿童中有 50%~85% 在 4 岁时产生 EBV 抗体[94~96]。儿童时期 EBV 感染不显著，但是青少年或者成人 EBV 却是 IM 的病因。病毒通过上呼吸道飞沫传播。IM 的症状和体征包括发热、淋巴结病、咽痛、肝炎、心包炎、多发性关节炎、肌炎和外周血涂片显示非典型淋巴细胞增多。

许多眼部疾病与 IM 相关，眼前段疾病包括滤泡性结膜炎、干眼综合征、结节性浅层巩膜炎、虹膜睫状体炎、眼-腺综合征、基质和上皮性角膜炎。EBV 相关视网膜炎[97]和多灶性脉络膜炎[98]也有报道。眼部神经表现有视神经乳头水肿、视觉神经炎和颅神经麻痹（表 7.5）[99]。

表 7.5　EBV 的诊断和治疗

眼部疾病	治疗
干眼综合征、滤泡性结膜炎、上皮性角膜炎	人工泪液
基质性角膜炎	轻症：人工泪液或观察 重症：外用皮质类固醇
视网膜炎或多发性脉络膜炎、视神经乳头水肿、视神经炎	不治疗或全身使用类固醇
颅神经麻痹	出现复视时闭上单眼

IM 的实验室确证以嗜异性抗体试验阳性或 EBV 特异性血清抗体滴度升高为基础[100,101]。因为 IM 通常是自限性的，所以 IM 的治疗主要为支持疗法。由于会出现脾肿大现象，因此应该限制剧烈的体力活动及涉及身体接触的体育运动。EBV 相关眼部疾病同样采用支持疗法。不必外用抗病毒治疗，全身性阿昔洛韦治疗的作用也不清楚。眼部炎症应考虑外用类固醇。基质性角膜炎的治疗取决于炎症的严重程度，轻症时使用人工泪液或不作处理，重症时推荐外用类固醇滴眼液。

在对任何一种非典型的眼部炎症进行鉴别诊断时都应该考虑到 EBV。当诊断结果不明确时，还应该考虑 EBV 感染的血清学试验。

巨细胞病毒

50 岁以上的美国人中，有一半以上可以检测到巨细胞病毒（cytomegalovirus，CMV）抗体[102]。它是最常见的先天性感染病毒，大约 2% 的新生儿被感染，但是大多数为亚临床症感染。感染的新生儿全身表现有肝脾肿大、黄疸、呼吸窘迫和颅内钙化，原发性眼部表现是脉络视网膜炎。众所周知，CMV 是造成子宫内和围产期感染的 5 种生物体之一（弓形虫、风疹、CMV、HSV 和梅毒，合称为 TORCHS）[99]。

CMV 可通过与感染者密切接触传播，少数情况下通过输血或感染器官移植传播。在大多数免疫功能正常个体中，CMV 感染可以无症状或呈现类似传染性单核细胞增多症的症状。在免疫抑制的个体中，CMV 可导致伴有终末器官损伤的严重临床疾病（图 7.5）。

CMV 是疱疹病毒科中的一员。CMV 和 HIV 之间的作用被认为是双向的。具体表现为，HIV-1 可增强 CMV 的产毒型感染，CMV 和 HIV-1 共感染单核细胞时会增强 HIV 的复制[103]。

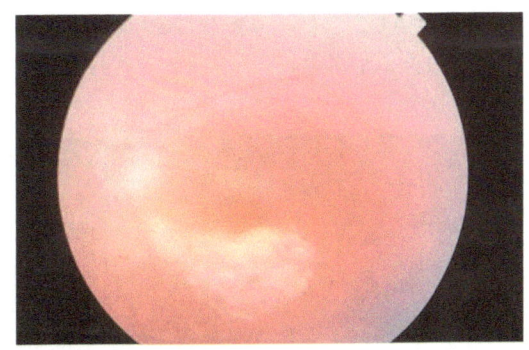

图 7.5 肾移植后经环孢霉素治疗的患者左眼的萎缩视网膜。随着免疫状态恢复和免疫抑制药物的减量，CMV 视网膜炎消退。

尽管 CMV 视网膜炎通常出现在 HIV 感染之前，但是它的出现可能是 AIDS 早期指标，约有 1.8% 的 HIV 感染者出现这一指标[104]。在高效抗逆转录病毒治疗（highly active antiretroviral therapy，HAART）时期，包括 CMV 视网膜炎、卡氏肺孢子虫肺炎和鸟分枝杆菌疾病在内的机会性感染病例有所下降，从 1994 年的 21.9 例/100（人·年）已经降低到 1997 年中期的 3.7 例/100（人·年）[105]。但是在一些经济条件有限或者难以实施 HAART 的地区，CMV 视网膜炎仍然是常见的眼部并发症。当 CD4 计数降低至 50 个细胞/mm^3 时，CMV 视网膜炎发生的可能性明显增加[106]。

尽管 CMV 的全身表现如肺炎、肠胃炎和脑炎难以诊断，但是由于具有特征性的眼底表现，所以可以通过临床检查对 CMV 视网膜炎进行鉴定。有些患者主诉的症状为视力模糊、漂浮物、幻视或盲点，而另一些可能完全无症状，尤其是当损伤很小或者位于外周视网膜时。

CMV 经血管进入视网膜，可导致视网膜损伤分布于血管周围。当黄斑区受累时，可观察到白色视网膜损伤和邻近视网膜出血及外周视网膜颗粒状损伤。损伤的后缘通常有多个小的圆形卫星状损伤环绕。CMV 视网膜炎也可能与脉管炎有关。如果不进行治疗，CMV 视网膜炎会蔓延到邻近区域的健康视网膜，造成视网膜萎缩、缺血和功能丧失。随着视网膜炎的蔓延，视觉区域缩小（图 7.6 和图 7.7）。如果不累及黄斑区或视神经，则中央视力可以保留。坏死视网膜的脱落也可以导致视力丧失。

在 CMV 视网膜炎中，位于视网膜中央的小损伤与 HIV 视网膜病类似。视网膜炎的鉴别诊断也包括其他病毒因素，如水痘带状疱疹或单纯疱疹。弓形虫、梅毒螺旋体和眼内

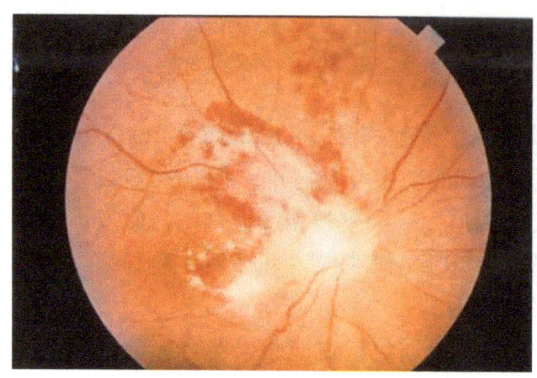

图7.6 在AIDS患者中诊断出CMV视网膜炎。CD4计数为20，并且视网膜中央出现视网膜炎相关的视力减弱。

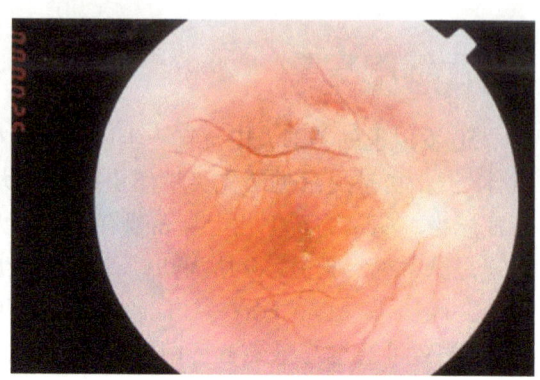

图7.7 这是与图7.6中同一个视网膜炎患者6周后的图片。患者出现进行性视觉区域丧失，并且在视网膜炎进程中视网膜上部出现飞蚊症。

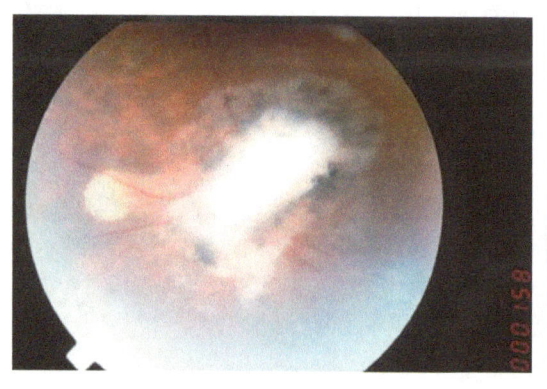

图7.8 CD4计数为120的HIV患者诊断出弓形体视网膜脉络膜炎。神经影像学检查确定已经累及中枢神经体统。由于已经累及黄斑区，所以视力下降到只能识别眼前手动。

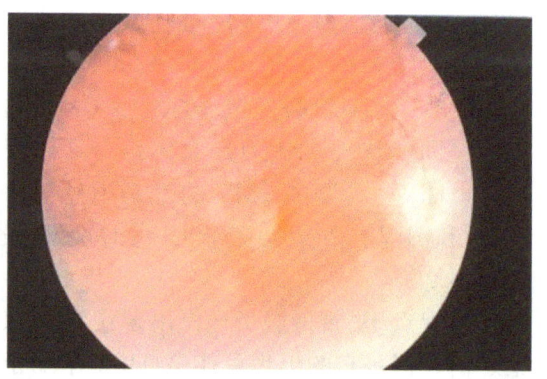

图7.9 AIDS和广泛性视网膜色素上皮萎缩患者的双眼患有梅毒性视网膜炎，且经过梅毒性视网膜炎治疗后，患者视力保持在右眼20/40、左眼20/30。

淋巴瘤也呈现相似的眼底表现（图7.8~图7.10）。弓形体病的视网膜损伤可能是颅内或弥散性弓形体病的最早迹象（表7.6）[107]。当患者出现密集、厚视网膜炎或者非典型CMV视网膜炎时应该考虑进行神经影像学检查。视网膜淋巴瘤浸润也类似于CMV视网膜炎。AIDS患者的眼内淋巴瘤可能与颅内疾病有关[108]。在不发生全身性淋巴瘤的情况下出现中枢神经系统（central nervous system，CNS）淋巴瘤非常罕见，且预后很差[109]。眼部梅毒很少表现为坏死性视网膜

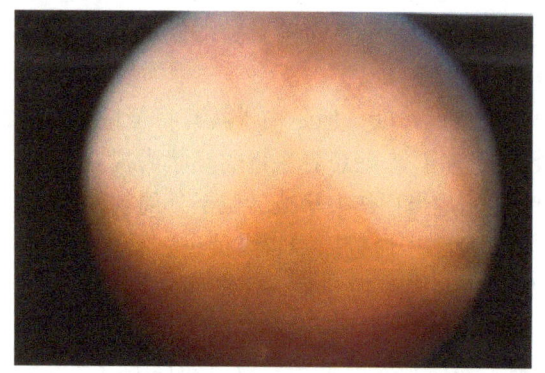

图7.10 AIDS患者、轻微玻璃体炎和视网膜脉络膜浸润。诊断性玻璃体切割术显示为大细胞淋巴瘤。

炎，应该与CMV视网膜炎进行鉴别诊断。眼部梅毒可能是HIV疾病的早期表现，并且需要采取针对神经梅毒的治疗方案[110]。

表 7.6　CMV 视网膜炎的鉴别诊断

HIV 视网膜病	早期 CMV 视网膜炎类似棉絮状斑点。与棉絮状斑点不同的是，未经治疗的 CMV 视网膜炎会继续发展。在 2 周内进行重复检查可区分这两种疾病
带状疱疹	带状疱疹性视网膜炎发展快速，其预后比 CMV 视网膜炎更差
弓形虫	典型的活动期弓形虫病与视网膜中心区域的坏死和玻璃体炎共存，同时可能伴随有中枢神经系统疾病
梅毒螺旋体	梅毒损伤表现为坏死性视网膜炎或奶油色小板状后段脉络膜视网膜炎
眼内淋巴瘤	与 CMV 视网膜炎相比，AIDS 相关的眼内淋巴瘤更加类似肺囊虫脉络膜炎或真菌性视网膜脉络膜炎。在一些病例中需要诊断性玻璃体切除术或视网膜活组织检查来区分

目前，CMV 的全身性药物治疗包括静脉注射更昔洛韦、膦甲酸和西多福韦（表7.7）[111~114]。每一种药物都需要两周的诱导剂量之后采取维持疗法。为了延缓病毒的活化或疾病进程，应该定期进行再诱导剂量的治疗。再诱导治疗的间隔随着疾病的进程而缩短。缬更昔洛韦是以口服形式使用的更昔洛韦的前体药物，在诱导治疗中，它与静脉注射更昔洛韦具有同样的疗效，对于 CMV 视网膜炎的长期治疗也有效[115]。

表 7.7　CMV 视网膜炎的诊断和治疗

眼科病变	治　疗
中央视网膜出血和外周视网膜颗粒状混浊相关的视网膜乳浊化和水肿	静脉注射：更昔洛韦、膦甲酸、西多福韦 玻璃体灌输：更昔洛韦 玻璃体注射：更昔洛韦、膦甲酸、福米韦生

1996 年 3 月，缓释更昔洛韦片（Vitrasert™）被批准用于局部眼内治疗[116]。这种埋入眼中的缓释剂与静注更昔洛韦相比，可将视网膜炎进展的风险降低 3 倍。然而，单独使用眼内埋入治疗时，未感染眼和全身性 CMV 病的风险更高。口服更昔洛韦与局部埋入联合使用可降低 CMV 新发疾病的风险，延缓手术后眼部 CMV 视网膜炎的发展，并降低卡波西肉瘤的风险[117]。

影响视网膜炎进程的因素包括眼内亚治疗药物水平、CMV 耐抗病毒药物株的产生及患者免疫力的进行性衰退。全身或眼部副作用也会影响药物的选择。更昔洛韦和缬更昔洛韦潜在的剂量限制性毒性包括中性粒细胞减少症、贫血和血小板减少症。西多福韦和膦甲酸均具有肾毒性，需要定期监测肾功能并调节用药剂量。

有研究报道了在经过延长治疗之后，CMV 对更昔洛韦或膦甲酸耐药性的研究结果[118]。福米韦生（Vitravene™）是 1998 年以来使用的一种反义化合物，可以降低其他抗 CMV 药物不能控制的视网膜炎患者的损伤活性[119]。已知的玻璃体腔给药的不良事件有前房炎症、眼内高压和可逆性中心黄斑病[120]。

随着 HAART 的发展，在 HIV 患者免疫恢复性葡萄膜炎中联合应用蛋白酶抑制剂和逆转录酶抑制剂，可以改变 CMV 视网膜炎的发病率和进程[121,122]。接受 HAART 治疗并且免疫系统得以重建的 AIDS 患者在经过 CMV 视网膜炎治疗之后会出现前、后葡萄膜炎，继而导致玻璃体炎、黄斑囊样水肿、视网膜前膜形成和视神经乳头炎的发生（图 7.11）。

轻症病例可停药观察，中度到严重病例可使用皮质类固醇眼周注射治疗[123~126]。随着 HAART 治疗后 CD4 水平的恢复，如果能够确保良好的后续治疗，停止维持性 CMV 治疗可有效预防免疫恢复性葡萄膜炎的发生[127]。

为了筛查 CMV 视网膜炎，建议 CD4 细胞计数高于 100 的患者每年进行一次扩张眼基底检查。CD4 细胞计数在 50~100 之间的患者应该每 6 个月检查一次，而 CD4 计数低于 50 的患者应该间隔 2~3 个月检查一次。如果患者诊断有全身性 CMV 疾病也应该接受检查。预防性筛查能够提高早期发现和治疗率，保护视力[128]。

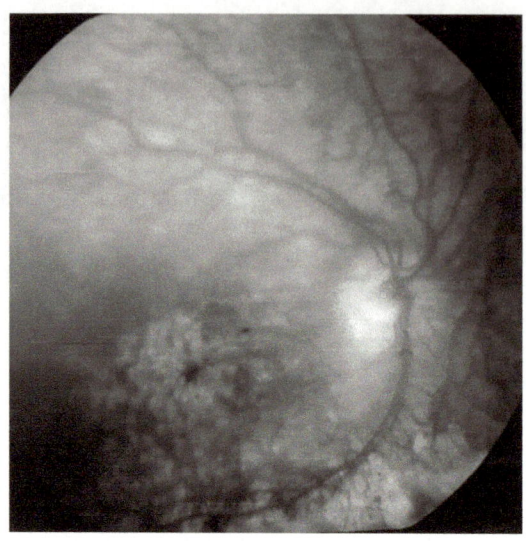

图 7.11 AIDS 患者中免疫恢复性葡萄膜炎黄斑囊样水肿导致视力下降后的眼底荧光素血管造影片。CMV 视网膜炎处于静止期。HAART 治疗后，CD4 计数是 180。

人类疱疹病毒 -8

人类疱疹病毒 -8 型（human herpes virus-8，HHV-8）DNA 序列是由 Chang 等[129]在 AIDS 相关卡波西肉瘤中鉴定发现的。HHV-8 引起恶性肿瘤的发病机理尚在研究中[130]。皮肤卡波西肉瘤是鉴定 HIV 的标志[131]。20%~30%AIDS 患者的眼部结构也会受到同样的皮肤肿瘤的影响[132,133]。尽管眼附属器也会受到影响，但眼部卡波西肉瘤通常发生在眼睑或结膜的位置（图 7.12 和图 7.13）。眼部卡波西肉瘤极少危及视力。结膜损伤与下结膜穹窿部结膜下出血症状相似。当这类损伤影响容貌，或伴随有睑内翻、倒睫、继发性溃疡或感染时，应采用局部治疗。治疗方法包括冷冻疗法、含或不含荧光素的血管造影外科切除术及局部放射治疗[133,134]。用化学疗法治疗内部组织损伤也会缩小眼内损伤的范围（表 7.8）。

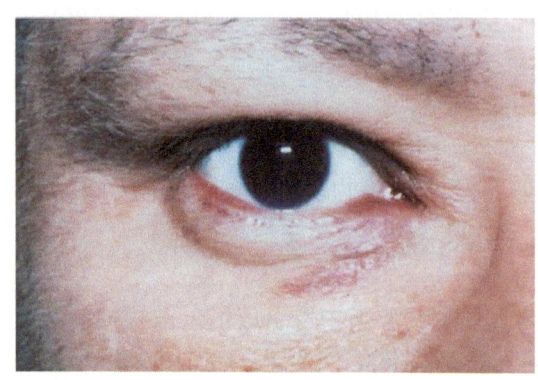

图 7.12 AIDS 患者右眼下眼睑的无痛紫罗兰色卡波西肉瘤。

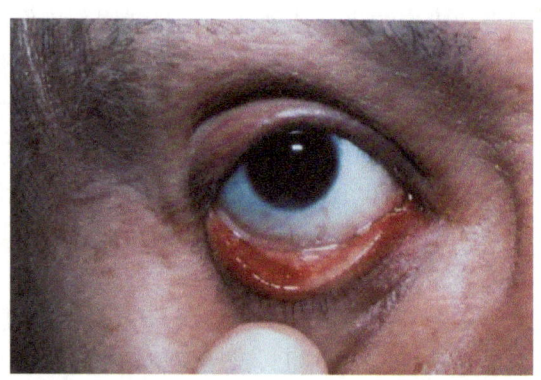

图 7.13 与图 7.12 是同一个患者。外翻下眼睑，发现卡波西肉瘤累及邻近结膜。眼睑与内部组织损伤在化学治疗后恢复。

表 7.8　HHV-8 的诊断和治疗

眼部疾病	治疗方法
眼睑或结膜出现紫罗兰色、红色至紫色的无症状损伤	化学疗法
眼窝卡波西肉瘤，极为罕见，发生在眼睑可影响视野	冷冻疗法、外科手术切除或者放射疗法

眼睑或结膜损伤的鉴别诊断疾病包括睑板腺囊肿、结膜下出血（图 7.14）、化脓性肉芽肿、淋巴瘤和转移性淋巴瘤（表 7.9）。卡波西肉瘤可通过组织活检来确证，但在 AIDS 患者中确证不是必需的（图 7.15）。

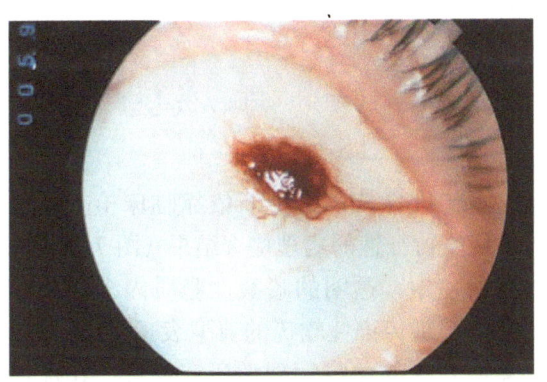

图 7.14　左眼眼球底部结膜处的椭圆形突起的卡波西肉瘤损伤。该损伤可误诊为结膜下出血。

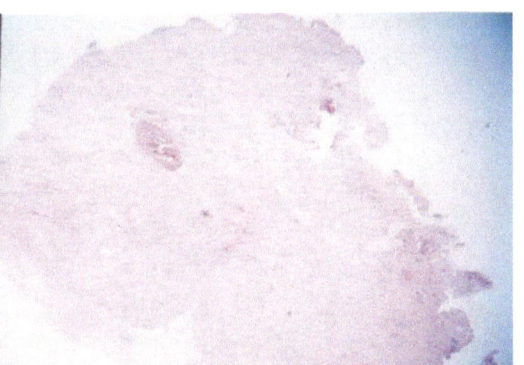

图 7.15　结膜卡波西肉瘤损伤的组织病理学。结膜表面和结膜下发生杯状细胞及下面单核细胞的炎性浸润。在更深的皮下基质处可见膨胀的脉管和众多特征性不规则的"锯齿状"管状区域，由胶原质束隔离 [苏木精和伊红染色（HE，10×）]。

表 7.9　HHV-8 的鉴别诊断

类　型	症　状
霰粒肿	睑板腺或脂肪腺阻塞后引起的脂肪肉芽肿性炎症
结膜下出血	发生在结膜下，与外伤、咽鼓管充气检查或隐匿性出血相关
化脓性肉芽肿	与外伤或手术相关的蒂状深红色病变
淋巴瘤	在 AIDS 患者中可见，多数是 B 细胞淋巴瘤，典型症状为逐渐扩大的平滑的鲑鱼色的损伤

传染性软疣

传染性软疣属于痘病毒家族中的 DNA 病毒。它在皮肤和黏膜上皮处增生后形成多发性脐状疣样损伤[135,136]。病毒通过直接接触损伤或污染物传播。

眼周软疣最初呈现出肉色、平滑、圆顶状的丘疹，然后变为中央凹陷的脐状（图 7.16）。损伤与慢性滤泡性结膜炎和浅表上皮性角膜炎有关（图 7.17）。角膜血管翳可转为慢性。损伤通常是无症状的，但曾经有过继发性细菌感染导致瘙痒的相关报道[137]。大多数患者的损伤少于 20 处，但也可能更多[138]。

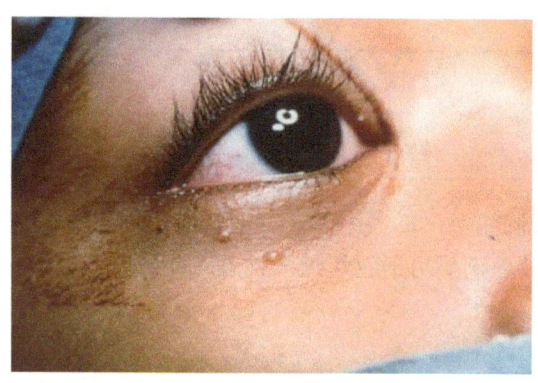

图7.16 传染性软疣。常见的受累部位是下眼睑，病变呈圆形、蜡色、脐状。在免疫缺陷患者中，病变有较高的复发率，并且更加难以治疗。

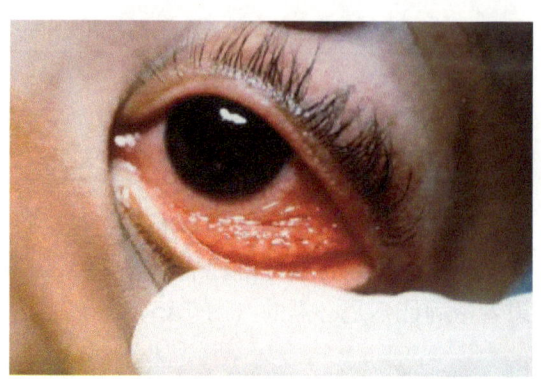

图7.17 眼睑病变处的病毒颗粒引起传染性软疣相关的滤泡性结膜炎。皮肤损伤治疗后，结膜炎可消退。

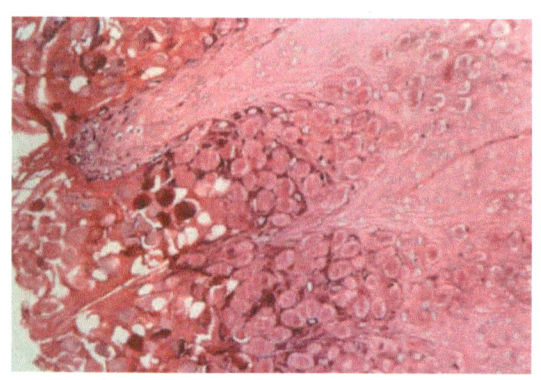

图7.18 传染性软疣组织病理学显示亨德森-帕特森嗜酸性透明的胞质内含物，或称之为软疣体，这种软疣体由很多病毒颗粒组成（HE，×64）。

传染性软疣的诊断依靠临床检查，确诊依据特征性的病理检查结果（图7.18）。在活检中，透明的嗜酸性胞质内含物或软疣体都是传染性软疣的典型表现[139]。对传染性软疣的免疫病理学研究发现，在疣体病变附近的表皮和真皮有T细胞介导的淋巴细胞反应[140]。

单纯累及结膜的眼周传染性软疣较难诊断，因为这种病变很容易与霰粒肿、异位泪腺组织、异物或上皮赘生物相混淆[141]。

软疣病变在AIDS患者中的发病率有逐渐增高的趋势[141,142]。这些患者可能会有多重病变融合，并且这些病变在治愈后6~8周可能复发[142]。HIV患者中这些病变不易自发性缓解。角膜结膜炎在HIV患者中不太常见。

若不进行治疗，眼周软疣病变通常会在数月内自愈，有效疗法包括刮除术、化学烧灼或冷冻疗法。软疣眼睑病变的鉴别诊断疾病包括睑腺炎、脂溢性角化病、乳头状瘤、痣及角化棘皮瘤（表7.10）。

表7.10 传染性软疣的鉴别诊断

鳞状上皮乳头状瘤	以纤维管为核心的指状病变
痣	不同皮肤层内典型的痣细胞形成的色素沉着的、界限明确的病变
角化棘皮瘤	生长迅速的脐状病变，可自愈
麦粒肿	急性发作，与睑缘炎相关的界限明确的眼睑病变，由睑板或皮脂腺阻塞引起
睑板腺囊肿	慢性，由阻塞的睑板或皮脂腺引起的脂肪肉芽肿性炎症
脂溢性角化病	脂肪过多的突起病变，老龄患者可见
化脓性肉芽肿	与外伤或外科手术相关的带状深红色病变
恶性肿瘤（如腺囊性基底细胞癌）	许多上皮肿瘤与正常皮肤的溃疡和炎症相关，可进行组织学诊断

人乳头瘤病毒

人乳头瘤病毒（human papilloma virus，HPV）是一种双链环形乳头状瘤多型空泡形DNA病毒，最初在生殖器病变中发现。至今已发现了80多种病毒亚型，每种亚型的病毒都具有感染部位或细胞类型特异性。一些亚型在特定器官导致疣，而其他亚型可能与恶性肿瘤相关[143,144]。

HPV与喉部[145]、口腔黏膜[146]、泪囊上皮细胞[147]和眼结膜部位[148]的肿瘤相关。在良性和恶性结膜病变中可见HPV-6、HPV-11和HPV-16亚型[148,149]。HPV-16和HPV-18亚型与宫颈癌相关[150,151]。在宫颈非典型增生患者的眼结膜中也发现了HPV-16[152]。

泪囊原发性上皮肿瘤虽然罕见，但是也有报道。HPV-11与良性泪囊肿瘤相关。HPV-18与泪腺上皮恶性肿瘤相关[147]，在眼结膜上皮瘤中可检测到HPV-16 DNA[153]。在眼结膜上皮内肿瘤标本中可检测到HPV-16和HPV-18 DNA及信使RNA（mRNA）[154]。但有报道称，在一系列眼结膜上皮恶性肿瘤患者中没有检测到HPV DNA[155]。

眼部HPV乳头状瘤好发于睑缘，其次为结膜，并且儿童和青少年较为常见。HPV通过自体传播或直接接触传播，病毒潜伏期长达数月至两年。眼睑乳头状瘤可单发，也可多发。发生在上眼睑的通常为亚急性乳头状结膜炎。患者主诉有异物感和畏光症状，某些患者可能会进一步发展为角结膜炎。儿童的眼睑病变容易复发。老龄患者的病变不具有传染性，但偶尔会发生恶性转化。

结膜乳头状瘤的发生频率要比眼睑低（图7.19和图7.20）。美国陆军病理研究所在1016例眼球病变检查中检测出126例乳头状瘤病例[156]。Mayo诊所在64年的时间里共切除了27例乳头状瘤[157]。

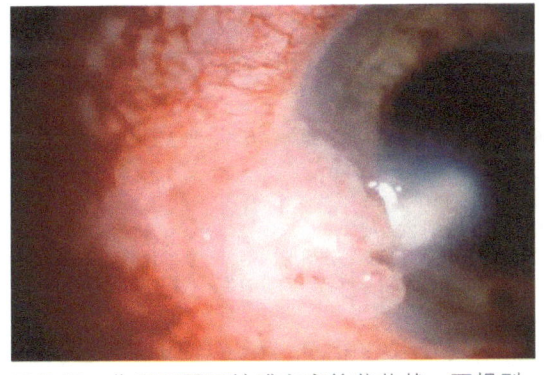

图7.19 位于眼颞下结膜穹窿的菜花状、不规则的乳突团。鳞状上皮细胞结膜乳头状瘤被认为是由乳多空病毒引起的，切除后可能会复发。

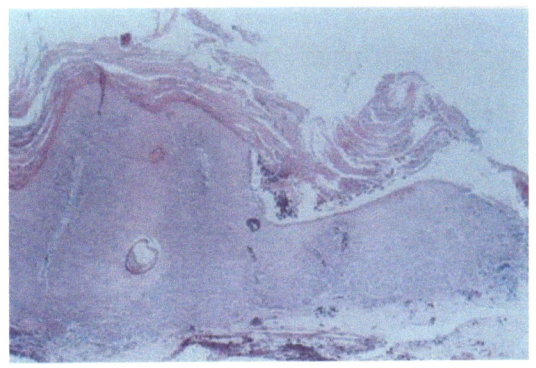

图7.20 鳞状上皮细胞结膜乳突状瘤的病理学特征。病变由棘层肥厚、角化过度、角化不全及角囊肿的鳞状上皮细胞组成。基质存在太阳改变和慢性炎症，但上皮细胞并没有发育不良（HE，×16）。

无症状的眼部小损伤可自愈，所以治疗以观察为主。由于手术切除后经常传播和复发，所以对儿童和青少年患者要考虑采取保守疗法。疑似恶性、病变进展迅速或因累及眼睑影响视力的患者都需要进行治疗。治疗方法包括手术切除、冷冻治疗或者两者联合。手术切除时建议将病变部位连同周边1mm内正常组织一同进行切除。其他治疗方法包括二氧化碳激光法、电干燥法和刮除术、二硝基氯苯及病灶内注射 IFN-α[158,159]。局部使用 IFN-α 对两例进行切除和冷冻疗法后复发的乳头状瘤患者有效[159]。

眼部乳头状瘤病变的鉴别诊断疾病包括良性和恶性病变（表7.11）。HPV 可通过 PCR、免疫组化染色和原位杂交进行检测[160]。

表 7.11　HPV 的鉴别诊断

化脓性肉芽肿	与创伤或外科手术相关的蒂状深红色病变
淋巴管瘤	多囊性肿块，成人期以前出现
卡波西肉瘤	紫红色或紫色病变，AIDS 患者可见
淋巴瘤	鲑鱼色病变，青年到中年人可见
淀粉样病变	光滑、蜡样肿块，主要出现在下穹窿
皮脂腺细胞癌	应该考虑用常规治疗方法（即切除，注射皮质类固醇）难以治愈的复发性霰粒肿患者

腺病毒

腺病毒为无包膜 DNA 病毒。腺病毒的整个复制过程发生在被感染细胞的细胞核内。全世界共发现了 47 种不同血清型的腺病毒，它们引起上呼吸道和眼部感染，常见症状包括咽结膜热（pharyngoconjunctival fever，PCF）、流行性角膜结膜炎（epidemic keratoconjunctivitis，EKC）、急性非特异性滤泡性结膜炎（nonspecifc follicular conjunctivitis，NFC）（表7.12）。PCF 主要与 1 型、3 型、4 型、5 型、6 型、7 型和 14 型有关；EKC 主要与 1 型、2 型、3 型、7 型、8 型、9 型、10 型、11 型和 19 型有关；NFC 与导致 EKC 或 PCF 的很多血清型有关[161]。PCF、EKC 和 NFC 的鉴别诊断见表7.13。

表 7.12　腺病毒的诊断与治疗

	症　状	治　疗
咽结膜热（PCF）	发热、咽炎、结膜炎、鼻炎、颈前和耳前腺病、瘙痒、发炎和流泪、眼睑水肿、瘀斑和角膜炎	PCF 能自愈 恰当的卫生保健对预防很有效；儿童应休学两周
角膜结膜炎（EKC）	结膜炎、角膜炎、无全身症状、疼痛、流泪、异物感、眼睑水肿、充血滤泡性结膜炎、结膜水肿、耳前淋巴结疼痛假膜及睑球粘连形成	EKC 能自愈 预防非常重要 支持治疗包括：血管收缩剂、冷敷或热敷、眼睛润滑剂及睫状肌麻痹剂，严重的角膜炎应使用局部皮质类固醇治疗
非特异性滤泡性结膜炎（NFC）	成年和儿童患者都未见角膜炎	非特异性滤泡性结膜炎临床症状轻微，可自愈

表 7.13　腺病毒的鉴别诊断

其他病毒性结膜炎：病毒培养有助于诊断
细菌性结膜炎：典型的症状是排出脓液，其他症状包括结膜充血水肿，细菌培养有助于诊断
毒性结膜炎：患者有化学药品接触史，包括外用滴眼液
过敏性结膜炎：患者通常有过敏史
眼瘢痕性类天疱疮：可观察到下眼睑睑球粘连，下眼穹窿缩短

咽结膜热

咽结膜热是儿童和青少年感染相对比较常见的综合征，其流行常发于家庭、学校或其他公共场所。病毒通过接触呼吸飞沫、受污染的游泳池水或污染物传播，潜伏期为5~12天。咽结膜热的症状包括发热、咽炎、滤泡性结膜炎、出血性结膜炎、鼻炎及颈前或耳前淋巴结病[161,162]。早期眼部症状包括轻微瘙痒和灼烧感，或明显的烦躁和流泪，随后出现眼睑水肿并伴有弥漫性充血。下眼睑症状则更为严重，通常还会出现瘀斑。典型症状为两只眼睛相差几天先后发作，出现症状的几天后，可能会出现点状上皮性角膜炎。荧光染色显示角膜炎开始于表层角膜上皮糜烂。糜烂进一步发展，在角膜中心形成皮上和皮下局部浸润。浸润物被认为是抗原-抗体免疫复合物。尽管疾病急性期会在几天到一个月内消退，但上皮下浸润可能会持续数月，并导致眩光或视力减退。

腺病毒的诊断主要依靠临床症状。实验室诊断方法包括直接荧光抗体染色法和酶联免疫吸附试验（enzyme-linked immunosorbent assay, ELISA）。病毒可在最初8~10天进行培养。

咽结膜热是一种自限性疾病。急性期症状可在数天到一个月内消退。应建议患者采取预防接触的措施和勤洗手，以防将疾病传染给他人。咽结膜热对氯化消毒处理有抵抗力，所以患者应避免去游泳池。病毒也对洗涤剂和低pH耐受。对病毒有效的消毒剂包括苯酚、福尔马林及10%家用漂白粉溶液。

流行性角膜结膜炎

EKC通常在秋冬季高发，成人较儿童更为常见。EKC通常亚急性发作，双眼可能都会感染并持续数周，随后的角膜炎可能会持续数月。这种疾病通过手-眼接触或受污染的医疗器械传播。最常见的引起EKC的腺病毒血清型为8型和19型[163]。从活动期EKC和宫颈炎妇女的子宫颈和眼中也能分离出19型，表明该病可通过性接触传播[164]。与PCF不同的是，EKC没有全身症状。经过大约8天的潜伏期后，患者表现出眼睑水肿、眼结膜充血、滤泡性和乳头状结膜炎及结膜水肿[161]，并可伴有结膜下出血和耳前淋巴结疼痛。患者主诉持续流泪、异物感或者轻微的畏光等症状。对侧眼通常会在4~5天后也被感染。最后，结膜结疤和睑球粘连的形成促使假膜的出现，角膜上皮细胞内病毒复制活跃。2~3周后，角膜皮下浸润继续发展，如果角膜中心受到影响，视力分辨能力将下降（图7.21）。

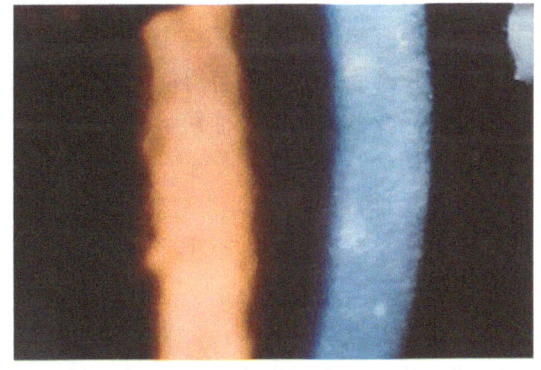

图7.21　裂隙灯观察腺病毒导致的流行性角膜结膜炎皮下浸润。浸润持续时间超过感染急性期，并妨碍视力。

双侧滤泡性结膜炎的患者应怀疑为EKC。实验室确诊需要从眼结膜拭子或刮片中进行腺病毒的细胞培养和分离。腺病毒在眼部疾病发作的第一周就能很容易分离到[165]。其他检测包括利用ELISA检测一组血清的抗体滴度或抗原含量[166,167]。鉴别诊断包括其他病毒、细菌、毒素、过敏原导致的结膜炎。如果有明显的假膜或睑球粘连存在，应考虑与眼部瘢痕性类天疱疮进行鉴别。

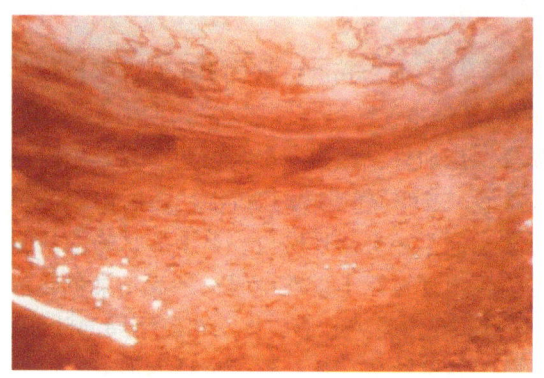

图 7.22 腺病毒引起的急性滤泡性结膜炎的特征包括结膜瘀斑、结膜滤泡、结膜下出血、眼睑水肿和大量流泪。在急性期,病毒很容易通过未清洗的双手和污染物传播。

与 PCF 一样,EKC 也需要采取严格的污染预防措施和洗手以预防感染的传播。支持疗法可用于缓解症状。冷敷或热敷及眼部润滑剂均有帮助,也可考虑外用血管收缩剂和睫状肌麻痹剂。不需要进行局部抗生素治疗,急性点状角膜炎不经治疗也可痊愈。数月至数年之后,角膜皮下损伤逐渐消退,视力逐渐恢复。严重的角膜炎病例可外用类固醇治疗,但类固醇可能会延迟角膜中病毒的清除,并促进排毒[168]。

非特异性滤泡性结膜炎

儿童和成人中的非特异性滤泡性结膜炎无角膜炎症状(图 7.22)。临床症状非常轻微,有的病例甚至没有症状,7~10 天内症状消退[169]。

人类免疫缺陷病毒

人类免疫缺陷病毒(human immunodeficiency virus,HIV)是逆转录病毒家族中的一员,导致获得性免疫缺陷综合征(acquired immune deficiency syndrome,AIDS)。HIV 可以从眼泪、结膜、角膜和视网膜等眼组织中分离得到。结膜感染后的临床体征包括毛细血管扩张和微动脉瘤。HIV 导致的最常见眼部疾病都集中在视网膜上。在 CD4 计数降低的 HIV 患者中,会有超过 50% 的发生视网膜病变,这也是疾病进一步发展的标志[170,171]。

HIV 视网膜病变中最有可能发生的是视网膜缺血,临床症状包括中央视网膜表面的点状缺血性病变(称之为"棉絮状斑")及外周视网膜内出血。这种微血管病变可能是由视网膜血管内的[172,173]或者来自被感染血管内皮细胞的免疫复合物沉积所致[174]。超高黏度/高丙球蛋白血症改变了血流速度,导致缺血性视网膜病变,这可能也是 HIV 视网膜病变的一种机制[175]。20 世纪 70 年代末,AIDS 第一次被确定为一种特殊的疾病。1978 年以前,在糖尿病、高血压或胶原蛋白血管病患者中也有类似的视网膜疾病。现在,对棉絮状斑的鉴别诊断应重点考虑 HIV 视网膜病变。

棉絮状斑类似于发生在中央视网膜的早期 CMV 视网膜炎(图 7.23)。HIV 视网膜病变可通过对病变的眼底成像来确诊,如果必要的话,可在随后两周内或更短时间内进行复查。由于 HIV 视网膜病变不需要治疗,而 CMV 视网膜炎如果未被发现和治疗的话,可能会导致严重的视力丧失,所以鉴别诊断非常重要。HIV 高危患者出现 HIV 视网膜病的临床症状时需要接受进一步的血清学检查。

机会感染也会影响 HIV 感染者的眼部结构。CMV 视网膜炎出现在 AIDS 终末期。AIDS 患者中能导致视力丧失的其他病毒包括上述的单纯疱疹病毒和带状疱疹病毒。

AIDS 相关的其他眼部机会性感染由细菌、真菌和寄生虫所致，包括梅毒螺旋体、分枝杆菌（图 7.24）、新型隐球菌、卡氏肺孢菌及刚第弓形虫[176]。梅毒螺旋体视网膜炎、刚第弓形虫视网膜炎和眼内淋巴瘤与 CMV 视网膜感染相似。新型隐球菌和卡氏肺孢菌眼部感染与脉络膜圆形多病灶损伤有关[177]（图 7.25 和图 7.26）。视神经乳头水肿与隐球菌脑膜炎有关。

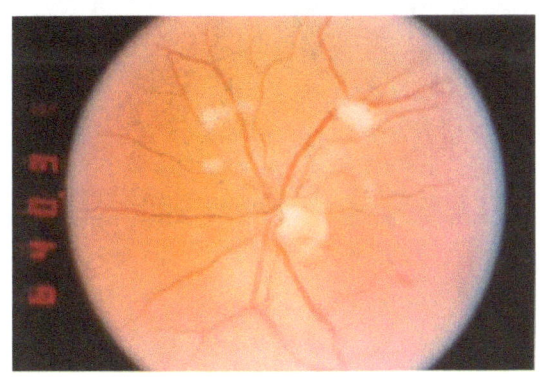

图 7.23 一位年轻的男性 HIV 感染者的视网膜病变，可见棉絮状斑和视网膜出血。这种视网膜微血管病变不影响视力，病变可在数周内消失。早期 CMV 视网膜炎可能会被误诊为棉絮状斑。如果不接受治疗，CMV 病变会在数周内加重。

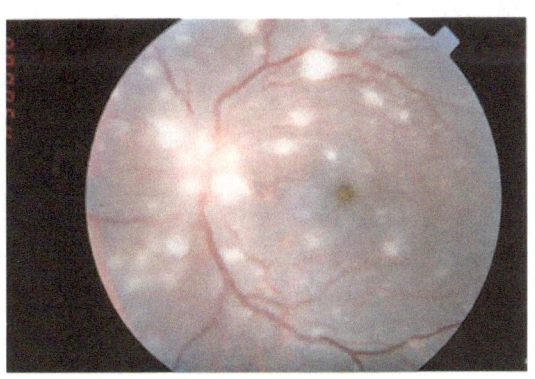

图 7.24 AIDS 患者的粟粒性结核。双眼都被诊断为多灶性视网膜脉络膜炎。使用结核药物治疗后病变和其他症状消退。

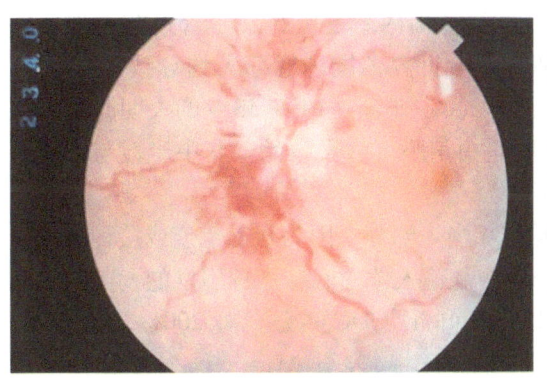

图 7.25 AIDS 患者出现视力模糊和视神经乳头水肿，诊断为隐球菌性脑膜炎和弥散性感染。

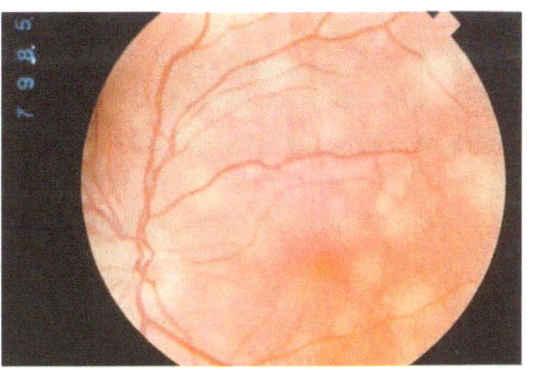

图 7.26 AIDS 患者中发生的多卡氏肺囊虫状脉络膜病变。患者接受过雾化潘他米丁预防性治疗。由于预防措施已经由雾化改为口服甲氧苄氨嘧啶/新诺明，所以这种眼部的机会性感染现在已经很少见到。

发生在 AIDS 患者身上的药物相关的眼部副作用包括利福布丁相关性葡萄膜炎（图 7.27）、西多福韦相关性葡萄膜炎和眼压过低（图 7.28）[178]、地达诺新相关性色素视网膜病[179]、福米韦生相关性葡萄膜炎、高眼压症和视网膜色素上皮细胞毒性。熟悉这些病症有助于区别药物相关副作用与病毒性眼科急症。

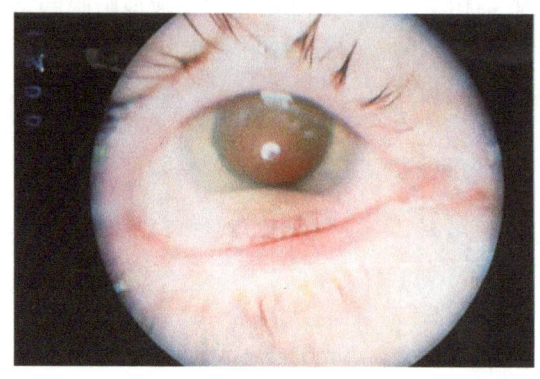

图 7.27 AIDS 患者中，炎症细胞堆积在眼前段下部。使用克拉霉素和利福布丁治疗期间视力减退。在使用局部类固醇滴眼药和停用克拉霉素及利福布丁后药物毒性消失。

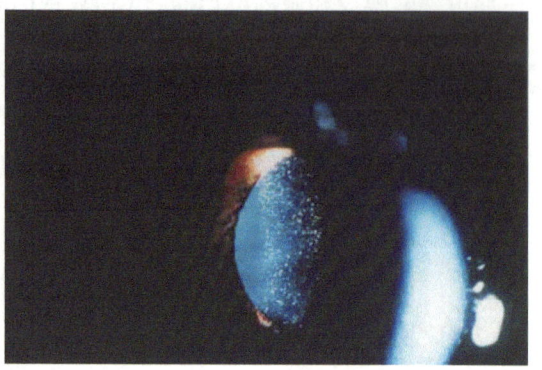

图 7.28 AIDS 患者诊断出西多福韦相关性眼部毒性。患者服用了治疗 CMV 视网膜炎的药物，出现畏光、双眼疼痛的症状。裂隙灯检查眼前室发现炎症细胞，眼内压降低（低眼压）。

麻疹

麻疹病毒是副黏病毒属的一种 RNA 病毒，通过呼吸道传播[180,181]。这种病毒具有高传染性，并且只感染人类。麻疹是一种急性热疹性疾病，主要感染儿童和青少年[182]。

在 1963 年麻疹疫苗出现以前，麻疹在全世界范围内暴发流行。尽管疫苗出现后麻疹发病率下降了，但是在 2000 年，WHO 估计在全世界范围内麻疹大约导致了 77.7 万个死亡病例，其中 45.2 万（58%）发生在非洲[183]。在非洲，14%~33% 的失明儿童可能是由麻疹导致的。在赞比亚，80% 的儿童失明是由角膜疾病导致的，其中半数与麻疹有关[184]。

虽然美国麻疹的发病率有所降低，但仍然有相当一部分人因为缺乏免疫或接种失败而成为麻疹易感人群[185~187]。在美国，绝大部分病例是输入性的麻疹毒株引发的。美国疾病预防控制中心（Centers for Disease Control and Prevention，CDC）报道称，2001~2003 年间，美国没有地方性麻疹毒株的流行[188]。

麻疹的临床表现包括持续 3 天或 3 天以上的全身性斑丘疹发作、发热及咳嗽、鼻炎和结膜炎三联症。麻疹常见的眼部症状为结膜炎和角膜炎。眼结膜及口腔黏膜表面会出现 1~2mm 有红晕的蓝白斑点，称为麻疹口腔黏膜斑（Koplik 氏斑）。其他眼部症状包括球结膜和睑板结膜充血和结膜下出血。荧光染色后，麻疹角膜炎表现为双侧对称性的点状的角膜上皮和皮下病变[189,190]。

在发展中国家，病毒性结膜炎混合细菌感染后引发角膜穿孔、全角膜炎和眼球结核，从而导致失明[191,192]。有报道称，麻疹引发的脉络膜视网膜炎和视神经炎可导致视力丧失[193,194]。在没有其他神经性症状表现的情况下，亚急性硬化性全脑炎可导致皮质盲[195]。

在发展中国家，麻疹可通过多种不同的致病机制导致角膜性失明。麻疹相关的营养不良使得维生素 A 缺乏，导致干眼症、角膜坏死或者角膜软化症[196]。眼睛表面发生细菌性或疱疹性角膜炎会导致角膜结疤或穿孔。发展中国家采用的有害的传统治疗方法也被认为是原因之一[197]。

麻疹的诊断依靠临床表现，从唾液、血液和黏膜中分离到副黏病毒可以作为辅助诊断依据，体液抗体反应也有助于进行确诊。

目前，对麻疹病毒还没有可行的治疗方法。可对全身和眼部症状进行支持治疗。尽管患者症状消失后角膜上皮损伤仍会存在，但是健康的患者在麻疹性角膜炎痊愈后通常不会留有后遗症。对营养不良的患者推荐使用角膜润滑剂。细菌性角膜炎可进行适当的抗生素治疗。维生素 A 治疗能减轻眼部和全身症状发病率，也能降低营养不良儿童的死亡率[198]。

腮腺炎

腮腺炎是属于副黏病毒科的另一种 RNA 病毒引起的。腮腺炎是一种全身性疾病，绝大部分患者为儿童，偶尔可见未免疫成年人患病。自从 1967 年出现腮腺炎减毒活疫苗后，发病率下降。1985 年，美国腮腺炎病例最低降至 2982 例。1987 年，报告发病 12 848 例，反映出腮腺炎在青少年人群中发病率上升[199]。这是由于这部分人群未进行免疫接种，并且存在 10%~25% 的免疫失败率[200]。

病毒传播途径为感染者唾液到其他人的呼吸道，接触 2~3 周后发病[201]。病毒感染后出现全身症状，包括腮腺炎、脑膜炎、耳聋、脑炎、附睾炎、睾丸炎、胰腺炎、心肌炎、肾炎及甲状腺炎[202]。

对腮腺炎缺乏免疫力的成人可能会出现唾液分泌增多症状。按发病率降序排列，眼部并发症依次为：泪腺炎（被称为泪腺腮腺炎）、结膜炎、巩膜炎、角膜炎、虹膜睫状体炎、视神经炎、视网膜炎及眼外肌肉瘫痪[203~205]。双侧泪腺炎一般需要数周才能痊愈。泪腺炎后期并发症为干燥性角膜炎综合征或严重的干眼症。成人腮腺炎的诊断基于临床症状、唾液和泪液中的病毒分离及抗体滴度的升高。成人腮腺炎的治疗建议采用支持疗法（表7.14）。可使用睫状肌麻痹滴眼液来缓解眼睑抽搐带来的不适，使用局部皮质类固醇治疗眼内炎症。视神经视网膜炎可使用全身类固醇治疗。免疫接种仍然是控制疾病传播的最佳手段。

表 7.14　腮腺炎的诊断和治疗

眼部症状	治疗
泪腺炎，结膜炎，巩膜炎，角膜炎，巩膜睫状体炎，视神经炎，视网膜炎，眼外肌瘫痪	接种疫苗预防感染 支持疗法 外用类固醇和睫状肌麻痹药 对视神经视网膜炎进行全身性类固醇治疗

风疹

风疹属于披膜病毒科的一种 RNA 病毒，通过呼吸道分泌物传播。风疹病毒通常引起发热性疾病，并伴随出疹、关节疼痛和淋巴结肿大。但如果孕妇在妊娠早期感染风疹，则

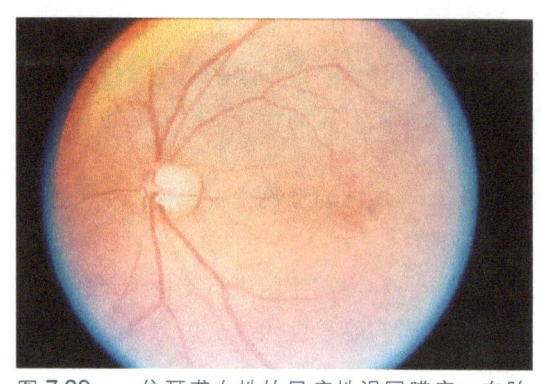

图 7.29 一位耳聋女性的风疹性视网膜病。在胎儿期由风疹感染导致的椒盐状视网膜色素改变。视觉仅略微受到影响。

出生婴儿将会出现严重的并发症[206~208]。

1941 年，有报道称风疹病毒的致畸作用为先天性心脏病、白内障和耳聋的同时发生。最常见的眼部症状为白内障，其他眼部症状包括角膜水肿、巩膜基质萎缩及由视网膜色素上皮细胞内色素分布不均导致的色素视网膜病变。风疹视网膜病变呈现椒盐状眼底，并在生命的最初几年内持续发展（图 7.29）。累及黄斑的视网膜下新血管生成可导致风疹视网膜患者视力下降[209~211]。发展为青光眼的先天性风疹儿童视力低下[212]。其他并发症包括小视网膜、小角膜、斜视、眼球震颤及眼性斜颈。成人风疹在接受全身皮质类固醇治疗时可能会导致视网膜炎[213]。

通过临床症状和抗体滴度测定可对风疹进行诊断。治疗风疹感染可用支持疗法，如有必要可对眼科症状进行治疗（如对先天性白内障实施白内障摘除术）。减毒活疫苗接种可预防这种疾病。接种风疹疫苗后很少见感觉异常、视神经炎和脊髓炎[214~219]。风疹视网膜病的鉴别诊断见表 7.15。

表 7.15 风疹的鉴别诊断

TORCHS 综合征：弓形虫病（TO）、风疹（R）、巨细胞包涵体病（C）、单纯疱疹（H）和梅毒（S）。
弓形虫病（TO）：对中枢神经系统和视网膜有特殊亲和力。患者的视网膜和玻璃体细胞将会发生白色到米色病变。如果前葡萄膜炎患者表现出症状，可使用局部类固醇和睫状肌麻痹剂治疗。
风疹（R）：健康个体也有外周视网膜病变，但是靠近视神经或黄斑区的病变应以乙胺嘧啶、亚叶酸、磺胺嘧啶或含有磺胺嘧啶的克林霉素治疗。也可用甲氧苄氨嘧啶/新诺明，添加或不添加克林霉素治疗。还可口服泼尼松。
巨细胞包涵体病（C）：CMV 属于疱疹病毒家族，对人体器官具有广泛的感染谱。视网膜脉络膜炎是最常见的眼部症状，表现为白色到米色病变且伴有出血。治疗药物包括更昔洛韦、膦甲酸、西多福韦、福米韦生和缬更昔洛韦。
单纯疱疹（H）：单纯疱疹引起角膜结膜炎，导致干眼症、角膜炎和葡萄膜炎。角膜炎具有典型的树枝状溃疡，可使用局部抗病毒制剂治疗，如阿糖腺苷、曲氟尿苷、疱疹净，也可利用清创术治疗。
梅毒（S）：梅毒螺旋体是感染源，性接触是最常见的传播方式。梅毒诊断方法包括性病研究实验室（venereal disease research laboratory, VDRL）的检测或 FTA-ABS 检测（fluorescent treponemal antibody absorption, FTA-ABS）；治疗可使用抗生素，如青霉素。

小核糖核酸病毒

柯萨奇病毒 A24（coxsackievirus A24, CA24）和肠道病毒 70（enterovirus 70, EV70）可引起急性出血性结膜炎（acute hemorrhagic conjunctivitis, AHC）。这些 RNA 病毒属于小核糖核酸病毒科[220]。AHC 因其高度传染的特性而被人所熟知。传播方式是人–人传播或通过污染物传播。

1969 年，在西非加纳发现了 AHC[221]。1980~1982 年，在加勒比海、南美洲北部、中美洲和佛罗里达州南部报告了超过 200 万病例[222]。2003 年春天，巴西开始暴发由 CA24

导致的 AHC，大约 20 万人受到感染，并且传播到了中美洲，最终导致波多黎各大约 49 万人受到感染。学龄儿童（5~18 岁）和城市密集居住区的居民都是最易感染的高危人群[223]。

经过 1~2 天的短潜伏期后，AHC 表现为骤发性眼皮肿胀、眼结膜出血、异物感、畏光及眼部疼痛（图 7.30）。累及双眼是其典型特点，一侧眼部感染后 24h 对侧眼部也感染[224]。感染的眼部可能会发展为上皮性角膜炎，甚至发生继发性细菌感染，导致视力丧失。全身症状包括不适、肌痛、发热、头痛、精神萎靡、有痰的上呼吸道症状及耳前淋巴结肿大，症状可持续 2~3 周。结膜炎发作后 10~20 天或 AHC 发作后 3 个月都可能会出现神经症状。万分之一的病例会出现神经性后遗症，其中 1/3 可能会出现永久性神经损伤，如面部或下肢的脊髓灰质炎样瘫痪、颅神经受累和原发性视神经萎缩症[225]。病毒在结膜和角膜上皮细胞内复制后导致表面缺损[226]。

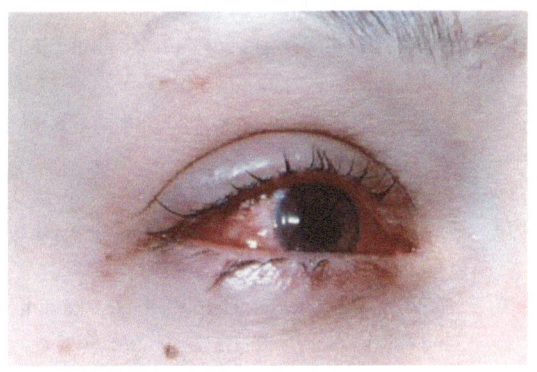

图 7.30　柯萨奇病毒和肠道病毒相关的 AHC。患者出现疼痛、瘙痒和畏光症状。眼睛因明显结膜下出血而发红。

急性、疼痛和出血性结膜炎可作为诊断依据。通过对结膜拭子中 EV70 或 CA24 的组织病理学鉴定进行确诊。在疾病活动期，69% 的患者血液中 EV70 IgM 抗体出现 4 倍及 4 倍以上升高[227]。鉴别诊断疾病包括眼损伤、其他病毒性感染、细菌性结膜炎和过敏性结膜炎。

AHC 的治疗是以冷敷为主的支持疗法，如果怀疑发生继发性细菌感染，可适量添加抗生素，不应局部使用皮质类固醇[228]。培养患者的卫生意识非常重要，包括严格的预防感染措施，勤洗手，避免共用毛巾、被褥和化妆品等。

总结

眼部是病毒感染的常见部位。病毒性眼部疾病范围广泛，从腺病毒结膜炎等自限性疾病，到可能损伤视力的疱疹性眼病并发症及可能危及生命的疾病，如免疫受损患者中的 CMV 感染。及时诊断和恰当治疗对降低病毒性眼部疾病视力损伤的发病率非常重要。由于某些病毒性眼病的症状非常复杂，所以可能需要各科医师进行会诊。

参 考 文 献

[1]　Faber DW, Wiley CA, Lynn GB, Gross JG, Freeman WR. Role of HIV and CMV in pathogenesis of retinitis and retinal vasculopathy in AIDS patients. Invest Ophthal Vis Sci 1992;33:2345–2353.

[2]　Leisegang TJ, Melton III LJ, Daly PJ, Ilstrup DM. Epidemiology of ocular herpes simplex. Incidence in Rochester, Minn, 1950 through 1982. Arch Ophthalmol 1989;107:1155–1159.

[3]　Nahmias A, Roisman B. Infection with herpes simplex viruses I and II. Part III. N Engl J Med 1973;289:781–789.

[4] O'Connor GR. Recurrent herpes simplex uveitis in humans. Surv Ophthalmol 1976;21:165–170.

[5] Nahmias AJ, Alford CA, Korones SB. Infection of the newborn with herpesvirus hominis.Adv Pediatr 1970;17:185–226.

[6] Cook SD, Hill JH. Herpes simplex virus: molecular biology and the possibility of corneal latency. Surv Ophthalmol 1991;36:140–148.

[7] Pepose JS.Herpes simplex keratitis: role of viral infection vs. immune response. Surv Ophthalmol 1991;35:345–352.

[8] Cook SD. Herpes simplex virus in the eye. Br J Ophthalmol 1992;76:365–366.

[9] Liesegang TJ. Biology and molecular aspects of herpes simplex and varicella-zoster virus infections. Ophthalmology 1992;99:781–799.

[10] Hyndiuk RA, Glasser. Herpes simplex keratitis. In:Tabbara KF, Hyndiuk RA, eds. Infections of the Eye, 2nd ed. Boston: Little, Brown, 1996:366.

[11] Pavan-Langston D. Viral disease of the cornea and external eye. In: Albert DM, Jakobiec FA, eds. Principles and Practice of Ophthalmology. Philadelphia:Saunders, 1994:122.

[12] Nahmias A, Roisman B. Infection with herpes simplex viruses I and II. Part III. N Engl J Med 1973;289:781–789.

[13] Blaum J. Morphogenesis of the dendritic figure in herpes simplex keratitis. A negative study. Am J Ophthalmol 1970;70:722–724.

[14] Paven-Langston D. Major ocular viral infections. In:Galasso G, Whitley R, Merrigan T, eds. Antiviral Agents and Viral Diseases of Man, 3rd ed. New York:Raven Press, 1990:183.

[15] Kaufman H, Raefield M. Viral conjunctivitis and keratitis:Herpes simplex virus. In: Kaufman H, Barron B, McDonald M,Waltman S, eds The Cornea. New York:Churchill Livingstone, 1988:299.

[16] Ostler HB. Herpes simplex: the primary infection.Surv Ophthalmol 1976;21:91–99.Figure 7.30. Acute hemorrhagic conjunctivitis associated with coxsackievirus and enterovirus. The patient has symptoms of pain, itching, and photophobia. The eye is red from prominent subconjunctival hemorrhage.

[17] Kimberlin D. Herpes simplex virus, meningitis and encephalitis in neonates. Herpes. 2004;11(suppl 2):65A–76A.

[18] Mommeja-Marin H, Lafaurie M, Scieux C, et al.Herpes simplex virus type 2 as a cause of severe meningitis in immunocompromised adults. Clin Infect Dis 2003;37:1527–1533.

[19] Wilhelmus KR, Coster DJ, Donovan HC, Falcon MG, Jones BR. Prognostic indicators of herpetic keratitis:Analysis of a five-year observation period after corneal ulceration. Arch Ophthalmol 1981;99:1578–1582.

[20] Hyndiuk RA, Glasser DB. Herpes simplex keratitis. In:Tabbara KF, Hyndiuk RA, eds. Infections of the Eye, 2nd ed. Boston: Little, Brown, 1996:367.

[21] You T, Paven-Langston D. Immune reactions in corneal herpetic disease. Int Ophthal Clin 1996;36:31–39.

[22] Abelson M, Pavan-Langston D. Viral uveitis. In:Schlaegel T, ed. Essentials of Uveitis. Int Ophthalmol Clin 1977;17:109–120.

[23] O'Connor GR. Recurrent herpes simplex uveitis in humans. Surv Ophthalmol 1976;21:165–170.

[24] Meyers JF. Immunology of herpes simplex virus infection.Int Ophthalmol Clin 1975;15:37–47.

[25] Sillis M. Clinical evaluation of enzyme immunoassay in rapid diagnosis of herpes simplex infections. J Clin Pathol 1992;45:165–167.

[26] Chichili GR, Athmanathan S, Farhatullah S, et al. Multiplex polymerase chain reaction for the detection of herpes simplex virus, varicella-zoster virus, and cytomegalovirus in ocular specimens. Curr Eye Res

2003;27:85–90.

[27] O'Day DM. Herpes simplex keratitis. In: Leibowitz H, ed. Corneal Disorders: Clinical Diagnosis and Management.Philadelphia: Saunders, 1984:387.

[28] LaLau C, Oosterhuis JA,Versteeg J, et al.Acyclovir and trifluorothymidine in herpetic keratitis—a multicenter trial. Br J Ophthalmol 1982;66:506–508.

[29] Wilhelmus KR. The treatment of herpes simplex virus epithelial keratitis. Trans Am Ophthalmol Soc. 2000;98:505–532.

[30] Kimura SJ, Okumoto M. The effect of corticosteroids on experimental herpes simplex keratoconjunctivitis in the rabbit. Am J Ophthalmol 1957;43:131.

[31] Ostler HB. Glucocorticoid therapy in ocular herpes simplex. I. Limitations. Surv Ophthalmol 1978;23:35–43.

[32] Sanitato J, Asbell P, Varnell E, Kissling GE, Kaufman HE. Acyclovir in the treatment of herpetic stromal disease. Am J Ophthalmol 1984;98:537–547.

[33] Schwab IR. Oral acyclovir in the management of herpes simplex ocular infections. Ophthalmology 1988;95:423–430.

[34] Teich SA, Cheung RW, Friedman AH. Systemic antiviral drugs used in ophthalmology. Surv Ophthalmol 1992;37:19–53.

[35] The Epithelial Keratitis Trial. The Herpetic Eye Disease Study Group A controlled trial of oral acyclovir for the prevention of stromal keratitis or iritis in patients with herpes simplex virus epithelial keratitis. Arch Ophthalmol 1997;115:703–712.

[36] Cohen EJ, Laibson PR. The use of corticosteroids in herpes simplex keratitis. In: Blodi FC, ed. Herpes Simplex Infections of the Eye. New York: Churchill Livingstone, 1984:109–116.

[37] Collum LMT, Logan P, Ravenscroft T. Acyclovir (Zovirax) in herpetic disciform keratitis. Br J Ophthalmol 1983;67:115–118.

[38] Barron BA, Gee L, Hauck WW, et al. Herpetic Eye Disease Study. A controlled trial of oral acyclovir for herpes simplex stromal keratitis. Ophthalmology 1994;101(12):1871–1882.

[39] The Herpetic Eye Disease Study Group. A controlled trial of oral acyclovir for iridocyclitis caused by herpes simplex virus. Arch Ophthalmol 1996;114(9):1065–1072.

[40] Herpetic Eye Disease Study Group. Oral acyclovir for herpes simplex virus eye disease: effect on prevention of epithelial keratitis and stromal keratitis. Arch Ophthalmol 2000;118:1030–1036.

[41] Herpetic Eye Disease Study Group. Acyclovir for the prevention of recurrent herpes simplex virus eye disease. N Engl J Med 1998;339(5):300–306.

[42] Foster CS, Barney NP. Systemic acyclovir and penetrating keratoplasty for herpes simplex keratitis. Doc Ophthalmol 1992;80:363–369.

[43] Young TL, Robin JB, Holland GN, et al. Herpes simplex keratitis in patients with acquired immune deficiency syndrome. Ophthalmology 1989;96:1476–1479.

[44] Weller TH.Varicella-herpes Zoster virus. In: Evans AS, ed. Viral Infections of Humans. Epidemiology and Control. New York: Plenum, 1976:457–480.

[45] Chang S, De Luise V. Varicella and herpes zoster ophthalmicus. In: Duane's Clinical Ophthalmology, vol 4.Philadelphia: JB Lippincott, 1996:1.

[46] Pavan-Langston D. Varicella-zoster ophthalmicus. Int Ophthalmol Clin 1975;15:171–185.

[47] Gershon A. Varicella in mother and infant. In:Krugman S, Gershon A, eds. Infections of the Fetus and the Newborn Infant. New York: Alan R Liss,1975:79.

[48] Charles NC, Bennett TW, Margolis S. Ocular pathology of the congenital varicella syndrome. Arch Ophthalmol 1977;95:2034–2037.

[49] Lambert S, Taylor D, Kriss A, Holzel H, Heard S. Ocular manifestations of the congenital varicella syndrome. Arch Ophthalmol 1989;107:52–56.

[50] Juel-Jensen BE, MacCallum FO. Herpes Simplex, Varicella and Zoster: Clinical Manifestations and Treatment. Philadelphia: JB Lippincott, 1972.

[51] Yamamoto S, Tada R, Shimomura Y, Pavan-Langston D, Dunkel EC, Tano Y. Detecting varicella-zoster virus DNA in iridocyclitis using polymerase chain reaction:a case of zoster sine herpete. Arch Ophthalmol 1995;113:1358–1359.

[52] Osler HB, Thygeson P. The ocular manifestations of herpes zoster, varicella, infectious mononucleosis and cytomegalovirus disease. Surv Ophthalmol 1976;21:148–159.

[53] Jones DB. Herpes Zoster Ophthalmicus. In: Golden B,ed. Ocular Inflammatory Disease. Springfield, IL:Thomas, 1974:198–209.

[54] Liesegang T. Corneal complications from herpes zoster ophthalmicus. Ophthalmology 1985;92:316–324.

[55] O'Brien JJ, Campoli-Richards DM. Acyclovir: an updated review of its antiviral activity, pharmacokinetic properties, and therapeutic efficacy. Drugs 1989;37:233–309.

[56] McKendrick MW, McGill JI, White JE, Wood MJ. Oral acyclovir in acute herpes zoster.Br Med J (Clin Res Ed) 1986;293:1529–1532.

[57] Cobo LM, Foulks GN, Liesegang T, et al. Oral acyclovir in the therapy of acute herpes zoster ophthalmicus. Ophthalmology 1985;92:1574–1583.

[58] Hoang-Xuan T, Buechi ER, Herbort CP, et al. Oral acyclovir for herpes zoster ophthalmicus. An interim report. Ophthalmology 1992;99:1062–1071.

[59] Herbort CP, Buechi ER, Piguet B, Zografos L, Fitting P. High-dose oral acyclovir in acute herpes zoster ophthalmicus: the end of the corticosteroid era. Curr Eye Res 1991;10(suppl):171–175.

[60] Aylward GW, Claou CMP, Marsh RJ, Yasseem N. Influence of oral acyclovir on ocular complications of herpes zoster ophthalmicus. Eye 1994;8:70–74.

[61] Tyring S, Barbarash RN, Nahlik JE, et al. (Collaborative Famciclovir Herpes Zoster Study Group). Famciclovir for the treatment of acute herpes zoster: effects on acute disease and postherpetic neuralgia: a randomized, double-blind, placebo-controlled trial. Ann Intern Med 1995;123:89–96.

[62] Acosta EP, Fletcher CV. Valacyclovir Ann Pharmacother 1997;31(2):185–191.

[63] Physicians' Desk Reference. 1997:1168.

[64] Wilson FM II.Varicella and herpes zoster ophthalmicus. In: Tabbara KF,Hyndiuk RA, eds. Infections of the Eye. Boston: Little, Brown, 1986:369.

[65] Sanfor E, Croxson T, Millner A, Mildvan D. Herpes zoster ophthalmicus in patients at risk for AIDS. N Engl J Med 1984;310:1118–1119.

[66] Kestelyn P, Stevens AM, Bakkers E, Rouvroy D,Van de Perre P. Severe herpes zoster ophthalmicus in young African adults: a marker for HTLV-III seropositivity. Br J Ophthalmol 1987;71:806–809.

[67] Margolis TP, Milner MS, Shama A, Hodge W, Seiff S. Herpes zoster ophthalmicus in patients with human immunodeficiency virus infection. Am J Ophthalmol 1998;125(3):285–291.

[68] Seiff SR, Margolis T, Graham SH, O'Donnell JJ. Use of intravenous acyclovir for treatment of herpes zoster ophthalmicus in patients at risk for AIDS. Ann Ophthalmol 1998;20:480–482.

[69] Engstrom RE Jr, Holland GN, Margolis TP, et al. The progressive outer retinal necrosis syndrome: a variant of necrotizing herpetic retinopathy in patients with AIDS. Ophthalmology 1994;101:1488–1502.

[70] Holland GN. The progressive outer retinal necrosis syndrome. Int Ophthalmol 1994;18:163–165.

[71] Perez-Blazquez E, Traspar R, Mendez MI, Montero M. Intravitreal ganciclovir treatment in progressive outer retinal necrosis. Am J Ophthalmol 1997;124:418–421.

[72] Ciulla TA, Rutledge BK, Morley MG, Duker JS. The progressive outer retinal necrosis syndrome: successful treatment with combination antiviral therapy. Ophthalmic Surg Lasers 1998;29:198–206.

[73] Fisher JP, Lewis ML, Blumenkranz M, et al. The acute retinal necrosis syndrome. Part 1: clinical manifestations. Ophthalmology 1982;89:1309–1316.

[74] Ludwiz IH, Zegarra H, Zakov ZN. The acute retinal necrosis syndrome: possible herpes simplex retinitis. Ophthalmology 1984;91:1659–1664.

[75] Duker JS, Nielsen JC, Eagle RC, Bosley TM, Granadier R, Benson WE. Rapidly progressive acute retinal necrosis secondary to herpes simplex virus, type 1. Ophthalmology 1990;97(12):1638–1643.

[76] Yeo JH, Pepose JS, Stewart JA, et al. Acute retinal necrosis syndrome following herpes zoster dermatitis. Ophthalmology 1986;93:1418–1422.

[77] Mitchell SM, Fox JD, Tedder RS, et al. Vitreous fluid sampling and viral genome detection for the diagnosis of viral retinitis in patients with AIDS. J Med Virol 1994;43:336–340.

[78] Guex-Crosier Y, Rochat C, Herbort CP. Necrotizing herpetic retinopathies. A spectrum of herpes virusinduced diseases determined by the immune state of the host. Ocul Immunol Inflamm 1997;5:259–265.

[79] Blumenkranz MS, Culbertson WW, Clarkson JG, Dix R. Treatment of the acute retinal necrosis syndrome with intravenous acyclovir. Ophthalmology 1986;93:296–300.

[80] Figueroa MS, Garabito I, Gutierrez C, Fortun J. Famciclovir for the treatment of acute retinal necrosis (ARN) syndrome. Am J Ophthalmol 1997;123:255–257.

[81] Luu KK, Scott IU, Chaudhry NA, et al. Intravitreal antiviral injections as adjunctive therapy in the management of immunocompetent patients with necrotizing herpetic retinopathy. Am J Ophthalmol 2000;129:811–813.

[82] Chau Tran TH, Cassoux N, Bodaghi B, Lehoang P. Successful treatment with combination of systemic antiviral drugs and intravitreal ganciclovir injections in the management of severe necrotizing herpetic retinitis. Ocul Immunol Inflamm 2003;11:141–144.

[83] Epstein MA, Achong BG, Barr YM. Virus particles in cultured lymphoblasts from Burkitt's lymphoma. Lancet 1964;1:702–703.

[84] Rickinson AB. On the biology of Epstein-Barr virus persistence: a reappraisal. In: Lopez C, ed. Immunobiology and Prophylaxis of Herpesvirus Infections. New York: Plenum, 1990:137–146.

[85] Klein G. Viral latency and transformation: the strategy of Epstein-Barr virus. Cell 1989;58:5–8.

[86] Henle W, Henle G. Epstein-Barr virus and infectious mononucleosis. N Engl J Med 1973;288:263–264.

[87] Henle G, Henle W, Diehl V. Relation of Burkitt's tumorassociated herpes-type virus to infectious mononucleosis. Proc Natl Acad Sci USA 1968;59:94–101.

[88] Lenoir GM. Role of the virus chromosomal translocations and cellular oncogens in the etiology of Burkitt's lymphoma. In: Epstein MA, Achong BG, eds. The Epstein-Barr Virus: Recent Advances. New York: John Wiley, 1986:184–207.

[89] Henle G, Henle W. Epstein-Barr virus-specific IgA serum antibodies as an outstanding feature of nasopharyngeal carcinoma. Int J Cancer 1976;17:1–7.

[90] Leyvraz S, Henle W, Chahinian AP, et al. Association of Epstein-Barr virus with thymic carcinoma. N Engl J Med 1985;312:1296–1299.

[91] Pflugfelder SC, Roussel TJ, Culbertson WW. Primary Sjogren's syndrome after infectious mononucleosis. JAMA 1987;257:1049–1050.

[92] Miyasaka N, Saito I, Haruta J. Possible involvement of Epstein-Barr virus in the pathogenesis of Sjogren's syndrome. Clin Immunol Immuopathol 1994;72:166–170.

[93] Alvarado JA, Murphy CG, Juter RP, Hetherington J. Pathogenesis of Chandler's syndrome, essential iris atrophy and the Cogan-Reese syndrome. II: estimate age at disease onset. Invest Ophthal Vis Sci 1986;27:873–882.

[94] Evans AS, Niederman JC, Cenabre LC, West B, Richards VA. A prospective evaluation of heterophile and Epstein-Barr virus-specific IgM antibody tests in clinical and subclinical infectious mononucleosis: specificity and sensitivity of the tests and persistence of antibody. J Infect Dis 1975;132:546–554.

[95] Henle W, Henle G. Observations on childhood infections with Epstein-Barr virus. J Infect Dis 1970;121:303–310.

[96] Niederman JC, Evans AS, Subrahmanyan L, McCullom RW. Prevalence, incidence and persistence of EB virus antibody in young adults. N Engl J Med 1970;282:361–365.

[97] Raymond LA, Wilson CA, Linnemann CC, Ward MA, Bernstein DI, Love DC. Punctate outer retinitis in acute Epstein-Barr virus infection. Am J Ophthalmol 1987;104:424–425.

[98] Tiedeman JS. Epstein-Barr Viral antibodies in multifocal choroiditis and panuveitis. Am J Ophthalmol 1987;103:659–663.

[99] Remington JS, JO Klein, eds. Infectious Diseases of the Newborn Infant. Philadelphia: WB Saunders, 1976.

[100] Matoba AY. Ocular disease associated with Epstein-Barr virus infection. Surv Ophthalmol 1990;35:145–150.

[101] Pflugfelder SC, Crouse CA, Atherton SS. Ophthalmic manifestations of Epstein-Barr virus infection. Int Ophthalmol Clin 1993;33:95–101.

[102] Krech U, Jung M, Jung F. Cytomegalovirus Infections of Man. New York: S Karger, 1971.

[103] Skolnik PR, Kosloff BR, Hirsch MS. Bidirectional interactions between human immunodeficiency virus type 1 and cytomegalovirus. J. Infect Dis 1988;157:508–513.

[104] Sison RF, Holland GN, MacArthur LJ, Wheeler NC, Gottlieb MS. Cytomegalovirus retinopathy as the initial manifestation of the acquired immunodeficiency syndrome. Am J Ophthalmol 1991;112:243–249.

[105] Palella FJ, Delaney KM, Moorman AC, et al. Declining morbidity and mortality among patients with advanced human immunodeficiency virus infection. N Engl J Med 1998;338:853–860.

[106] Drew WL. Cytomegalovirus infection in patients with AIDS. J Infect Dis 1988;158:449–456.

[107] Cochereau-Massin I, LeHoang P, Lautier-Frau M, et al. Ocular toxoplasmosis in human immunodeficiency virus-infected patients. Am J Ophthalmol 1992;114:130–135.

[108] Schanzer MC, Font RL, O'Malley RE. Primary ocular malignant lymphoma associated with the acquired immune deficiency syndrome. Ophthalmology 1991;98:88–91.

[109] Levine AM. Epidemiology, clinical characteristics, and management of AIDS-related lymphoma. Hematol Clin North Am 1991;5:331–342.

[110] Aldave AJ, King JA, Cunningham ET Jr. Ocular syphilis. Curr Opin Ophthalmol 2001;12:433–441.

[111] Jabs DA, Newman C, De Bustros S, Polk BF. Treatment of cytomegalovirus retinitis with ganciclovir. Ophthalmology 1987;94:824–830.

[112] Lehoang P, Girard B, Robinet M, et al. Foscarnet in the treatment of cytomegalovirus retinitis in acquired

immune deficiency syndrome. Ophthalmology. 1989; 96:865–873; discussion 873–734.

[113] Jacobson MA, Drew WL, Feinberg J, et al. Foscarnet therapy for ganciclovir-resistant cytomegalovirus retinitis in patients with AIDS. J Infect Dis. 1991;163:1348–1351.

[114] Lalezari JP, Stagg RJ, Kuppermann BD, et al. Intravenous cidofovir for peripheral cytomegalovirus retinitis in patients with AIDS. A randomized, controlled trial. J Acquir Immune Defic Syndr Hum Retrovirol. 1998;17:339–344.

[115] Martin DF, Sierra-Madero J, Walmsley S, et al. A controlled trial of valganciclovir as induction therapy for cytomegalovirus retinitis. N Engl J Med 2002;346:1119–1126.

[116] Musch DC, Martin DF, Gordon JF, et al. Treatment of cytomegalovirus retinitis with a sustained-release ganciclovir implant. N Engl J Med 1997;337:83–90.

[117] Martin DF, Kuppermann BD, Wolitz RA, Palestine AG, Li H, Robinson CA. Oral ganciclovir for patients with cytomegalovirus retinitis treated with a ganciclovir implant. N Engl J Med 1999;340:1063–1070.

[118] Proceedings on meeting of drug resistance in cytomegalovirus: current knowledge and implications for patient management. J Acquir Immune Defic Syndr Hum Retrovirol 1996;2(suppl 1):1–22.

[119] Perry CM, Balfour JA. Fomivirsen. Drugs 1999;57(3):375–380.

[120] Stone TW, Jaffe GJ. Reversible bull's-eye maculopathy associated with intravitreal fomivirsen therapy for cytomegalovirus retinitis. Am J Ophthalmol 2000;130(2):242–243.

[121] Deeks SG, Smith M, Holodniy M, Kahn JO. HIV-1 protease inhibitors. A review for clinicians. JAMA 1997;277:145–153.

[122] Nguyen QD, Kempen JH, Bolton SG, et al. Immune recovery uveitis in patients with AIDS and cytomegalovirus retinitis after highly active antiretroviral therapy. Am J Ophthalmol 2000;129:634–639.

[123] Henderson HW, Mitchell SM. Treatment of immune recovery vitreitis with local steroids. Br J Ophthalmol 1999;83:540–545.

[124] El-Bradey MH, Cheng L, Song MK, et al. Long-term results of treatment of macular complications in eyes with immune recovery uveitis using a graded treatment approach. Retina 2004;24:376–382.

[125] Arevalo JF, Mendoza AJ, Ferretti Y. Immune recovery uveitis in AIDS patients with cytomegalovirus retinitis treated with highly active antiretroviral therapy in Venezuela. Retina 2003;23:495–502.

[126] Karavellas MP, Azen SP, MacDonald JC, et al. Immune recovery vitreitis and uveitis in AIDS: clinical predictors, sequelae, and treatment outcomes. Retina 2001;21:1–9.

[127] Jabs DA, Bolton SG, Dunn JP, Palestine AG. Discontinuing anticytomegalovirus therapy in patients with immune reconstitution after combination antiretroviral therapy. Am J Ophthalmol 1998;126:817–822.

[128] Kupperman BD, Petty JG, Richman DD, et al. Correlation between CD4+ counts and prevalence of cytomegalovirus retinitis and human immunodeficiency virus-related noninfectious retinal vasculopathy in patients with acquired immunodeficiency syndrome. Am J Ophthalmol 1993;115:575–582.

[129] Chang Y, Cesarman E, Pessin MS, et al. Identification of herpes virus-like DNA sequences in AIDS associated sarcoma. Science 1994;266:1865–1869.

[130] Levy JA. Three new human herpesviruses (HHV6, 7, and 8). Lancet 1997;349:558–563.

[131] Hatcher VA. Mucocutaneous infections in acquired immune deficiency syndrome. In: Friedman-Kien AE, Laubenstein LJ, eds. AIDS: The Epidemic of Kaposi's Sarcoma and Opportunistic Infections. New York: Masson, 1984:245–251.

[132] Dugel PU, Gill PS, Frangieh GT, Rao NA. Ocular adnexal Kaposi's sarcoma in acquired immunodeficiency syndrome. Am J Ophthalmol 1990;110:500–503.

[133] Shuler JD, Holland GN, Miles SA, Miller BJ, Grossman I. Kaposi's sarcoma of the conjunctiva and

eyelids associated with the acquired immunodeficiency syndrome. Arch Ophthalmol 1989;107:858–862.

[134] Dugel PU, Gill PS, Frangieh GT, Rao NA. Treatment of ocular adnexal Kaposi's sarcoma in acquired immune deficiency syndrome. Ophthalmology 1992;99:1127–1132.

[135] Epstein WL. Molluscum contagiosum. Semin Dermatol 1992;11:184–189.

[136] Charteris DG, Bonshek RE, Tullo AB. Ophthalmic molluscum contagiosum: clinical and immunopathological features. Br J Ophthalmol 1995;79:476–481.

[137] Deoreo GA, Johnson HH Jr, Binkey GW. An eczemous reaction associated with molluscum contagiosum. Arch Dermatol 1956;74:344–348.

[138] Margo C, Katz NNK. Management of periocular molluscum contagiosum in children. J. Pediatric Ophthalmol Strabismus 1993;20:19–21.

[139] Pepose JS, Esposito JJ. Molluscum contagiosum, orf, and vaccinia. In: Pepose JS, Holland GN, Wilhelmus KR, eds. Ocular Infection and Immunity. St. Louis:Mosby, 1986:846–856.

[140] Charteris DG, Bonshek RE, Tullo AB. Ophthalmic molluscum contagiosum: clinical and immunopathological features. Br J Ophthalmol 1995;79(5):476–481.

[141] Charles NC, Friedberg DN. Epibulbar molluscum contagiosum in acquired immune deficiency syndrome, case report and review of the literature. Ophthalmology 1992;99:1123–1126.

[142] Robinson MR, Udell IJ, Garber PF, Perry HD, Streeten BW. Molluscum contagiosum of the eyelids in patients with acquired immune deficiency syndrome. Ophthalmology 1992;99:1745–1747.

[143] Miller DM, Bredell RT, Levine MR. The conjunctival wart: report of a case and review of treatment options. Ophthalmic Surgery 1994;25(8):545–548.

[144] de Villiers EM. Heterogeneity of the human papilloma virus group. J Virol 1989;63:4898–4903.

[145] Quick CA, Watts SL, Krizyzek RA, Faras AJ. Relationship between condylomata and laryngeal papillomata:clinical and molecular biological evidence. Ann Otol Rhinol Laryngol 1980;89:467–471.

[146] de Villiers EM, Weidauer H, Otto H, Zur Hausen H. Papillomavirus DNA in human tongue carcinomas. Int J Cancer 1985;36:575–578.

[147] Madreperla SA, Green WR, Daniel R, Shah KV. Human papillomavirus in primary epithelial tumors of the lacrimal sac. Ophthalmology 1993;100(4):569–573.

[148] McDonnell PJ, McDonnell JM, Kessis T, Green WR, Shah KV. Detection of human papillomavirus type 6/11 DNA in conjunctival papillomas by in situ hybridization with radioactive probes. Hum Pathol 1987;18:1115–1119.

[149] McDonnell JM, Mayr AJ, Martin WJ. DNA of human papillomavirus Type 16 in dysplastic and malignant lesions of the conjunctiva and cornea. N Engl J Med 1989;320:1442–1446.

[150] Brescia RJ, Jenson AB, Lancaster WD, Kurman RJ. The role of human papillomaviruses in the pathogenesis and histological classification of precancerous lesions of the cervix. Hum Pathol 1986;17:552–559.

[151] Bonfiglio TA, Stoler MH. Human papillomavirus and cancer of the uterine cervix. Hum Pathol 1988;19:621–622.

[152] McDonnell JM, Wagner D, Bernstein G, Sun YY. Human papillomavirus type 16 DNA in ocular and cervical swabs of women with genital tract condylomata. Am J Ophthalmol 1991;112:61–66.

[153] McDonnell JM, McDonnell PK, Sun YY. Human papillomavirus DNA in tissues and ocular surface swabs of patients with conjunctival epithelial neoplasia. Invest Ophthalmol Vis Sci 1992;33:184–189.

[154] Scott IU, Karp CL, Nuovo GJ. Human papilloma virus 16 and 18 expression in conjunctival intraepithelial neoplasia. Ophthalmology 2000;109:542–547.

[155] Eng HL, Lin TM, Chen SY, Wu SM, Chen WJ. Failure to detect human papillomavirus DNA in malignant epithelial neoplasms of conjunctiva by polymerase chain reaction. Am J Clin Pathol 2002;117:429–436.

[156] Ash JE. Epibulbar tumors. Am J Ophthalmol 1950;33:1203.

[157] Erie JC, Campbell RJ, Liesegang TJ. Conjunctival and corneal intraepithelial and invasive neoplasia. Ophthalmology 1986;93:176–183.

[158] Petersen CS, Nurnberg BM. Carbon dioxide laser vaporization combined with perilesionally injected interferon alfa-2b in the treatment of a hyperkeratotic verruca vulgaris on the upper eyelid. Arch Dermatol 1994;130:1369–1370.

[159] de Keizer RJ, de Wolff-Rouendaal D. Topical alphainterferon in recurrent conjunctival papilloma. Acta Ophthalmol Scand 2003;81(2):193–196.

[160] Nakamura Y, Mashima Y, Kameyama K, Mukai M, Oguchi Y. Detection of human papillomavirus infection in squamous tumours of the conjunctiva and lacrimal sac by immunohistochemistry, in situ hybridization, and polymerase chain reaction. Br J Ophthalmol 1997;81:308–313.

[161] Pavan-Langston D. Viral disease of the cornea and external eye. In: Albert DM, Jakobiec FA, eds. Principles and Practice of Ophthalmology, Clinical Practice, vol. 1. Philadelphia: WB Saunders, 1994.

[162] Duke-Elder S. The adenoviruses. In: Duke-Elder S, ed. System of Ophthalmology, vol. 8. St. Louis: CV Mosby, 1965:348.

[163] O'Day D, Guyer B, Hierholzer J. Clinical and laboratory evaluation of epidemic keratoconjunctivitis due to adenoviruses type 8 and 19. Am J Ophthalmol 1976;81:207–215.

[164] Harnett. Newnham W. Isolation of adenovirus type 19 from the male and female genital tracts. Br J Vener Dis 1981;57:55–57.

[165] Gibson J, Darougar D, McSwiggan D, Thaker U. Comparative sensitivity of a cultural test and the complement fixation test in the diagnosis of adenovirus ocular infection. Br J Ophthamol 1979;63:617–620.

[166] Schwartz H, Vastine D, Yamashiroya H, West CE. Immunofluorescent detection of adenovirus antigen in EKC. Invest Ophthalmol 1976;15:199–207.

[167] Rodrigues M, Lennette D, Arentsen J, Thompson C. Methods for rapid detection of human ocular viral infections. Ophthalmology 1979;86:452–464.

[168] Romanowski EG, Yates KA, Gordon YJ. Topical corticosteroids of limited potency promote adenovirus replication in the Ad5/NZW rabbit ocular model. Cornea 2002;21:289–291.

[169] Vastine V. Adenoviruses and miscellaneous viral infections. In: Smolin G, Thoft R, eds. The Cornea, 2nd ed. Boston: Little, Brown, 1987:266.

[170] Freeman WR, Chen A, Henderly DE, et al. Prevalence and significance of acquired immunodeficiency syndrome-related retinal microvasculopathy. Am J Ophthalmol 1989;107:229–235.

[171] Jabs DA, Green WR, Fox R, Polk BF, Bartlett JG. Ocular manifestations of acquired immune deficiency syndrome. Ophthalmology 1989;96:1092–1099.

[172] Newsome DA. Microvascular aspects of acquired immune deficiency syndrome retinopathy. Am J Ophthalmol 1984;98:590–601.

[173] Pepose JS, Holland GN, Nestor MS, Cochran AJ, Foos RY. Acquired immune deficiency syndrome. Pathogenic mechanisms of ocular disease. Ophthalmology 1985;92:472–484.

[174] Pomerantz RJ, Kuritzkes DR, de la Monte SM, et al. Infection of the retina by human immunodeficiency virus type 1. N Engl J Med 1987;317:1643–1647.

[175] Engstrom RE, Holland GN, Hardy WD, Meiselman HJ. Hemorrhagic abnormalities in patients with

human immunodeficiency virus infection and ophthalmic microvasculopathy. Am J Ophthalmol 1990;109:153–161.

[176] Jabs DA, Green WR, Fox R, Polk BF, Bartlett JG. Ocular manifestations of acquired immune deficiency syndrome.Ophthalmology 1989;96:1092–1099.

[177] Rosenblatt MA, Cunningham C, Teich SS, Freidman AH.Choroidal lesions in patients with AIDS.Br J Ophthalmol 1990;74:610–614.

[178] Fraunfelder FW, Rosenbaum JT. Drug induced uveitis. Drug Safety 1997;17(3):197–207, 199.

[179] Whitcup SM, Dastgheib K, Nussenblatt RB, Walton RC, Pizzo PA, Chan CC. A clinical pathologic report of the retinal lesion associated with didanosine. Arch Ophthalmol 1994;112(12):1594–1598.

[180] Ray CG. Measles (rubeola). In: Thorn GW, et al., eds. Harrison's Principles of Internal Medicine, 8th ed., vol.1. New York: McGraw-Hill, 1977.

[181] Katz SL. Measles. In: Rudolph AM, Barnett HL, Einhord AH, eds. Pediatrics, 16th ed. New York:Appleton-Century-Crofts, 1977.

[182] Bergstrom TJ. Measles infection of the eye. In: Darrell RW, ed. Viral Diseases of the Eye. Philadelphia: Lea & Febiger, 1985:233–238.

[183] Measles mortality reduction—West Africa, 1996–2002.MMWR 2004;53:28–30.

[184] Awdrey PN, Cobb B, Adams PCG. Blindness in the Luapula Valley. Central Afr J Med 1967;13:197–201.

[185] Hinman AR, Brandling-Bennett AD, Nieburg PI. The opportunity and obligation to eliminate measles from the United States. JAMA 1979;242:1157–1162.

[186] Hinman AR, Brandling-Bennett AD, Bernier RH, Kirby CD, Eddins DL. Current features of measles in the United States. Epidemiol Rev 1980;2:153–170.

[187] Measles—United States, 1977–1980. MMWR 1980;29:598–599.

[188] Epidemiology of measles—United States, 2001–2003.MMWR 2004;53:713–716.

[189] Kayikcioglu O, Kir E, Soyler M, Guler C, Irkec M. Ocular findings in a measles epidemic among young adults. Ocul Immunol Inflamm 2000;8:59–62.

[190] Deckard PS, Bergstrom TJ. Rubeola keratitis. Ophthalmology 1980;88:810–813.

[191] Furgiuele FP, Hiles DA, Cignetti FE. Measles. In:Harley RD, ed. Pediatric Ophthalmology. Philadelphia:WB Saunders, 1975.

[192] Fedukowicz HB. Measles In External Infections of the Eye, 2nd ed. New York: Appleton-Century-Crofts,1978.

[193] Caruso JM, Robbins-Tien D, Brown WD, Antony JH, Gascon GG. Atypical chorioretinitis as an early presentation of subacute sclerosing panencephalitis. J Pediatr Ophthalmol Strabismus 2000;37:119–122.

[194] Azuma M, Morimura Y, Kawahara S, Okada AA. Bilateral anterior optic neuritis in adult measles infection without encephalomyelitis. Am J Ophthalmol 2002;134:768–769.

[195] Senbil N, Aydin OF, Orer H, Gurer YK. Subacute sclerosing panencephalitis: a cause of acute vision loss. Pediatr Neurol 2004;31:214–217.

[196] Sommer A. Xerophthalmia, keratomalacia and nutritional blindness. Int Ophthalmol 1990;14:195–199.

[197] Gilbert C, Awan H. Blindness in children. BMJ 2003;327:760–761.

[198] Hussey CD, Klein M. Measles-induced vitamin A deficiency. Ann NY Acad Sci 1992;669:188–194.

[199] Centers For Disease Control. Mumps—United States, 1985–1988. Leads from the MMWR. JAMA 1989;261:1702.

[200] Kim-Farley R, Bart S, Stetler H, et al. Clinical mumps vaccine efficacy. Am J Epidemiol 1985;121:593.

[201] Wilfert CM. Mumps. In: Joklik WK, ed. Principles of Animal Virology.New York: Appleton-Century-

Crofts, 1980.

[202] Foster ER, Lowder CY, Meisler DM, Kosmorsky GS, Baetz-Greenwalt B. Mumps neuroretinitis in an adolescent. Am J Ophthalmol 1990;110:91–93.

[203] Katavisto M.Ocular complications of epidemic parotitis. Acta Ophthalmol 1956;34:208.

[204] Bang HO, Bang J. Involvement of the central nervous system in mumps. Acta Med Scand 1943;113:487.

[205] Al-Rashid RA. Cress C. Mumps: uveitis complication the course of acute leukemia. J Peidatr Ophthal 1977;14(2):100–102.

[206] Yanoff M. The retina in rubella. In: Tasman W, ed. Retinal Disease in Children. New York: Harper and Row, 1971:223–232.

[207] Walff SM. The ocular manifestations of congenital rubella. A prospective study of 328 cases of congenital rubella. J Pediatr Ophthalmol 1973;10:101–141.

[208] Franceschetti A, Francois J, Babel J. Chorioretinal Heredodegenerations. Springfield, IL: Charles C. Thomas, 1974:1069.

[209] Slusher MM, Tyler ME. Rubella retinopathy and subretinal neovascularization. Ann Ophthalmol 1982;14(3):292–294.

[210] Orth DH, Fishman GA, Segall M, Bhatt A, Yassur Y. Rubella maculopathy. Br J Ophthalmol 1980;64:201–205.

[211] Frank KE, Purnell EW. Subretinal neovascularization following rubella retinopathy. Am J Ophthalmol 1978;86:462–466.

[212] Wolff SM. The ocular manifestations of congenital rubella. Trans Am Ophthal Soc 1972;70:577–614.

[213] Hayashi M, Yoshimura N, Kondo T. Acute rubella retinal pigment epitheliitis in an adult. Am J Ophthalmol 1982;93:285–288.

[214] Speier JE. Complications of rubella vaccination. JAMA 1970;213:2272.

[215] Kilroy AW, Schaffner W, Fleet WF, Lefkowitz LB Jr, Karzon DT, Fenichel GM. Two syndromes following rubella immunization. JAMA 1970;214:2287–2292.

[216] Gilmartin RC, Jabbour JR, Duenas DA.Rubella vaccine myeloradiculoneuritis. Pediatrics 1992;80:406–412.

[217] Rubella Surveillance Report. Atlanta: Center for Disease Control, August 1970.

[218] Rubella Surveillance Report. Atlanta: Centers for Disease Control, August 1976.

[219] Kline LB, Margulies SL, Oh SJ. Optic neuritis and myelitis following rubella vaccination. Arch Neurol 1982;39:443–444.

[220] Patriarca PA, Onorato IM, Sklar VEF, et al.Acute hemorrhagic conjunctivitis. investigation of a large-scale community outbreak in Dade County, Florida. JAMA 1983;249:1283–1289.

[221] Wright PW, Strauss GH, Langford MP. Acute hemorrhagic conjunctivitis.Am Fam Physician 1992;45:173–178.

[222] Patriarca PA. Clinical experience with acute hemorrhagic conjunctivitis in the United States. In: Uchida Y, Ishii K, Migamura K, Yamazaki S, eds. Acute Hem-orrhagic Conjunctivitis: Etiology, Epidemiology, and Clinical Manifestation. New York: Karger Press, 1989:49–56.

[223] Acute hemorrhagic conjunctivitis outbreak caused by Coxsackievirus A24—Puerto Rico, 2003. MMWR 2004;53:632–634.

[224] Uchida Y. Clinical features of acute hemorrhagic conjunctivitis due to enterovirus 70. In: Uchida Y, Ishii K, Miyamura K, Yamazaki S, eds. Acute Hemorrhagic Conjunctivitis: Etiology, Epidemiology, and Clinical Manifestation. New York: Karger Press, 1989:213–224.

[225] Chopra JS, Sawhney IM, Dhand UK, et al. Neurological complications of acute haemorrhagic conjunctivitis.J Neurol Sci 1986;73:177–191.

[226] Langford MP, Yin-Murphy M, Barber JC, Heard HK, Stanton GJ. Conjunctivitis in rabbits caused by enterovirus type 70 (EV 70). Invest Ophthalmol Vis Sci 1986;27:915–920.

[227] Wulff H, Anderson LJ, Pallansch MA, de Souza Carvalho RP. Diagnosis of enterovirus 70 infection by demonstration of IgM antibodies. J Med Virol 1987;21:321–327.

[228] Sklar VE, Patriarca PA, Onorato IM, et al. clinical findings and results of treatment in an outbreak of acute hemorrhagic conjunctivitis in southern Florida. Am J Ophthalmol 1983;95:45–54.

索 引

词条	页码
Buschke 和 Llöwenstein 巨大湿疣	17
Castleman 氏病	124
EB 病毒	112, 220
Heck 氏病	112, 124, 126~127, 144
HBGA	80
Toll 样受体	6, 11, 26
察内克试验	114
癌症	1, 16, 118, 123, 128
白色念珠菌	132~134
杯状病毒	59, 75~76, 78~79, 80~81, 84~85, 88, 91
鼻病毒	189~190, 198~200, 204
鼻相关淋巴组织	8~9, 32, 204
鼻咽癌	112, 121, 123, 220
鞭毛蛋白	11, 26, 30~31, 42
癣疽	117~119
病原体相关分子模式	11
肠道病毒-70	213
肠道细菌	23, 30, 36, 38, 43, 46, 50
肠道相关淋巴组织	8, 72
肠套叠	67, 73
出血	75, 82, 213, 221, 223~225, 229~230, 232, 234~235
川崎病	67
传染性单核细胞增多	112, 121~123, 220~221
传染性疾病	87, 136, 145, 213
传染性软疣	8, 18~19, 131, 149, 212~213, 225~226
唇疱疹	112~113, 115~118
大肠杆菌	2, 26, 44, 46, 49~50, 145
带状疱疹	112, 116, 119~120, 131, 144~145, 216~219, 221, 223, 230
带状疱疹病毒	112, 216, 219, 230
带状疱疹性眼病	216~219
单纯疱疹病毒	3, 7, 111, 213~215, 230
德国麻疹	128
痘病毒科	213
多发性骨髓瘤	124
防御素	3, 28, 203
肺部黏膜免疫	189, 202~203, 205
肺炎克雷伯菌	145
封闭蛋白	24~25
干扰素	24, 29, 66, 71, 194
杆状病毒	63, 74, 76~77, 87~88
肛门与生殖道	7
弓形体病	222
宫颈癌	1, 227
固有层	9, 13, 26, 32~38, 41, 42, 67, 72, 81, 91
固有免疫应答	7, 12, 23, 27~28, 35, 42, 46, 49
冠状病毒	189~190, 192~194
归巢	9, 13, 19, 23, 31, 38, 73
黑猩猩鼻炎病毒	200
红斑	113, 115~117, 121, 123, 128~133, 135~136, 145, 148
虹膜角膜内皮综合征	213
呼肠孤病毒科	60
呼吸道	1~2, 7, 66, 71, 75, 113, 128, 189~205, 216, 220, 228, 232, 233, 235
呼吸道合胞病毒	128, 189~190, 200
弧菌	2, 44~45, 47
花生过敏	48
坏死	25, 66~67, 120, 128, 131, 135~136,

	141~142, 145~148, 196, 200~201, 218~223, 233
环状病毒	193
获得性免疫缺陷综合征	230
霍乱弧菌	2, 44~45
霍乱疫苗	2
脊髓灰质炎病毒疫苗	2, 59
季节性	71, 85, 238, 189~191, 199
尖锐湿疣	18, 112, 124~127, 131, 143~144
睑板腺囊肿	225, 226
角化棘皮瘤	226
角膜结膜炎	212~213, 226, 228~229, 234
接合菌病	131, 146
结核病	140
结核分枝杆菌	131, 140
结膜下出血	224~225, 229, 232, 230, 235
结膜炎	212~214, 218, 220, 225~230, 232~235
进行性外层视网膜坏死	219
精子	4
局灶性上皮增生症	124, 131, 144
巨细胞病毒	112, 212, 219, 221
卡波西肉瘤	112, 123, 131, 136~139, 142, 145, 148, 213, 223~225, 228
卡氏肺孢子虫	221
抗微生物肽	27, 50, 189
抗原漂移	3, 195~196
抗原转换	195~196
柯萨奇病毒	112, 129~131, 234~235
麻疹口腔黏膜斑	232
克罗恩病	43, 49
口腔癌	128
口腔表现	111~113, 121, 123~124, 126~132, 144, 148
口腔毛状白斑	112, 121, 123, 134~135
口腔炎	135~136, 141~142
溃疡	16, 40~44, 112, 114~116, 119~120, 128~131, 139~142, 145~148, 214~219, 224, 226, 234
泪囊肿瘤	227
淋巴瘤	9, 40, 43, 112, 121~124, 131, 138~140, 220, 222~223, 225, 228, 231
流感病毒	2~3, 128, 189~190, 194~198, 204
轮状病毒	2, 31, 38, 59~60, 62~64, 66~67, 70~72
猫抓病	131, 145
毛霉菌病	131, 146
梅毒	221~223, 231, 234
梅毒螺旋体	221, 223, 231, 234
棉絮状斑	223, 230~231
免疫受损个体	87, 90, 214
免疫系统	1~2, 4, 6~9, 11~13, 16~19, 23, 26, 28~32, 37~39, 43~44, 46~47, 49~51, 75, 84, 135, 189, 204, 213, 223
免疫抑制	24, 111~114, 117~118, 120~121, 123, 131~134, 140~142, 144~148, 201, 219, 221
模式识别受体	30, 46, 50
囊泡病毒	75
脑膜炎	67, 146, 214, 231, 233
脑炎	3, 67, 88, 128~129, 214, 221, 232~233
逆转录病毒科	213
黏附分子	9, 13, 26~27, 198, 204
黏膜免疫	1, 4, 6, 8, 9, 12~13, 19, 23, 26, 30, 32, 37~39, 43~44, 47, 49~51, 204
黏膜免疫系统	1, 4, 6, 8, 9, 12~13, 19, 23, 26, 30, 32, 37~39, 43~44, 47, 49~51, 204
黏膜相关淋巴组织	6, 8, 30
念珠菌病	131~134
鸟分枝杆菌	221
疟疾	1
诺如病毒	2, 75, 81~83, 86~88
诺如病毒疫苗	87
诺瓦克病毒	59, 75~78, 80~83, 88
诺瓦克样病毒	75~76, 84~85
派尔集合淋巴结	8~9, 30, 33, 88, 91
疱疹病毒	3~4, 7, 12~13, 111~112,

	118~119, 121,124, 145, 148, 212~216, 219~221, 224, 230, 234	水痘	112, 116, 120~121, 144, 216~218
疱疹性咽峡炎	112, 129~131	水痘-带状疱疹病毒	112, 216
披膜病毒	128, 213, 233	体液因子	24, 27, 47
皮肤棘层松解	113, 114	兔病毒属	75
皮区	13~14, 16, 217	兔出血症病毒	75
热病疱疹	117	唾液腺疾病	123, 128, 131, 141~142
人类免疫缺陷病毒	3, 7, 131, 212	外周免疫系统	1~2, 7, 13
人类疱疹病毒	212, 224	委内瑞拉马脑炎	88
人乳头瘤病毒	7, 212, 227	胃癌	40
病毒样颗粒	12	胃肠道病毒学	59
溶菌酶	29, 203	胃肠道黏膜免疫	23, 60
肉芽肿	140~141, 225~226, 228	细胞毒性T细胞	34, 47, 72~73, 191
乳铁蛋白	28~29, 203	细胞介导免疫	15
乳头瘤病毒	1, 7~9, 13, 16~17, 112, 124, 212~213, 227,	细菌	85, 87, 216, 218, 225, 228~229, 231~233, 235
腮腺炎	8, 112, 128~129, 212, ~213, 233	细菌感染	24~28, 30, 49, 190, 197, 216, 218, 225, 232, 235
三叉神经	131, 147, 213, 216~218	腺病毒	86, 189~192, 212~213, 228~229, 235
色素沉着	131, 141~142, 226	小肠结肠炎耶尔森氏菌	44
沙门氏菌	26, 44~47	小肠三叶因子	24
上皮	6, 8, 10, 13, 18~19, 23~42, 45, 49, 64, 66, 67, 69~70, 72, 80, 82, 90~91, 189~192, 194, 196~200, 202~203, 214~219, 220, 222, 225~227, 229, 232~235	小核糖核酸病毒	129, 198, 212~213, 234
		效应部位	9, 13, 19, 23, 32~35, 37~38
		新型隐球菌	131, 146, 231
		星形病毒	59, 86, 88~92
		星形病毒疫苗	92
上皮内淋巴细胞	8, 19, 23, 33, 72	性传播感染	16
上皮细胞	64, 66~67, 69, 72, 80, 82, 90, 189~192, 194, 196~200, 202~203	胸腺癌	220
		血管瘤	131, 137~138, 142, 145
神经氨酸苷酶	195~196, 200	血管生成素	29
神经痛	120, 131, 147, 218	血凝素	62, 193, 196, 198, 200
生殖器疱疹	4, 9, 11, 13	血源性传播	7
食物过敏	24, 47~48	寻常疣	124~126, 131, 144
食物耐受不良	47	牙周病	136
视网膜病	213, 221, 223, 230~231, 234	咽结膜热	189, 228~229
适应性免疫	6~8, 10, 12~14, 18~19, 23~25, 27~28, 31~33, 36~37, 39, 42~43, 47, 51	眼部表现	148, 212~214, 221
		眼部疾病	212, ~214, 216~217, 220, 225, 229~230, 235
手足口病	112, 129~130	药物反应	121, 131, 145
鼠诺如病毒1型	81		

耶尔森氏菌外膜蛋白	45	诱导部位	8~9, 23, 32~34, 36~38
胰腺炎	67, 233	藻菌病	146
阴茎癌	18	札幌样病毒	75
龈口炎	112~115, 117	札如病毒	75~77
隐球菌病	146	真菌感染	131~133, 146~147
隐窝小结	32, 34	支气管相关淋巴组织	8~9, 204
婴儿猝死综合征	67, 201	志贺氏菌	2, 26, 43~47, 49
疣	8, 12, 16~19, 112, 124~127, 131, 143~144, 212~213, 225~227	紫癜	128, 131, 142~143
幼儿急疹	112	组织胞浆菌病	146~147